COUNSELING AND PSYCHOTHERAPY WITH CHILDREN AND ADOLESCENTS:

THEORY AND PRACTICE FOR SCHOOL AND CLINIC SETTINGS

(Second edition)

COUNSELING AND PSYCHOTHERAPY WITH CHILDREN AND ADOLESCENTS:

THEORY AND PRACTICE FOR SCHOOL AND CLINIC SETTINGS

(Second edition)

Douglas T. Brown
James Madison University

H. Thompson Prout
State University of New York at Albany

(Editors)

CPPC 4 Conant Square
Brandon, Vermont 05733

Published 1983. Second Edition 1989. Fifth Printing 1995.

Library of Congress Catalog Card Number: 89-62094
ISBN: 0-88422-104-0

CPPC 4 Conant Square
Brandon, Vermont 05733

Cover Design: Tom Hannan

Printed in the United States of America.

Preface

Few volumes have been published which attempt to apply theory and research in psychotherapy to settings in which children and adolescents receive service. The first edition of *Counseling and Psychotherapy with Children and Adolescents* was designed to fill this void. This new, second edition of the book is also designed to provide a detailed theoretical and empirical analysis of the major therapeutic techniques which can be employed with children and adolescents. The second edition, however, has been expanded to include systemic theoretical approaches (family and group applications). The other chapters have been revised to reflect trends in research and practice. Thus, seven therapeutic schools of thought have been chosen on the basis of their relevance to children and adolescents. These include psychoanalytic therapy, Adlerian therapy, person-centered therapy, behavior therapy, rational-emotive therapy, reality therapy, and systemic therapy. In addition, Chapter 10 deals with counseling and psychotherapy applied to handicapped children and adolescents. In this chapter an attempt has been made to relate relevant therapeutic approaches to exceptional children.

The general objective in each of the seven chapters that cover therapeutic approaches is to provide an overview of that given theoretical approach and relate it to the utilization of specific techniques with children and adolescents. Thus, the book is intended to provide a review and an analysis similar to that found in more adult-oriented texts such as Corsini's *Current Psychotherapies* and Patterson's *Theories of Counseling and Psychotherapy.* The intended audience includes students and practitioners in school psychology, counseling and guidance, child/clinical psychologists, psychiatric nurses, clinical social workers, and special educators. Although the chapters dealing with major therapeutic theories were chosen to provide an adequate theoretical basis, each one is directed more specifically at issues in the application and practice of a given therapy. Each chapter is divided into 12 sections. These sections include an introduction to the therapy, an overview of the theory, applications with children under 12 years of age, applications with adolescents, group procedures with children and adolescents, classroom and educational applications, parenting skills applications, family intervention techniques, efficacy, conclusions, case study material, and an annotated bibliography comprising several major references related to the particular therapeutic approach. We have provided a separate chapter on ethical and legal issues relating to psychotherapeutic interventions with children and adolescents. This chapter provides detailed information on the law as it relates to the practice of therapy with children and adolescents as well as ethical guidelines promulgated by various national associations.

In the selection of authors for each of the chapters, our intention was to identify persons who are leaders in advocating a given therapeutic approach and *who have significant applied experience in relating the particular approach to school and clinic settings.* Chapter 1 was designed to provide a historical reference for child and adolescent psychotherapy and to integrate current knowledge across various therapeutic techniques. In Chapter 11, the editors summarize and critique each of the therapeutic techniques discussed on the basis of operationalized criteria. Further, strengths and weaknesses of each therapy are presented together with an analysis of the current efficacy data available as presented in each chapter.

The contributors to this volume deserve special thanks for their cooperation and timeliness in the preparation and revision of manuscripts. The scholarly manner in which they developed their chapters is sincerely appreciated. We would like to thank Jane Todorski for her thoughtful and comprehensive editing of the manuscript. We would also like to thank Jerry Fuller for his support throughout this project. Finally, special thanks go to Elizabeth F. Rooney for her invaluable editorial assistance.

DTB
HTP

About the Authors

CONSTANCE BENOIT, M.S.W. Constance Benoit is a psychiatric social worker in the Department of Psychiatry at the Montreal General Hospital and is a field instructor in the School of Social Work at McGill University. In addition, she maintains a private practice and consults with social service agencies in the Montreal community. Her research interests focus on psychotherapeutic treatment modalities for psychiatric patients, and she has published in the area of community-based alternatives to hospitalization.

JOHN D. BOYD, Ph.D. John Boyd practices full-time as an independent clinical psychologist. He has also taught for 14 years at the university level in the areas of counseling and clinical psychology. At present he is an Associate Clinical Professor in Behavioral Medicine and Psychiatry at the University of Virginia in Charlottesville. His current areas of interest are in hypnotherapy and rational-emotive therapy, in which he has published numerous articles and books. He has also published in the area of counselor supervision.

DOUGLAS T. BROWN, Ph.D. Doug Brown is Professor of Psychology and Coordinator of the School Psychology Program at

James Madison University in Virginia. He is also a Fellow of the American Psychological Association. His research interests include counseling and psychotherapeutic interventions, assessment and test development, and mental retardation. He has an extensive array of publications in school psychology.

HARRIET C. COBB, Ed.D. Harriet Cobb is an Associate Professor of Psychology in the School Psychology Program at James Madison University in Virginia. She has extensive experience at the state and national level as a child advocate. Her research interests include child psychotherapy, psychotherapeutic interventions with handicapped children, and therapeutic interventions for adolescents. She has a variety of publications in child psychotherapy interventions.

RICHARD A. DEMARTINO, Psy.D. Rick DeMartino, a school psychologist with the Saratoga Springs, New York, school system, works with the drug prevention program. He specializes in working with clients who are sexual abuse victims, juvenile sex offenders, and with families experiencing separation and divorce.

DON DINKMEYER, JR., Ph.D. Don Dinkmeyer, Jr. is a faculty member at the Alfred Adler Institute of Chicago. He is also an editor for Communication and Motivation Training Institute Press (CMTI). His research interests are in school guidance, counseling, and educational materials development. He has a variety of publications in the areas of affective curriculum and Adlerian counseling and psychotherapy.

DON DINKMEYER, SR., Ph.D. Don Dinkmeyer, Sr. is president of the Communication and Motivation Training Institute in Coral Springs, Florida. He is also a Diplomate of the American Psychological Association and an American Association of Marriage and Family Therapy Supervisor. His current area of interest is in marriage and family counseling, and he has an extensive publication record in the areas of parent training and family therapy.

SUSAN FERBER, Ed.S. Susan Ferber is a school psychologist with the Schalmant Central Schools in New York. Her interests are in school-based interventions and issues in delivery of school psychological services. She has extensive experience in school psychology and special education in a variety of settings.

BARBARA L. FISHER, PH.D. Barbara Fisher is currently Co-Director of the Rocky Mountain Marriage and Family Center in Fort Collins, Colorado. She conducts groups, supervises group leaders, and does marriage and family therapy. She has been an associate professor at Purdue University and Colorado State University and has written extensively in the area of marriage and family enrichment programs.

DIANE L. FULLER, M. A. Diane Fuller is a clinical psychologist currently in private practice. She also teaches for Central Michigan University. Her research interests are in the areas of therapeutic interventions and health psychology.

GERALD B. FULLER, Ph.D. Jerry Fuller is Director of Research and Development for Clinical Psychology Publishing Company and adjunct professor at Central Michigan University. He is the editor of *Psychology in the Schools.* His current research interests include therapeutic interventions, psychopathology, and differential diagnosis. He has written extensively on both assessment and psychopathology and is the author of the *Minnesota Percepto-Diagnostic Test.*

RUSSELL M. GRIEGER, Ph.D. Russ Grieger is a licensed clinical psychologist in private practice and Clinical Director of Performance Seminars, Inc. His research interests are in the areas of theory and application of rational-emotive therapy and the use of rational-emotive therapy in business settings. Dr. Grieger has published extensively in the area of rational-emotive therapy.

WILLIAM B. GUNN, JR., Ph.D. William Gunn is a clinical associate professor of family medicine at the Fort Collins Family Medicine

Center, Padre Valley Hospital. He has extensive experience as a school psychologist and is an approved supervisor of the American Association for Marriage and Family Therapy. Currently, he supervises psychology interns and medical residents providing collaborative care to families. His clinical and research interests are in the areas of physician-family interaction and effective interventions with adolescent mothers.

HELEN B. MOORE, Ed.D. Helen Moore is Professor of Psychology and Coordinator of the Counseling Psychology Program at James Madison University in Virginia. She maintains a private practice and has worked as a counselor, consultant, social worker, and teacher in school and agency settings. She has numerous publications in diverse areas including meditation, child abuse, and psychotherapy. Her current interest is in the use of creative arts in counseling and therapy.

H. THOMPSON PROUT, Ph.D. Tom Prout is Associate Professor of School Psychology at the State University of New York-Albany. His research interests are in the areas of therapeutic interventions with children and adolescents, child psychopathology, personality assessment, mental retardation, and developmental disabilities. He has published extensively in the areas of therapeutic interventions, personality assessment, and mental retardation.

FREDERICK WEISZ, Ph.D. Frederick Weisz is a practicing psychologist in the Minneapolis/St. Paul area. Previously he was a staff psychologist at Montreal Children's Hospital and has had a faculty appointment at the Department of Psychiatry at Mineola University. His research interests are in the areas of social cognition and personality assessment. He has published a number of articles on temperamental characteristics in children.

DEDICATION

To Adam, Alex, and Lauren
our children

Table of Contents

Chapter 1

Counseling and Psychotherapy with Children and Adolescents: An Overview[1]

H. Thompson Prout, Ph.D.

The psychological treatment of children's problems is the focus of a variety of professions and is carried out in a variety of settings and situations. Although theoretical viewpoints are wide-ranging and essentially rooted in adult-based theories, the child or adolescent presents a unique challenge to the child mental health worker. Children are not simply "little adults." Their treatment cannot be viewed as scaled-down adult therapy—their developmental stages, environments, reasons for entering therapy, and other relevant factors necessitate a different, if not creative, approach to therapy. The child/adolescent therapist must have an expanded knowledge base of the human condition and a different perspective of what constitutes therapy or counseling.

This book is about psychotherapy and mental health counseling with children and adolescents. The intent of the book is to bring together in a comparative format the major theoretical views of psychological treatment of children. There are, however, a number of issues that cut across the theories and are relevant to any provision of mental health services to children. The purpose of this introductory chapter is to highlight some of these

[1]The terms *counseling* and *psychotherapy* will be used interchangeably throughout this chapter.

issues. Historical perspectives, the current mental health needs of children and adolescents, developmental issues, the adolescent phase, the unique aspects of child and adolescent therapy, psychotherapy with adolescents, a multimodal view of treatment, practitioner concerns, and research/efficacy issues will be discussed.

HISTORICAL PERSPECTIVES ON THE MENTAL HEALTH NEEDS OF CHILDREN AND ADOLESCENTS

Many of the major advances in clinical mental health work can, in some way, be traced to Freud. The area of mental health work with children is no exception. Freud's classic case study of "Little Hans" in 1909 is generally viewed as the first reported attempt to psychologically explain and treat a childhood disorder (Freud, 1909/1955). Although Freud did not directly treat Little Hans' phobia, he offered a psychoanalytic explanation of the problems and guided the father in the treatment of Hans. This case study is recognized as providing the base for Freud's theories on the stages of psychosexual development. Freud's interest in childhood disorders apparently waned at this point, and it was not until 1926 that his daughter, Anna, presented a series of lectures entitled "Introduction to the Technique of Psycho-analysis of Children" to the Vienna Institute of Psychoanalysis. These lectures generated considerable interest and established Anna Freud as a pioneer in child psychotherapy (Erickson, 1978). Shortly thereafter, Melanie Klein (1932), emphasizing the symbolic importance of children's play, introduced free play with children as a substitute for the free association technique utilized with adults, thus inventing play therapy. Although these two camps disagreed on a number of issues, they have remained the dominant voices in the child psychoanalytic field, with most analytic work being a spin-off of either Anna Freud or Klein.

At approximately the same time, the early twentieth century, a number of other forces were beginning to put more emphasis on work with children. In France in 1905, Alfred Binet completed initial work on his intelligence test that was used for making educational placement decisions in the Paris schools. This work provided the base for the psychometric study of individuals and had great impact on child study and applied psychology (Schwartz & Johnson, 1981). In the United States, Witmer had established a clinic for children at the University of Pennsylvania in 1896 which focused on school adjustment (Erickson, 1978), and in 1909 Healy founded what is now the Institute for Juvenile Research in Chicago (Schwartz & Johnson, 1981). These events provided the base for the child guidance movement, emphasizing a multidisciplinary team approach to the diagnosis and treatment of children's adjustment and psychological difficulties. The child guidance model involved treating both the child and his or her parents. The increased interest in clinical and research work on children's problems led to the founding of the American Orthopsychiatric Association in 1924, an organization of psychologists, social workers, and psychiatrists concerned with the mental health problems of children (Schwartz & Johnson, 1981).

Through the 1940s and into the 1950s, psychoanalytic psychotherapies were used almost exclusively in the treatment of children. In 1947, Virginia Axline published *Play Therapy,* describing a nondirective mode of treatment utilizing play. Nondirective play therapy was, in effect, a child version of Carl Rogers' adult-oriented client-centered therapy. Both nondirective play therapy and client-centered therapy represented the first major departures from psychoanalytic thought, differing in conceptualization of the therapeutic process and content in the role of the therapist. Rogers' impact on adult psychotherapy was paralleled and followed by Axline's impact on child therapy. The next major movement in psychotherapy was the rise of the behaviorally based approaches to treatment. Although the principles and potential applications of behavioral psychology were long known, it was not until the 1960s that behavior modification and therapy began to be used frequently in clinical work with children (Graziano, 1975).

The mental health treatment of children and adolescents has also been affected by two policy and legislative mandates. First, the community mental health movement was strongly influenced by the passage in 1963 of the federal program to construct mental health centers in local communities and to begin a move away from large institutional treatment. This movement grew not only because it was mandated by a federal program but because it represented a philosophy that mental health interventions are more likely to be successful when carried out in the community where the maladjustment is occurring. The new programs also included an emphasis on early intervention and prevention of mental disorders. The second mandate, with a similar philosophical base, involved the provision of special education services to all handicapped children, including those emotionally disturbed and behavior-disordered children and adolescents. Exemplified by Public Law 94-142 (Education for All Handicapped Children Act), this movement has not only expanded the role of public education in provision of services to these children but has also allowed more children to remain in their home communities. Psychotherapy and mental health treatment, if deemed a part of the total educational program of a child, have become by law and policy an education service.

THE NEED FOR CHILD AND ADOLESCENT SERVICES

The estimates of the numbers of children who are experiencing significant mental health problems are staggering. In a study of public school children, Bower (1969) estimated that at least three students in a typical classroom (i.e., 10% of school-age children and adolescents) are suffering from moderate to severe mental health problems, many children disturbed enough to warrant special educational services for the emotionally handicapped. In 1968, Nuffield, citing an estimate of 2.5 to 4.5 million children under the age of 14 in need of psychiatric treatment, found indices of only 300,000 receiving treatment services. This figure represents services to roughly 10% of those in need. Berlin estimated in 1975 that each year 6 million school-age children have emotional problems serious enough that professional intervention is indicated. Cowen (1973) noted a smaller group (1.5 million) in need of immediate help but estimated that fewer than 30% of these children were receiving this help. The incidence of juvenile delinquency is rising steadily, with approximately 4% of all children coming into contact with juvenile courts

(Schwartz & Johnson, 1981). Regardless of the estimate of incidence, it is clear that many children and adolescents with problems are not identified by educational, mental health, and social service institutions as having emotional difficulties and thus are not referred for or provided treatment services.

The Joint Commission on Mental Health of Children (1973) published the results and recommendations of an interdisciplinary task force study on children's mental health needs and the service delivery system. The Commission concluded that, even using conservative estimates, the unmet mental health and social service needs of children would continue to present a serious problem through the 1980s. The manpower to meet these needs did not exist at that time and would require considerable changes in the output of traditional training programs to meet these needs in the future. The Commission was also critical of the service delivery system as a whole: "Focusing on what we have described as the system of services to nonnormal-stream children, there is a dramatic mismatch between the character of these services and the demands and needs of children. The system is in need of drastic restructuring" (p. 174). The Commission cited fragmented services, a remedial orientation rather than preventative services orientation, and an arbitrary system of determining with whom and when to intervene. The Commission emphasized the need for more preventive services, as have other child professionals (e.g., Clarizio, 1979). The Commission report, among others, has consistently pointed to the lack of trained, qualified mental health professionals. Cummings (1979), reviewing a more recent report of the President's Commission on Mental Health, has noted that the lack of trained professionals still exists. A related issue is the quality of the training of professionals in our traditional programs. For example, Nathan (1979), commenting on graduate training in clinical psychology, has noted, "I realize that most clinical training programs provide their students with little or no training with children beyond a few WISC's and observation of an occasional family in treatment" (p. 967). This training pattern exists despite the obvious differences between child and adult psychological disorders. Although more programs are now geared to training professionals to work with children (e.g., school psychology programs, child/clinical psychology programs, child psychiatry residency programs), the lack of child-focused training is often paralleled in generic psychiatry and social work training. In general, it is safe to say that children and adolescents can be regarded as critically underserved populations, despite the continued recognition at the national level of the need (Cummings, 1979). The mental health needs of children present an enormous service delivery problem that is currently not keeping up with demand. With fiscal austerity being forecast for the coming decade, the gap between need and available services is likely to widen. Preventive services may be a cost- and resource-efficient mode for dealing with part of this problem, but the provision of quality counseling and psychotherapeutic services will be a crucial component in the total mental health system.

DEVELOPMENTAL ISSUES

The child/adolescent mental health worker must be familiar with human development for a number of reasons. With the exception of severe psychopathology or extreme behaviors, much of what may be presented as problematic in children may simply be normal developmental deviation. What is considered pathological behavior in adults may not be abnormal in children or adolescents. Knowledge of development and the behavioral ranges that are considered normal at different ages is crucial to making the discrimination between truly deviant behavior and minor developmental crises. Development in children and adolescents may follow sequences. The specific order for the appearance of certain behaviors and characteristics, however, tends to be highly variable. Children's personalities are quite unstable when compared to expectations of stability in adults. Related to this instability factor is evidence indicating that normal development is often marked by the appearance of a number of behavior problems. The classic developmental study by MacFarlane, Allen, and Honzik (1954) clearly pointed to a number of behaviors that were considered problems by parents yet were normative at different age levels. The child/adolescent therapist must be able to sort out these "normal" problems from those that may represent more serious disorders.

Awareness of development will also aid the therapist in clinical decision making at various points in the treatment process. Appropriate goal setting is important to any therapeutic venture. It provides a direction for our work, allows us to monitor progress, and tells us when we are done. The child/adolescent therapist must set these goals within a developmental framework. We would not expect an average 8-year-old to acquire, in the course of therapy, the cognitive abilities to problem-solve or the moral judgment of a 10-year-old. To set goals above developmental expectations is almost insuring that the intervention will fail. This knowledge of development also allows the therapist to choose appropriate content and to decide what level of therapeutic interaction is best suited for the child. Within these developmental age expectations, the therapist must also be sensitive to developmental delays in children. Not only do delays, particularly in cognition and language, dictate goal setting, but also they must be distinguished from behavioral or emotional disorders. These delays may also be major contributing factors in the development of disorders. For example, learning-disabled and mentally retarded children often display poor self-concepts and negative self-images as well as other socioemotional difficulties (Clarizio & McCoy, 1976). On the other end of the spectrum, we need to be cautious not to set limited goals for developmentally advanced children. Although we are not advocating psychological assessment as a prerequisite for treatment, the child/adolescent therapist will, in most cases, need to assess developmental levels of their clients early in the intervention.

The study of development can be broken down into essentially two types of information that are relevant for counseling or psychotherapy. The first involves an understanding of the developmental stage theorists, with the works of Freud, Piaget, Kohlberg, and Erikson most notable. Freud's psychoanalytic view of human development emphasizes the psychosexual aspects and pleasure-seeking drives that affect the child and adolescent. Development is seen as a series of crises that result in psychosexual conflicts which must be resolved in order for the individual to move on to the next phase (Neubauer, 1972). Athough obviously most consistent with the psychoanalytic approach to treatment, Freud's description of the developmental phases and parent-child relationship provides a useful base for assessing socioemotional development. Similarly, Piaget's theory of cognitive development provides a parallel base for assessing intellectual development. Piaget suggested that maturation, physical experience, social interaction, and equilibration (i.e., the internal self-regulating system) all combine to influence cognitive development. At different periods the type of information that can be processed and the cognitive operations that can be performed vary. Cognitive development is a coherent and fixed sequence with certain cognitive abilities expected at certain ages (Wadsworth, 1971). Piaget allows us to select developmentally appropriate modes of interacting with the child and to set appropriate goals for cognitive change in the child. For example, a child in the concrete operations stage solves problems involving real or observable objects or events. He or she has difficulty with problems that are hypothetical and entirely verbal, making verbally oriented or more abstract counseling interventions inappropriate for the child in this developmental stage.

Kohlberg (1964, 1973) has focused on the development of the understanding of morality, or what the individual believes would be the morally correct response to various problem situations. Moral judgment is seen as a developmental, age-bound variable similar to the cognitive and psychosexual stages. At different ages, the individual has certain beliefs about the reasons for displaying moral behavior, the value attached to a human life, and the reasons for conforming to moral standards. Awareness of the stages of moral development can provide insights into the behavior of the child, provide content for therapy sessions, and also allow therapy to be conducted at levels commensurate with current moral development levels. Lowered stages of moral development have been hypothesized to be related to child deviance, particularly delinquency (Quay, 1979).

Erikson's (1963) developmental theory is based in psychoanalytic theory and emphasizes a series of psychosocial crises. At each stage, the individual encounters a crisis which he or she must resolve by acquiring a new phase of social interaction. An unsuccessful resolution of a psychosocial crisis impedes further development and can have a negative effect on the individual's personality. Although his work is psychoanalytically based, Erikson places more emphasis on socialization and the demands of society. Erikson's work, along with the work of Havighurst (1951), is viewed by many as being particularly useful in understanding adolescent development. Taken together, these developmental stage theories provide the therapist with a comprehensive framework to view the child's current developmental levels.

The other child development information relevant to the child/adolescent therapist comes from the study of specific developmental variables. These variables are personality factors that are essentially developmental in nature. In many cases, these factors are components of the major personality theories. Although the list of variables that have been studied is almost infinite, Clarizio and McCoy (1976) have described several that are particularly relevant for child and adolescent therapy in that they can often be the focus of a referral concern or they interact with the problem. These developmental characteristics often follow developmental sequences similar to the stage theories. Certain periods will present behaviors that may be perceived as bothersome by parents or teachers but are, in actuality, part of the normal growth pattern.

Clarizio and McCoy (1976) cite dependency, anxiety and insecurity, aggressiveness, and achievement motivation as factors that are commonly involved in child and adolescent problems. In looking at each factor, one finds a developmental pattern, behavioral manifestations, contributing factors to problematic instances of the factor, and adaptive and maladaptive outcomes. For example, dependency may involve child-adult relationships in which the child is often seeking help and physical contact, engaging in attention-seeking behavior, and maintaining close physical proximity to the adult. These behaviors are relatively normal and expected with young children and their parents. As the child gets older, both the intensity of the dependency and the object of emotional dependence change. The maturing child becomes less dependent on his or her parents, with a resulting decrease in the dependent behaviors, and becomes more dependent on peers for approval and attention. Certain parental patterns (e.g., overpermissiveness, overprotection) are seen as contributing to a child's being overly dependent and as interfering with the move toward greater independence. The child who makes adequate progress in this area develops a sense of trust, is responsive to social reinforcers, and is able to display warmth toward others. The overly dependent child is more likely to become a passively dependent individual, submissive, and mistrusting of others. For dependency and other personality factors, a normal developmental progression is viewed as important to successful adult adjustment. Knowledge of these variables can be used in treatment planning and goal setting, in determining whether excessive or pathological behaviors are occurring at different ages, and in assessing contributing factors to problematic behaviors.

THE ADOLESCENT PHASE

Probably no single developmental period provides more confusion and consternation for parents, teachers, and clinicians than the adolescent period. Adolescence is characterized more by a developmental phase than by a set, sequenced series of stages. A variety of behaviors, many of them disturbing, seem to "possess" the adolescent. Weiner (1970) notes that many people view normal adolescence as a disturbed state. He notes that "normal adolescent development will be characterized by distressing, turbulent, and unpredictable thoughts, feelings, and actions" and that "as a consequence of such storm and stress, adolescents will normatively display symptoms that in an adult would suggest definitive psychopathology" (p. 41). In a similar vein, Schecter, Toussieng, and Sternlof (1972) have concluded "we view normal adolescence as a disruptive, sometimes awkward stage of life. Its very disorderliness defines its normality" (pp. 40-41). These views yield two important aspects of adolescent psychotherapeutic work. First, the adolescent therapist must be cautious not to overinterpret typical and, perhaps, seemingly bizarre behavior, thoughts, or feelings as being indicative of severe psychopatholgy. Second, the therapist should not be surprised or upset by a rocky, unpredictable, and frustrating course of treatment.

The adolescent is, in fact, at the crossroads of his or her life. He or she is making the transition from childhood to adulthood.

Havighurst's (1951) classic list of adolescent developmental tasks provides much insight into the pressures and demands faced by the adolescent. According to Havighurst, the mastery of nine developmental tasks is critical to adolescent adjustment:

1. Accepting one's physique and sexual role.
2. Establishing new peer relationships with both sexes.
3. Achieving emotional independence of parents.
4. Achieving assurance of economic independence.
5. Selecting and preparing for an occupation.
6. Developing intellectual skills and concepts necessary for civic competence.
7. Acquiring socially responsible behavior patterns.
8. Preparing for marriage and family life.
9. Building conscious values that are harmonious with one's environment.

The adolescent's response to much of this developmental stress leads to a number of what Copeland (1974) has described as "adolescent idiosyncrasies" that are not necessarily indicative of any pathological process. Copeland describes both the characteristics of adolescent thinking and the characteristics of adolescent affect and behavior. The characteristics of adolescent thought include:

1. *Preoccupation with Self.* The adolescent's thought represents an intense involvement with the self at this stage. This involvement may be narcissistic in nature, but it may also be coupled with self-doubt and crises of self-confidence.

2. *Preoccupation with Fantasy.* A rich fantasy life is a result of the intense drives and feelings the adolescent is experiencing. The fantasies provide a means of controlling these drives as well as some degree of gratification.

3. *Preoccupation with the Need for Self-Expression.* "Doing your own thing," as Copeland calls it, reflects the

adolescent's struggle to establish an independence free from parental supervision and consent. Being unique also is involved in the adolescent's attempts to develop a sense of identity.

4. *Preoccupation with Philosophical Abstraction, Theories, and Ideals.* The adolescent is preoccupied with such philosophical questions as "absolute truth" and "ultimate reality." The adolescent develops his or her own theories and views about the world, often strongly rejecting the established ideas of those in authority. Copeland attributes this perspective to Piaget's work. Piaget saw egocentrism in adolescence as a normal stage of cognitive development, when the adolescent becomes possessed with his or her newly found powers of logical thought. The adolescent is unable to differentiate between his or her own idealistic thought and the "real" world (Wadsworth, 1971).
5. *Preoccupation with Sexuality.* The adolescent is extremely interested in sexual matters, with initial heterosexual relationships often intense and overidealized. The adolescent may become overconcerned with appearance and dress, spending considerable time preening and grooming.
6. *Hedonism and/or Ascetisim.* Because of the intensity of drive states, the adolescent is virtually forced to respond to them. This response tends to be extreme—either hedonistic, with the adolescent fully pursuing instinctual gratification, or ascetic, where he or she renounces the drive out of fear and guilt.
7. *Conformism.* The adolescent, as part of the struggle for independence, shifts his or her identity patterns from parents and family to a chosen peer group. The behaviors and characteristics, often shown through dress and other interests, usually are antithetical to and criticized by the adults from whom the adolescent is attempting to become independent.

According to Copeland, the adolescent also tends to display certain characteristic affective states and behaviors:

1. *Heightened Sensitivity.* The adolescent experiences life intensely and passionately, sometimes overreacting. Minor concerns can become major issues, with the adolescent being indifferent to very little.

2. *Mood Swings.* Emotional reactions of joy and sadness can occur suddenly and almost concurrently. The shifts in affect are quick and intense.

3. *Propensity to Act Out.* Impulsive behavior often causes trouble both for the adolescent and for others. Rebelliousness may be common, and in some extreme cases delinquency and other antisocial behavior may occur.

4. *Inhibition of Behavior.* The adolescent may have episodes of inhibition and may withdraw socially at times.

The child/adolescent therapist will find much in theory and research in child and adolescent development that pertains to psychological interventions with these groups. In fact, one wonders how it would be possible to develop and carry out treatment plans without a firm grounding in these areas. Developmental theory and research provide us with a framework to work with children and adolescents systematically, if not scientifically, and to gauge our therapeutic progress with them more objectively.

UNIQUE ASPECTS OF PSYCHOTHERAPY WITH CHILDREN AND ADOLESCENTS

In addition to the developmental issues discussed above, there are a number of other issues related to the child's development and situation that have an impact on the nature of the psychotherapeutic relationship. These factors relate to the direct work with the child or adolescent and stem from some of the differences between child/adolescent psychotherapy and adult psychotherapy.

Clarizio and McCoy (1976) have offered an overview of some of the unique aspects of the child/adolescent therapeutic relationship. Children and adolescents bring a different motivation for treatment into the counseling situation. Whereas the adult is usually aware that a personal problem exists, the child may not agree or recognize that there are problems or concerns. Although he or she may be encouraged by others, the adult will in most cases make the decision to enter treatment. The child is unlikely to seek help and initiate entering into therapy voluntarily. This decision is usually made by an adult within the child's environment, with some varying degree of acceptance/compliance/resistance from the child. The "involuntary" nature of the child/adolescent client in many cases may yield little or no motivation on the part of the client to engage in a relationship with the therapist nor even an admission that any change is necessary. Thus, the first step in many interventions may simply be to establish some type of relationship with the child and to come to some agreement that change is necessary. Without developing some motivation in the client at least to examine the current situation, even if done nonjudgmentally, it will be difficult to make significant progress.

An aspect related to motivation is the child/adolescent's lack of understanding of both the therapeutic process and the treatment objectives. The adult is likely to recognize the need to "get something out of therapy" and to have certain expectations of what is supposed to happen in the counseling situation. The adult usually will be able to verbalize some expectations and goals and to engage in some role-appropriate "client behaviors," e.g., talking, reflecting, responding to questions. The child may have no clear view of what the therapy situation presents. This blurred view may range from total misinformation to seeing the therapist as an agent of his or her parents, the school, the courts, or some other individual or institution that forced the initiation of treatment. Initially the therapist may simply have to educate the child about therapy, explaining what it is and what it is not. Children may bring in very distorted or stereotyped ("Oh, so you're the shrink. Where's your couch?") perceptions of therapists. This author is reminded of one extremely anxious 12-year-old boy who failed to respond to the usual reassuring techniques in an initial therapy session. After some gentle probing, it was learned that the young man had watched one too many late-night horror movies in which the fiendish doctor had done bizarre things to his subjects. Somehow the boy had associated coming to the mental health clinic with the scenes in movies where the hero gets wired to a machine and is never the same again. When I reassured him that the use of electrodes was not part of my approach and that we were simply going to talk about problems he was having at home and school, he visibly relaxed and began to volunteer all sorts of information.

Even as therapy progresses, it is necessary to monitor these perceptions. The child who views the therapist as the person he plays games with once a week is unlikely to focus on the tasks necessary to facilitate change. Similarly, there may be little agreement as to what changes are needed and what mutually acceptable treatment objectives are to be established. The therapist is likely to be faced with the predicament of reconciling, on the one hand, the goals of those who initiated treatment (e.g., parents, teachers) and, on the other hand, the child or adolescent client's own view of what is needed. A parent-referred adolescent who has been arrested three times for shoplifting may verbalize a goal of having his parents "get off my case." Although this position may be a factor in the acting out, it is not likely to produce an appropriate therapy objective, given the referral problem. Thus, the therapist must negotiate with the client appropriate goals, objectives, and topics or content for the counseling. These goals may not necessarily be totally in agreement with the referral source's or therapist's view of appropriate goals, but they will provide a starting point. Objectives can always be renegotiated as the relationship develops. Further, the therapist needs to demonstrate to the child or adolescent client that the client will get something out of counseling. Initially, this demonstration may take a form as simple as providing a format that is interesting to the child. This accomplishment can lead to the establishment of a more congruent set of objectives.

Another major difference between child and adult therapy is the child's more limited verbal and linguistic development, which is also related to the limitations in cognitive development. Children may be unable to think in more abstract terms and may have even more difficulty verbally describing and discussing their thoughts and emotions. This limited verbal ability is one of the main reasons play has been used as a medium of therapy. Play and other nonverbal techniques allow expression without creating anxiety or frustration for the child because of an inability to find the correct verbal description. Further, the child may not have the receptive vocabulary to understand fully what is being asked in the interview situation. This author once observed a psychiatric interview of a 7-year-old girl in which the resident asked the child if she ever had any "hallucinations." The little girl, obviously not knowing what was meant by the word "hallucination," happily responded, "Oh, yes, all the time," whereupon the resident made note of this finding and continued the interview along other lines. Therapy must be geared at the appropriate developmental level for both the child's expressive and receptive language capabilities. Although not deemphasizing the worth of "talk therapy," alternative modes of expression should be investigated for use in conjunction with verbal interactions. The therapist may also find it useful to teach the child labels and verbal mediators for emotional experiences. This course of action can involve using the traditionally accepted labels for feelings or using the child's own terminology. An 8-year-old girl once accurately described several symptoms consistent with "feeling depressed." The girl, however, felt more comfortable generally describing the state as one of "yuckiness."

Children also differ from adults in terms of their dependence on environmental forces and changes. Children are reactors to changes in their living situations rather than initiators of change. They have relatively little power to take action to eliminate or prevent environmental causes of stress. They react to parental divorces, family moves, and school and peer pressures. The child's disturbance may actually be a relatively normal reaction to upheaval or stress in the environment. Yet, the child cannot divorce his or her parents, change schools, or move at will. Because the child is dependent on the environment, it is more important for those in the environment to be involved in treatment. Where the adult is more likely to seek treatment independently, the child is less likely to be treated in isolation. Even if the child makes significant progress in individual therapy, he or she still does not have the options open that an adult has in dealing with the environment. In some cases, therapy may even proceed on the notion of helping the child cope with a stressful situation, rather than assuming that change will be forthcoming in that environment. For example, an 11-year-old may be able to have little impact on the drinking and resulting behavior of an alcoholic parent yet may be assisted in finding ways of dealing with the problem in order to make that stress more manageable.

Another factor that contributes to the difference between child therapy and adult therapy is the fact that the child's personality is less likely to be set than the adult's. The child, whose defenses are not as well established, is more pliable and amenable to therapeutic influence, once the relationship and cooperation are established. The personality is still rapidly developing and changing, yielding a greater potential for change. But at the same time this situation presents a somewhat more labile client and can result in inconsistent responses in therapy sessions. The child has a greater range of normal emotional and behavioral reponses as a result of the unformed nature of the personality. The therapist, therefore, is freed to be more flexible and must anticipate and not be discouraged by seemingly broad swings of emotion and behavior in the course of treatment. The plasticity of the child's personality is also an asset in working out a preventive model in that disturbing patterns may be prevented with appropriate intervention prior to the crystallization of the personality.

PSYCHOTHERAPY WITH ADOLESCENTS

As unpredictable as the adolescent's behavior is to those in his or her environment, a similar unpredictability exists in the therapeutic relationship. Weiner (1970) notes, "Psychotherapy with disturbed adolescents is a demanding task that is sought by some clinicians, approached with trepidation by many, and eschewed by most" (p. 349). Adolescents entering the therapy situation are characteristically impatient, intolerant, and uncommunicative. They may fail to elaborate on any details of the current situation or difficulties presented. They may deny any responsibility for the current problems, preferring to place blame elsewhere, or may actually have almost no insight into the reasons why they have been referred for treatment. This uncooperativeness is frustrating and anxiety-arousing for the therapist and may even discourage attempts to build a therapeutic relationship. Picture a 16-year-old male sitting in your office, slouched in a chair, a cap and long hair covering his averted eyes. His first words and only complete sentence for the next hour are: "I don't want to talk to no f--king shrink." A reflective statement on your part noting that he must be upset about something only brings a muffled grunt. Your best open-ended questions elicit only a series of unelaborated "Yes's," "No's," "I don't know's," "Maybe's," and "It's the damn teachers." Your feeble attempts at humor or to discuss "safe" topics bring only more grunts, a few eye rolls, or no response at all. His posture throughout the seemingly never-ending hour remains essentially unchanged. This initial session represents the base upon which your therapeutic relationship with the young man will be built. It is little wonder why many therapists avoid this type of interaction. Despite our best rationalizing that the adolescent is reacting to the situation and not to us, it is often difficult to come out of such an unproductive session feeling as though we had made progress and that our skills were up to the task of helping the adolescent.

Although the adolescent may be a difficult client, Weiner (1970) feels that most disturbed adolescents are accessible to psychotherapeutic intervention. Depending on the level of development and maturity, work with the adolescent may range from more gamelike approaches utilized with younger children to therapy that resembles interventions with an adult presenting similar problems. Most adolescents will not be candidates for insight-oriented, in-depth therapy involving the reworking of previous experiences. According to Weiner, defenses may be serving a relatively useful function during this period of personality development, and attempts to strip these defenses away may be unproductive or actually conterproductive to the overall therapeutic plan. Goals may range from better self-understanding with some personality reorganization to simple stabilization and improved functioning without major personality change.

Weiner (1970) notes that adolescents differ from both adults and children in their view of treatment. Although most children are initially unaware of the significance of therapy and most adults have begun treatment by choice, adolescents are clearly aware that they have been brought to treatment by others who can force continual attendance at sessions. Commenting on the beginning of treatment, Weiner (1970) states: "A swift, incisive launching of the treatment relationship is vital to successful psychotherapeutic work with the adolescent, often more so than with other age groups" (p. 354). Initially, the therapist must attempt to put the adolescent at ease, explaining what to expect and taking steps to suppress apprehensions. Unstructured probing, queries about deep personal feelings, or challenging the adolescent to explain his or her misbehavior will likely produce further uncooperativeness or yield a strong emotional response. Beginning with factual information in a nonjudgmental manner will help allay initial anxieties. The therapist needs to explain how the relationship will differ from those with parents, teachers, peers, and others. The goal at this level is to achieve engagement with the adolescent so that the initial seeds for establishing a motivation can be implanted. The initial agreement from the adolescent may simply be to return for another session.

Weiner (1970) states that continuing to build the relationship involves maintaining a flow of communication, fostering a positive identification with the therapist, and dealing with the adolescent's concern about how therapy might affect his or her independence. The adolescent therapist will be more active in comparison with the adult therapist. Long silences, noncommittal responses, and long periods of formulating answers to the adolescent's concerns should be avoided. The adolescent therapist may find himself or herself talking relatively more than with an adult client. Explaining thoughts explicitly, phrasing questions concretely, being willing to explain himself or herself, and, in general, using a direct approach will facilitiate work with the adolescent. Many of the interpretive leads and nondirective probes that are utilized with adults may be perceived by the adolescent as trickery and may add to his or her resistance. The therapist needs to present himself or herself as genuine. A spontaneous, conversational approach that is more akin to talking with a casual friend is recommended. The adolescent is likely to be curious about the therapist's "real life," and the therapist's responses to such questions should be matter-of-fact and nonevasive. Although not attempting to influence values, the therapist should be willing to share his or her personal opinions and attitudes with the adolescent. Acknowledgment of the adolescent's feelings about various issues and situations is helpful, particularly being aware of the current teenage values, fads, slang, and so on, and being sensitive to the particular pressures related to adolescents' social and emotional developmental levels. The therapist needs to communicate his or her liking of and interest in the adolescent. This is best done indirectly because the adolescent will recognize the artificiality of an "I like you." A sincere commitment to engage with the adolescent in mutual problem solving and other concrete gestures and expressions of interest are most helpful. Finally, the therapist must work at maintaining a balance along the continuum of independence-dependence. The adolescent should not be treated like a child yet should not be given signals that he or she is entirely free to make all of his or her own life decisions.

Meeks (1971), in a book aptly entitled *The Fragile Alliance,* has also written about therapeutic work with adolescents. The important components in a successful therapeutic alliance with an adolescent involve (1) the adolescent being genuinely concerned about some aspect of his or her psychological functioning, (2) the adolescent being able to observe his or her own functioning accurately and honestly and report it to the therapist, and (3) the extent to which the family will be supportive of the therapeutic endeavor. The key to establishing this alliance, according to Meeks (1979), involves the "careful and systematic interpretation of affective states" (p. 136) presented by the adolescent in therapy. Signals or cues of changes in affect from the adolescent may be masked or quite subtle, and the therapist must be sensitive to the implications of these changes. Copeland (1974) in a similar vein has provided a list of prognostic indicators for a favorable outcome of adolescent psychotherapy: (1) sincere self-referral, (2) acceptance of the concept of personal problems, (3) presence of psychological pain, (4) motivation for change,

(5) economic independence, (6) history of accomplishments, (7) sense of responsibility, (8) ability to form a working relationship with the therapist, (9) acceptance of rules and other limits, and (10) positive relationships to family or other surrogates (p. 109). Motivation to change and a history of positive accomplishments are viewed as the two most important determiners of potential therapeutic success. Although Copeland's list may be useful in developing a prognostic prediction or even deciding whether to attempt therapy with an adolescent, one wonders what an adolescent who presents all or most of these indicators would be doing in therapy. It is likely that most of those referred adolescents would not present a positive prognostic picture given these guidelines.

A MULTIMODAL VIEW OF TREATMENT

This book borrows (and somewhat paraphrases) the term *multimodal* from Lazarus (1976) to describe the overall philosophy implicit in the subsequent chapters. Lazarus presented his BASIC ID, an acronym for seven interactive modalities which are investigated as potential points of intervention for problems. The modes are Behavior, Affect, Sensation, Imagery, Cognition, Interpersonal relationships, and Drugs-Diet. This approach presents a comprehensive method of identifying problems and then deciding the most effective way to intervene. Keat, in *Multimodal Therapy with Children* (1979), expanded on this approach with his own acronym, BASIC IDEAL, by adding E for Education or school pursuits, A for Adults in the child's life (parents, teachers, relatives), and L meaning Learn the client's culture.

This book takes a very broad view of what is "psychotherapeutic" for a child or an adolescent. By multimodal, we refer to the many varied types of interventions to help troubled children and adolescents. Barker (1979), noting that child psychiatric disorders are multifactorial in origin, lists a variety of treatment approaches that may need to be used, including "psychotherapy with the child, casework help for the family, family therapy, group therapy for children or parents, behavior therapy, drug treatment, in-patient treatment, day patient treatment, alternative families, educational measures, speech therapy, and other measures including removal from parental care" (p. 216). Although this list is not exhaustive, it does point to the many interventions we have available to facilitate therapeutic change with children and adolescents. There also exists a range within each alternative. Educational measures, for example, can range from resource room help to a full-time structured placement. Parental interventions may involve parenting classes or perhaps therapy for the parents. In most cases, a multimodal, or combined, approach will be used. For example, a child may receive individual therapy, his or her parents may receive counseling, and the teacher may conduct a behavior management program. Although it is desirable to intervene in the most efficacious and cost-efficient manner, we do not make assumptions that one technique is preferable to or more therapeutic than others. At this point, neither research nor clinical experience is able to tell us whether a child with a low self-concept, for example, is helped more by 2 hours a week of individual therapy or by having a teacher who is trained to provide a consistent, positive, successful school experience. We do not know whether group social skills training is more beneficial than family therapy. What we do know is that there is a variety of types of intervention that have some benefit for children and adolescents. The more interventions and systems that can be combined, i.e., the more modalities involved in the treatment, the more likely it is that our overall therapeutic goals will be realized. This approach is not a "let's try everything" one. It involves careful assessment of problems, selection of appropriate interventions, and coordination and communication among those providing services. As long as our treatment programs are not excessively costly or time-consuming, interventions involving several modalities are indicated.

This multimodal view also implies two other basic assumptions. First, a variety of professionals with a variety of backgrounds is involved in child "treatment." A teacher with a B.A. in Special Education may be working with a child who is receiving individual therapy from a psychiatrist who has completed a child psychiatry fellowship program. A high school guidance counselor may work individually with an adolescent whose family is in therapy with a Ph.D. psychologist. A further assumption here is that one does not have to be called a therapist to have therapeutic impact on a child. The second, related assumption involves the settings where "treatment" takes place. Troubled children and adolescents receive "treatment" in, among other places, classrooms, schools, agencies, clinics, group homes, and hospitals. In this book, we do not make the artificial distinction between counseling and psychotherapy. We assume that a similar core of principles and techniques can be adapted to a variety of settings. Although the presenting problems may vary in different settings, we make the assumption, for example, that an Adlerian-trained school counselor will function in a manner relatively similar to an Adlerian-trained psychiatrist in an inpatient setting. The overriding concern is that effective, coordinated, and multifaceted interventions are developed.

RESEARCH AND EFFICACY

Since publication of Eysenck's (1952) classic and much-debated study on the effectiveness of psychotherapy with adults, researchers and clinicians have pondered the question, "Does psychotherapy work?" Eysenck's study, generally recognized as having spawned considerable research in psychotherapy, reviewed a number of studies of psychotherapy outcome with neurotic adults. His evaluation concluded that the percentage of treated clients who improved was not substantially different from the spontaneous remission rate (i.e., those individuals who improved without psychotherapy). He found that roughly two-thirds of each group, treated and untreated, reported improvement. Eysenck concluded that there was little evidence to support the effectiveness of psychotherapy with adult neurotics. Eysenck's data and methodology have been cited, reanalyzed and reinterpreted, criticized, and condemned ever since. Despite its controversiality, his study is important for the discussion, research, and examination of the therapeutic venture it has fostered.

Systematically and carefully studying the psychotherapy effectiveness question is one of the most difficult research areas in the behavioral sciences. Understanding the process of psychotherapy and its relationship to behavior change is an extremely complex proposition. The three volumes of the *Handbook of Psychotherapy and Behavior Change* (Bergin & Garfield, 1971; Garfield & Bergin, 1978, 1986) point to both the methodological complexity and the enormity of the issues. These volumes have attempted to bring together current empirical knowledge and data on psychotherapy. To utilize current research findings or to attempt research in this area, one must be aware of the numerous problems facing the researcher:

1. Psychotherapy represents a wide variety of techniques, in some ways preventing a clear, unambiguous definition of psychotherapy. Psychotherapy differs depending on the theoretical orientation of the therapist, the length of time of the treatment, and the format (i.e., individual, group, marital, parent, family, consultation).
2. The clinical definition of client populations may be ambiguous and thus limit generalizability. Clear definition of symptomatology and the client characteristics may vary in studies and be somewhat a result of the setting. Would two studies of treatment of anxious children produce similar results if one were conducted in a school and one at a clinic? Similarly, there are various subgroups that might be studied separately (e.g., males vs. females, blacks vs. whites, the disadvantaged, children).
3. Therapists vary in age, sex, training, orientation, competency, style and personality characteristics. Outcome could be affected by any one of these. Some research has studied the client-therapist match issue, i.e., whether a certain type of therapist works best with a certain type of client.
4. Research can focus on process or content variables. Process studies examine what goes on in therapy, typically some client-therapist interaction variable. Outcome studies examine whether the person has improved or whether there is behavior or affective change following intervention. Although some studies attempt to

relate process to outcome, both have been and continue to be studied extensively.

5. In outcome studies, what represents appropriate measures to gauge "therapeutic change"? Do rating scales, personality tests, client report, therapist rating, or the reports of a significant other validly and reliably reflect genuine change? What represents improvement?
6. Various other methodological issues exist. Are single subject research designs appropriate for studying the general effectiveness of techniques? What represents an appropriate control group for those who receive treatment? Both those people on waiting lists for treatment and defectors (those who fail to return to the clinic for therapy) have been used in comparison studies. Do these groups represent ones that are clinically comparable to the experimental group?
7. Psychotherapy does not occur in isolation. How do we account for other extraneous variables that may affect our results?
8. What are the long-term effects of our interventions? Does a 1-year positive follow-up on clients treated for depression mean that these individuals will also suffer fewer problems with depression in the subsequent 5 or 10 years?

Psychotherapy research with children and adolescents presents some special research problems. Levitt (1971) notes that because the child is a developing organism, many of the symptomatic manifestations of essentially normal children tend to disappear as a function of development. Some problems like temper tantrums, enuresis, specific fears, and sleep disturbance tend to go away in time. Levitt notes that "there is some reality in the common-sense notion that children 'grow out' of certain behavior problems" (p. 477). This makes it difficult to sort out the effects of therapy versus the effects of maturation. Similarly, some problems that are indicative of underlying emotional disturbance may disappear as a function of development yet reappear in another form, what Levitt calls "developmental symptom substitution" (p. 477). For example, a child successfully treated for enuresis at age 8 might be classified, for research purposes, as "cured" or "improved" yet present serious problems as an adolescent. Extending this view somewhat, research on the effects of childhood psychological treatment on later adult adjustment is difficult to do, yet this issue is an important one. Levitt also notes that, although the child may be the identified patient in clinical studies, persons other than the child may actually be the direct focus of treatment, thus making the isolation of treatment effects difficult.

In reviewing psychotherapy research studies, one is left with certain impressions. Because of the difficulty in conducting research in this area, it is possible to examine critically almost any single study and dismiss its results or offer alternative explanations of the findings on methodological grounds. The orthodox experimental psychologist who spends his or her day in a rat laboratory might smirk at some of our research conclusions. But because we work with humans who have difficulties in living and because the alleviation of these difficulties is a complex process, we must take a somewhat softer view of the research. We must examine the literature with the understanding that few, if any, studies are going to answer absolutely the question "Does psychotherapy work?" Rather, we must continue to examine critically the data and conclusions and to glean from the research those implications which relate most directly to our clinical work. This proposal is made not to support "sloppy" research or blanket acceptance or rejection of findings but to support a flexible and open-minded view of the current literature and status of the psychotherapy venture. The question of whether psychotherapy works remains essentially unanswered at this point.

The effectiveness of psychotherapy with children has been chronicled in reviews by Levitt in 1957, 1963, and 1971, and in a review by Barrett, Hampe, and Miller in 1978. Levitt's 1957 study was modeled after Eysenck's (1952) study of the effectiveness of adult psychotherapy. Surveying reports of evaluations made both at the close of therapy and at follow-up and comparing them with similar evaluations of untreated children, Levitt found that two-thirds of the evaluations at close and three-fourths at follow-up showed improvement. Roughly the same percentages were found in the untreated control groups. Levitt wrote: "It now appears that Eysenck's conclusion concerning the data for adult psychotherapy is applicable to children as well; the results do not support the hypothesis that recovery from neurotic disorder is facilitated by psychotherapy" (p. 193). Levitt noted, however, that his evaluation "does not prove that psychotherapy (with children) is futile" (p. 194) and recommended "a cautious, tongue-in-cheek attitude toward child psychotherapy" (p. 194) until additional evidence became available. The 1963 study utilizes a similar methodology and again concluded that the hypothesis that psychotherapy facilitated recovery from emotional problems could not be supported. Some of the 1963 data did suggest that comparisons should be made within diagnostic categories. Levitt also found that improvement rates tended to be lowest for cases of antisocial acting-out and delinquency and highest for identifiable behavioral symptoms like enuresis and school phobia. The 1971 review departed slightly from the previous reviews and looked at a wider range of modalities rather than just examining child psychopathology. These included the effects of inpatient vs. outpatient treatment, drug therapy, type of special class placement, and the use of mothers as therapists. Although individual studies showed some effectiveness, the overall conclusion again pointed to a lack of proof that these interventions are generally helpful. Levitt also focused on two identifiable diagnostic classifications, juvenile delinquency and school phobia, for further examination. School phobia tended to respond favorably to treatment, but Levitt questioned whether treatment was simply removing the symptoms of more serious underlying core problems which would surface in some other form later. Conventional psychotherapy with delinquents generally appeared to be ineffective, but some moderately positive results were found in examining more comprehensive treatment programs for delinquents. In addition to still questioning the effectiveness of child psychotherapy, Levitt was able to provide some preliminary conclusions. He noted that many of the principles upon which traditional psychoanalytically based child guidance treatment have been founded are now being challenged by research. The evidence at that time did not support the necessity of involving the mother in treatment, the relative insignificance of father involvement, the relationship of outcome to intensity of treatment, the desirability of encouraging the expression of negative feeling, ignoring undesirable behavior, or the notion that the home or family situation is likely to be more therapeutic than other child care settings. In other words, many of the principles that had guided, and probably still do guide, much of traditional child treatment simply are not supported in the research. Rigid orthodoxies are not empirically supported, although few of the innovative treatments are definitely supported either. Levitt calls for more studies of treatment of specific diagnostic classifications and more long-range follow-up studies.

Barrett, Hampe, and Miller (1978) present a historical and methodological review in which they focus more on the research issues rather than providing clinical guidelines. Noting that their review found little progress in this area of research, they again indicate that the issue of efficacy of child treatment remains unresolved. They do pose a number of important questions for both future research and clinical work. They recommend abandoning the research questions of whether psychotherapy works and asking the more appropriate question: "Which set of procedures is effective when applied to what kinds of patients with which sets of problems and practiced by which sort of therapists?" (p. 428). Although this specific question complicates the issue, the answer is likely to be more productive in the long run than the answer to the general question. Further, they found current (i.e., 1978) classification systems to be inadequate and better systems to be needed for classifying childhood disorders. The efficacy of the DSM-III-R, which more clearly delineates childhood disorders, is yet to be established. Finally, research and practice both must focus more closely on the child's developmental level and the systems with which the child must interface.

Two other reviews of treatment bear mentioning. First, Abramowitz (1976) reviewed efficacy studies of group psychotherapy with children, reaching a conclusion similar to the reviews of individual therapy. Definitive conclusions are not possible at this point, and, based on available data, favorable responses to group therapy are not indicated. However, if a group therapy approach is indicated, the feasibility of using a behavioral approach might be considered first. Second, Tramontana (1980) has reviewed psychotherapy outcome research with adolescents and offered conclusions not much different from other reviews. Noting a sparseness in the adolescent literature, Tramontana found no clear evidence of effectiveness but found the area to be fraught with research methodology problems.

The reviews noted above all could be classified as evaluating the child psychotherapy research literature through the traditional critical literature review approach. More recently, the systematic approach of meta-analysis has been used as a mode of summarizing the efficacy literature in a variety of areas including that of psychotherapy. This approach combines the results of efficacy studies by evaluating the magnitude of the effect of treatments. Smith and Glass (1977) popularized this statistical approach in the psychotherapy literature. In a meta-analysis, each outcome result in a controlled study is treated as one unit of magnitude of effect or "effect size" (ES). The effect size is calculated by subtracting the mean of the control group (M_c) from the mean of the treated group (M_t) and then dividing the difference by the standard deviation of the control group (SD_c), i.e., ES = $M_t - M_c/SD_c$. The effect sizes are averaged to determine effects across and between treatments. The effect size is a standard score that indicates how many standard deviation units a treatment group differs from an untreated control group. A positive effect size indicates improvement or the beneficial effects of treatment. For example, an effect size of 1.00 indicates that an untreated subject at the mean of his or her group (i.e., the 50th percentile) would be expected, on average, to rise to the 84th percentile (i.e., a one standard deviation improvement) with treatment.

Evaluating across all types of counseling and psychotherapy, Smith and Glass (1977) found an average effect size of .68. Similar replications by Shapiro and Shapiro (1982) and by Landman and Dawes (1982) found overall effect sizes of .93 and .78, respectively. All three of these meta-analyses utilized primarily adult intervention studies, but all were generally supportive of the effectiveness of psychotherapy. Smith and Glass' analysis suggested that behavioral and nonbehavioral treatments were roughly equal in effectiveness, whereas Shapiro and Shapiro's finding suggested that behavioral and cognitive therapies were somewhat more effective than other therapies. The meta-analysis approach remains somewhat controversial and has met with some harsh criticism (e.g., Eysenck, 1978). Nonetheless, it does provide an option for more systematically and objectively summarizing research findings.

Two meta-analyses have been completed on the effectiveness of child/adolescent counseling and psychotherapy. Casey and Berman (1985) analyzed studies done primarily with younger children (under the age of 13) who received some form of psychotherapy, whereas Prout and DeMartino (1986) evaluated studies of children and adolescents who received interventions for school-based or school-related problems. Respectively, they found effect sizes across treatments of .71 and .58. These overall effect sizes are generally consistent with the meta-analyses done primarily with adult subjects. Using a model for evaluating the relative size of treatment effects proposed by Schroeder and Dush (1987), these effect sizes fall into the "moderate" effect size category.

More specifically, Casey and Berman (1985) found that behavioral and cognitive therapies were more effective than nonbehavioral (client-centered and dynamic) therapies with respective effect sizes of .91 and .40. Individual therapies were somewhat more effective than group interventions, .82 to .50. Similarly, Prout and DeMartino (1986) found behaviorally based treatments somewhat more effective than other approaches, .65 to .40, but found that school-based group interventions were superior to individual interventions, .63 to .39. Prout and DeMartino found only a small difference between interventions with elementary students vs. secondary students, .52 vs. .65. Both studies also found some differences in outcome related to the type of treatment targets and outcome measures. Casey and Berman (1985) note, however, that many of these comparisons are not meaningful because the various categorizing schemes also break the outcome studies into other classifications. For example, despite the differences they found between behavioral therapies and nonbehavioral therapies, the respective studies were often evaluating different problems with different targets and outcome measures. Thus, the treatment foci are frequently not equivalent, and it is not possible to make direct efficacy comparisons. It is best to view the various differences noted above cautiously.

Casey and Berman (1985) conclude that the evidence in their analysis indicates that psychotherapy with children is as effective as therapy with adults. Despite some continued shortcomings in the diagnostic and methodological areas, they feel that the available outcome studies demonstrate the efficacy of treatment across a range of therapeutic approaches and problems. They note: "clinicians and researchers need not be hesitant in defending the merits of psychotherapy with children" (p. 397). Similarly, Prout and DeMartino (1986) conclude that there is evidence to support counseling and psychotherapeutic efforts in the schools and for school-related problems.

In the first edition of this book it was noted that the outcome research on child and adolescent psychotherapy left one with a somewhat unclear and confusing impression (Prout, 1983). The available reviews at the time did not clearly support effectiveness, nor clearly prove the ineffectiveness, of child/adolescent therapeutic interventions. Yet, at the same time, they pointed to the complexity of the issue and the methodological problems in conducting research in this area. Although there are still many unresolved issues concerning the efficacy of child and adolescent therapeutic interventions, the recent meta-analyses of Casey and Berman (1985) and Prout and DeMartino (1986) do present systematic reviews suggesting at least some benefit to these interventions. Further, there are some preliminary data to support the greater efficacy of certain types of interventions, notably those interventions falling in the broad category of cognitive-behavioral interventions. Generally, there is now support that therapeutic interventions with children and adolescents are a viable clinical activity. Nonetheless, we continue to recommend a cautious, thoughtful, and examining approach to child and adolescent treatment.

SUMMARY

This chapter has attempted to provide an overview of the broad area of the psychological treatment of children and adolescents. We find a number of issues that are important to those who do clinical work with children. The mental health needs of children are an enormous problem and represent a need that has not yet been met by the social service and mental health delivery system. The child/adolescent therapist must be aware of developmental issues and must plan and conduct treatment accordingly. Further, the therapist must be aware of the unique aspects of the therapeutic relationship with children and adolescents. It has become somewhat clearer since the first edition of this book that a multimodal, combined approach to treatment is of efficacy. There is now moderate but clear support for the general effectiveness of child and adolescent therapeutic interventions.

REFERENCES

Abramowitz, C. V. (1976). The effectiveness of group psychotherapy with children. *Archives of General Psychiatry, 33,* 320-326.

Axline, V. (1947). *Play therapy.* Boston: Houghton Mifflin.

Barker, P. (1979). *Basic child psychiatry* (3rd ed.). Baltimore: University Park Press.

Barrett, C. L., Hampe, I. E., & Miller, L. (1978). Research on psychotherapy with children. In S. L. Garfield & A. D. Bergin (Eds.), *Handbook of psychotherapy and behavior change* (2nd ed.). New York: John Wiley and Sons.

Bergin, A. E., & Garfield, S. L. (Eds.). (1971). *Handbook of psychotherapy and behavior change.* New York: John Wiley and Sons.

Berlin, I. M. (Ed.). (1975). *Advocacy for child mental health.* New York: Brunner/Mazel.

Bower, E. M. (1969). *The early identification of emotionally handicapped children in school* (2nd ed.). Springfield, IL: Charles C. Thomas.

Casey, R. J., & Berman, J. S. (1985). The outcome of psychotherapy with children. *Psychological Bulletin, 98,* 388-400.

Clarizio, H. F. (1979). Primary prevention of behavioral disorders in the schools. *School Psychology Digest, 8,* 434-445.

Clarizio, H. F., & McCoy, G. F. (1976). *Behavior disorders in children* (2nd ed.). New York: Thomas Y. Crowell.

Copeland, A. D. (1974). *Textbook of adolescent psychopathology and treatment.* Springfield, IL: Charles C. Thomas.

Cowen, E. (1973). Social and community interventions. *Annual Review of Psychology, 24,* 423-471.

Cummings, N. A. (1979). Funding for children's services. *American Psychologist, 34,* 1037-1039.

Erickson, M. T. (1978). *Child psychopathology.* Englewood Cliffs, NJ: Prentice-Hall.

Erikson, E. H. (1963). *Childhood and society* (2nd ed.). New York: Norton.

Eysenck, H. J. (1952). The effects of psychotherapy: An evaluation. *Journal of Consulting Psychology, 16,* 319-324.

Eysenck, H. J. (1978). An exercise in meta silliness (Comment). *American Psychologist, 33,* 517.

Freud, S. (1955). *Analysis of a phobia in a five-year-old boy.* London: Hogarth Press. (Original work published 1909)

Garfield, S. L., & Bergin, A. E. (1978). *Handbook of psychotherapy and behavior change.* (2nd ed.). New York: John Wiley.

Garfield, S. L., Bergin, A. E. (1986). *Handbook of psychotherapy and behavior change.* (3rd ed.). New York: John Wiley and Sons.

Graziano, A. M. (Ed.). (1975). *Behavior therapy with children.* Chicago: Aldine.

Havighurst, R. J. (1951). *Developmental tasks and education.* New York: Longmans.

Joint Commission on Mental Health of Children. (1973). *The mental health of children: Services, research, and manpower.* New York: Harper and Row.

Keat, D. B. (1979). *Multimodal therapy with children.* New York: Pergamon Press.

Klein, M. (1932). *The psychoanalysis of children.* London: Hogarth Press.

Kohlberg, L. (1964). Development of moral character and moral ideology. In M. L. Hoffman & L. W. Hoffman (Eds.), *Review of child development research* (Vol. 1). New York: Russell Sage Foundation.

Kohlberg, L. (1973). Continuities in childhood and adult moral development revisited. In P. B. Baltes & K. W. Schaie (Eds.), *Lifespan developmental psychology: Personality and socialization.* New York: Academic Press.

Landman, J. T., & Dawes, R. M. (1982). Psychotherapy outcome: Smith and Glass' conclusions stand up under scrutiny. *American Psychologist, 37,* 504-516.

Lazarus, A. A. (1976). *Multimodal behavior therapy.* New York: Springer.

Levitt, E. E. (1957). The results of psychotherapy with children: An evaluation. *Journal of Consulting Psychology, 21,* 186-189.

Levitt, E. E. (1963). Psychotherapy with children: A further evaluation. *Behavior Research and Therapy, 60,* 326-329.

Levitt, E. E. (1971). Research on psychotherapy with children. In A. E. Bergin & S. L. Garfield (Eds.), *Handbook of psychotherapy and behavior change.* New York: John Wiley and Sons.

MacFarlane, J., Allen, L., & Honzik, M. (1954). *A developmental study of the behavior problems of normal children between twenty-one months and fourteen years.* Berkeley: University of California Press.

Meeks, J. E. (1971). *The fragile alliance: An orientation to the outpatient psychotherapy of the adolescent.* Baltimore: Williams and Wilkins.

Meeks, J. E. (1979). The therapeutic alliance in the psychotherapy of adolescents. In J. R. Novello (Ed.), *The short course in adolescent psychiatry.* New York: Brunner/Mazel.

Nathan, P. E. (1979). Diagnostic and treatment services for children: Introduction to the section. *American Psychologist, 34,* 967-968.

Neubauer, P. (1972). Normal development in childhood. In B. B. Wolman (Ed.), *Manual of child psychopathology.* New York: McGraw-Hill.

Nuffield, E. J. (1968). Child psychiatry limited: A conservative viewpoint. *Journal of the American Academy of Child Psychiatry, 7,* 210-212.

Prout, H. T. (1983). Counseling and psychotherapy with children and adolescents: An overview. In H. T. Prout & D. T. Brown (Eds.), *Counseling and psychotherapy with children and adolescents: Therory and practice for school and clinic settings.* Tampa, FL: Mariner.

Prout, H. T., & DeMartino, R. A. (1986). A meta-analysis of school-based studies of psychotherapy. *Journal of School Psychology, 24,* 285-292.

Quay, H. C. (1979). Classification. In H. D. Quay & J. S. Weery (Eds.), *Psychopathological disorders of childhood* (2nd ed.). New York: John Wiley and Sons.

Schecter, M. D., Toussieng, P. W., & Sternlof, R. E. (1972). Normal development in adolescence. In B. B. Wolman (Ed.), *Manual of child psychopathology.* New York: McGraw-Hill.

Schroeder, H. E., & Dush, D. M. (1987). Relinquishing the placebo: Alternative for psychotherapy outcome research. *American Psychologist, 41,* 1129-1130.

Schwartz, S., & Johnson, J. H. (1981). *Psychopathology of childhood.* New York: Pergamon Press.

Shapiro, D. A., & Shapiro, D. (1982). Meta-analysis of comparative therapy outcome studies: A replication and refinement. *Psychological Bulletin, 92,* 581-604.

Smith, M. L., & Glass, G. V. (1977). Meta-analysis of psychotherapy outcome studies. *American Psychologist, 32,* 752-760.

Tramontana, M. G. (1980). Critical review of research on psychotherapy with adolescents: 1967-1977. *Psychological Bulletin, 88,* 429-450.

Wadsworth, B. J. (1971). *Piaget's theory of cognitive development.* New York: David McKay.

Weiner, I. B. (1970). *Psychological disturbance in adolescence.* New York: John Wiley and Sons.

Chapter 2

Ethical and Legal Issues in Psychological Interventions with Children and Adolescents

Susan Ferber, Ed.S.
Richard A. DeMartino, Psy.D.
H. Thompson Prout, Ph.D.

The practice of child psychotherapy has been in existence for several decades but unlike its adult counterpart has had comparatively few research, development, and classification systems designed specifically for it (Johnson, Rasbury, & Siegal, 1986). Similarly, the professional, ethical, and legal considerations which pertain to therapy services for children have also been deficient. The primary emphasis has been on adult psychotherapy and on the therapist's role in relation to the adult client. However, different issues arise, both ethically and legally, when children are the recipients of therapeutic interventions. According to Ross (1980, p. 62), "the ethical implications of treating an individual's psychological problems increase in magnitude as an inverse function of that individual's freedom of choice."

Ethical considerations, by nature, do not have simple, straightforward, or black-and-white solutions; nevertheless, they are critical to child clinicians and mental health service providers. It is important that each therapist understand his or her role as it pertains to children's legal rights as well as the ramifications, both negative and positive, of therapeutic interventions with minors.

The purpose of this chapter is to discuss the legal and ethical considerations involved with the provision of therapeutic services to children and adolescents. This chapter will present a brief review of general ethical principles, followed by a discussion of special considerations in working with child/adolescent populations. Legal issues related to definitions of treatment, confidentiality and privileged communication, informed consent, records and privacy, and special considerations in schools will be discussed.

ETHICAL ISSUES

General Ethical Principles

Virtually all human service, educational, and medical associations have some type of ethical code or set of ethical principles to guide the professional behavior of their practitioners. These codes or principles are not legally binding, although their foci may overlap with some statutes. This is perhaps one of the major distinctions between ethical and legal principles. A violation of an ethical principle, when no related statute exists, can result only in censure, probation, or expulsion by the respective professional organization. Evidence of unethical practice may support documentation in a legal case but by itself has consequences related only to the professional organization.

The ethical guidelines of the major helping service professions (e.g., American Association for Counseling and Development, 1988; American Psychological Association, 1981; National Association of School Psychologists, 1985) provide codes that relate in part to ethical considerations in conducting psychological interventions with children and adolescents. A number of similarities and consistent themes tend to occur across these various sets of ethical principles. Additionally, many of these principles are interrelated. Some of the general ethical themes relevant to the practice of child/adolescent therapy will be reviewed below. It should be noted that more focused sets of ethical guidelines also exist. For example, Allen, Sampson, and Herlihy (1988) note that several of the divisions (e.g, mental health, career development) of the American Association for Counseling and Development have their own sets of professional codes.

The purpose of the following section will be to provide an overview of several of the ethical principles related to therapeutic intervention with children and adolescents. Although not all of the ethical principles of the various associations can be presented here, the following are included: responsibility and client welfare, confidentiality, professional relationships, competence, public statements and presentations, and private practice issues.

Responsibility and *client welfare* refer to the general concept of professionals' assuming responsibility for their position of influence with clients and recognizing the consequences of their actions and professional activities. In doing so, they promote foremost the welfare of their client or clients. With regard to psychological interventions, professionals use techniques that have the likelihood of promoting therapeutic gain in their clients and accept the responsibility of the consequences/results/changes of the use of the various techniques. Professionals should avoid conflicts of interest regarding their clients, clarifying allegiances between their clients, employers, agencies, and other persons directly involved. Clients should be fully informed about the nature of the services offered by the professional. When a client is clearly not benefiting from services, the professional should alter or terminate the therapeutic relationship.

Professionals have the responsibility to protect the *confidentiality* of information gathered in the context of a therapeutic relationship. The ethical principle of confidentiality should be distinguished from the legal concept of confidentiality which is discussed later in this chapter. Information should be released only with the permission of the client, with special provisions to protect those clients who cannot give informed consent. Professional cases should be discussed only with directly concerned colleagues. Both this information and the client's identity should be disguised if it is to be used in other contexts (i.e., teaching, training, case examples, etc.), or the client's consent should be obtained. Confidentiality also relates to the proper maintenance, storage, and disposal of notes or records of counseling or therapeutic interventions.

Issues related to *professional relationships* involve a variety of relationships with other colleagues, clients, and other concerned parties. Professionals should develop and maintain relationships with other colleagues in the human service area. They should also be aware of the traditions and practices of those in other professional disciplines and groups in order to cooperate with and utilize the resources of these other professionals. Therapeutic services should not be offered to a client who is receiving services from another professional. Professionals should be aware that there may be multiple parties concerned with the welfare of a client. Again, the professional's allegiances should be clarified.

Professionals are obligated to practice within the limits of their *competence.* They should recognize the limits of their skills, the techniques they utilize, and the range of clinical problems with which they are equipped to deal therapeutically. They should function within the sphere of their education, training, and professional experiences and accurately present their qualifications and backgrounds to clients. In conjunction with this ethic, it is incumbent upon professionals to participate in continuing education and other forms of professional development to maintain and improve upon their level of competency. If personal problems, conflicts, or other factors interfere with their therapeutic effectiveness and competence, they should take steps to protect their clients' welfare.

Issues related to *public statements and presentations* concern the presentation of materials in advertising, public lectures, and the print and electronic media. Announcements of services should present accurate, factual information about professional background and services offered and avoid testimonials or guarantees. Public presentations about psychological topics should focus on scientifically accurate information. Therapeutic and other professional services should be conducted not in a public forum, but rather in the context of a professional relationship.

There are aspects of *private practice* that could be problematic for both client and professional. Those practitioners in private practice should fully inform their clients about financial requirements and considerations in that relationship. If also employed in an institution, it is unethical to use one's institutional affiliation to solicit clients. In some situations, clients should be informed of services available through public institutions (e.g., schools).

A report from the Ethics Committee of the American Psychological Association (1988) found a large increase in both the number of inquiries (with intent to file) about ethical violations and the number of formal complaints actually filed. Ethical violations are classified by the specific principle and section(s) of principles found to have been violated. In terms of actual adjudicated complaints, the largest numbers of violations were found involving the principles of dual relationships, adherence to professional standards, governmental laws and institutional regulations, and confidentiality. "Dual relationships" refers to any relationship a psychologist might have with a client that might impair professional judgment and/or present the risk of exploitation. This could include the assessment and treatment of clients' friends, relatives, or employees, for example, as well as sexually intimate relationships with clients. The majority of complaints in this area dealt with psychologists' being sexually involved with their clients. Complaints regarding adherence to standards, laws, and regulations most often dealt with violation of a law or other formal legal (civil or criminal) adjudication. In particular, psychologists have had problems related to fee policies and practices, most often involving fraudulent third-party billing practices. Problems in confidentiality have involved both breaking confidentiality in violation of the law *and* refusing to break confidentiality where required by law, as in the case of mandated reporting of child abuse. Failure to follow informed consent procedures has posed problems in this area.

Special Considerations with Children and Adolescents

There are several ethical considerations with which all individuals in the helping professions must be concerned. However, there are also issues specific to those who provide services to children and adolescents. The issues to be discussed are client identification (child, parent/family, agency/school) and concomitant therapist responsibilities, child and parental rights, confidentiality, and general professional ethics with respect to service delivery and retraining.

CLIENT IDENTIFICATION. A major issue confronting child/adolescent therapists is identification of the client; the child, the parent(s), and in the case of educational personnel, the school. Ideally, there is minimal if any conflict between the triad or any combination within it.

According to the National Association of School Psychologists' (NASP, 1985) Principles of Professional Ethics, the pupil is the primary client. It is, therefore, the responsibility of the school psychologist to place the needs and rights of the child as the client first. However, it cannot always be assumed that professionals are necessarily child advocates or that they automatically recommend what is most appropriate for the child (Koocher, 1976). Koocher (1976) further states that a therapist is morally obligated to serve as a child advocate, because children cannot "serve as . . . their own advocate due to psychological or physical factors, immaturity, or legal statute" (p. 30).

Although it "makes sense" in theory that a clinician would relegate the child to the role of client, because it is the child who is being treated, practically and legally the role of the parent must also be considered. Because parents have legal responsibility for the well-being of their children under the age of 18 according to most state statutes, therapists have a responsibility to them. However, this factor can be confusing and conflictual at times for the service provider. Gumaer (1984) stated that because parents are legally responsible for their children, they need to be informed of and approve of any therapy or interventions. Most often parents are the primary referral agents for their child, and children frequently become involved in therapy because of parental referral rather than a personal request for help. They have usually been identified as having a "problem" based on adult perception (Ross, 1980). According to Koocher (1976), therapists infrequently refuse to consider a child as a client at the onset based upon his or her unwillingness to participate. Therefore, an agreement of sorts has been made with the parents, regardless of the child's wishes, which identifies the parent(s) as also having some client characteristics. Parental input is also critical to the therapeutic process concerning background information, problem identification, and goal setting.

Koocher (1976) and Ross (1980) raise the issue of whether parental rights are stymied when a child refuses treatment and a therapist accepts this decision. Several factors should be considered by a therapist when making this decision. According to

Johnson et al. (1986), the specific factors to be considered are "age and level of cognitive development of the child, the child's degree of disturbance, the degree of disturbance noted in the parents, and the degree to which the therapist feels that treatment is warranted." Wagner (1981) suggests that the younger the child's age, the greater the responsibility a therapist has to the parents. It appears that it is the role and responsibility of a counselor to view both the child and parent(s) as clients and ascertain the most appropriate means to meet the needs of both parties (Gelfand & Hartman, 1975; Ross, 1980).

An additional factor to be considered is the relationship of the therapist to the agency for which he or she works. Because many school psychologists, counselors, and social workers have been hired by educational agencies to provide therapy and counseling services to children within the school system, they have subsequent employer responsibilities. According to Huey (1986), acceptance of a staff position in an educational setting implies general agreement with the institution's objectives and principles. He further states that a counselor should not be perceived as more concerned with school rules than child rights, but should seek solutions to protect these rights in addition to advocating school policies to further them. Parents are seen as a third part of the triad of child and school, in which a cooperative relationship among the three is critical, albeit difficult, conflictual, and ambiguous at times. However, Huey (1986) sees ambiguity and ethical conflicts among the triad components as an inherent part of the school counselor/psychologist's role. It is a role that requires professional decision making based on ethical values and legal restraints in conjunction with a willingness to accept responsibility for judgments made concerning a child.

CHILD AND PARENTAL RIGHTS. The majority of the literature which discusses child and parental rights emphasizes that both parties are to be considered clients, but that it is the primary responsibility of the therapist to protect the rights of the child (Huey, 1986; Hughes, 1986; Koocher, 1976; Ross, 1980). This statement of ethical values provides what on the surface is an appropriate goal. However, in reality it is not necessarily easily obtained nor specific. Duncan and Moffett (1974) state that ethical guidelines do not apply to all situations and that their interpretation is affected by the therapist's values and attitudes. It is important when protecting the rights of parents and children for the therapist to be careful not to allow personal beliefs to interfere, but rather to assist parents and children in making appropriate decisions (Huey, 1986).

A summary of key rights for children and parents as described by several authors in the ethics literature (Huey, 1986; Koocher, 1976; Ross, 1980; Simmonds, 1976) follows.

Some of the key *rights of children* are that a child in therapy has the:

1. Right to be informed about the evaluation process and reasons and results in understandable terms;
2. Right to be informed about therapeutic interventions and rationale in understandable terms;
3. Right to be informed about confidentiality and its limitations;
4. Right to control release of information;
5. Right not to be involved in therapy if uncomfortable or unsuccessful (this is not always possible when it is mandated, i.e., by court order or Individual Education Plan);
6. Right to be treated with respect and told the truth;
7. Right to participate with the therapist and/or parents(s) in decision making and goal setting;
8. Right not to be labeled the scapegoat in a dysfunctional family.

Some of the key *parental rights and responsibilities* include the:

1. Legal responsibility to provide for their child's welfare;
2. Right to access to information (educational, medical, therapeutic) that pertains to their child's welfare;
3. Right to seek therapy and/or treatment services for their child;

4. Right to be involved in therapeutic decision making and goal setting for their child—right to give permission for treatments;
5. Right to release confidential information concerning their child.

It is evident from these lists of child and parental rights that there is overlap and interface between the two. The parental rights mentioned are for the most part also legal rights, unless legal guardianship has been removed by the courts. However, several of the child's rights are ethical values and not mandated or dictated by law. They have been presented by the abovementioned authors as recommendations to protect a child's rights during counseling or therapeutic interventions. A professional must make decisions and recommendations, particularly where the child's rights are concerned, depending upon variables, such as age, as were previously mentioned.

A factor that bears ethical consideration in the area of child rights is one discussed by Simmonds (1976) that involves a child referred for therapy when the family is the presenting problem. For example, a child is referred for counseling and identified by his or her parents as "problematic" when interviews and other disclosures reveal a family/parental dysfunction that would warrant a family counseling/systems approach (Simmonds, 1976). The child may be labeled as "dysfunctional" for insurance purposes, for example, due to the fact that he or she has no recourse or legal rights. Such a procedure may be prejudicial to the child in later years, according to Simmonds.

Additionally, a conflict in values may arise between parent and child when a treatment goal is based on parental request but the behavior causes no personal difficulties for the child. Ross (1980) raises the issue of whether, in such a situation, parental rights are violated if a child, particularly a young child, has the right to refuse treatment.

Ultimately rights for children and parents will be affected by the individual situation. Professional decisions will vary from client to client as a therapist strives to protect both child's and parents' rights, while advocating for the child.

CONFIDENTIALITY. Another ethical issue that regularly confronts therapists in private practice, mental health agencies, and school settings is that of confidentiality. The American Psychological Association guidelines (1981) state that client information is confidential unless the client gives permission to reveal or discuss it. However, as Johnson et al. (1986) state, it is common for professionals to share reports with other professionals involved with the child, such as teachers, private psychologists, and counselors. However, this is done with permission of the child's parent or legal guardian, rather than that of the child. It appears that the child's permission to share this information should ethically be obtained as a matter of routine.

There are also legal limitations to confidentiality such as the Family Educational Rights and Privacy Act and court-ordered evaluation and/or counseling. In these situations, information obtained specifically must be available to parents and to judicial or social services personnel. These issues are discussed in the Legal Issues section of this chapter.

Additional confidentiality issues that are less specifically defined, such as those which occur during individual or group counseling, should also be considered by mental health providers. Because parents, as a child's legal guardians, in many states have access to therapy records (Ehrenreich & Melton, 1983), it seems logical to search for a level of communication that is acceptable to both parents and the child. For example, a child should be told initially in therapy what information (i.e., statements of a suicidal nature or those that involve danger to others) will be shared with parents without his or her permission. Johnson et al. (1986) recommend that therapists seek a balance between a.child's and parents' rights, such as discussing general topics which arise during therapy but not the specific details.

Counseling provided in a group setting also involves protection of a child's rights of confidentiality. Gumaer (1984) recommends this be explained to the children at the onset of the counseling session in understandable terms (i.e., "What is talked about in group is not talked about outside of group" "You may talk to others about topics discussed, but do not mention names"). Consequences of breaking the confidentiality agreement can be decided by group members. Because of the nature of the school setting, groups in these settings may be particularly prone to problems of breaking confidentiality.

Confidentiality is designed to protect the child's privacy. Again, the therapist may find himself or herself in situations that will involve decision making that may alienate or upset either the child/client or parent when an acceptable compromise cannot be made.

PROFESSIONAL ETHICAL RESPONSIBILITIES. In addition to the previously mentioned ethical considerations which are primarily concerned with the protection of child and parental rights, the issues to be discussed pertain to the service provider. A major issue is that of professional competence or expertise in the areas of treatment the psychologist provides. For example, a therapist trained in adult psychopathology ethically should not treat children, or a child specialist treat adults, without specific training. According to Johnson et al. (1986), general training in "clinical psychology, psychiatry, or social work does not necessarily qualify one to offer psychological services to children, as many training programs do not provide didactic and clinical experience in working with younger age groups" (p. 94). Professional ethics would warrant a referral to another appropriately trained therapist under these circumstances.

A related concern involves obtaining a second professional opinion in situations where a treatment recommendation is controversial (i.e., aversive treatment) or unacceptable to parents (Koocher, 1976).

Continuing education and professional growth and development are also ethically critical, particularly to ensure that a therapist is providing up-to-date treatment and therapy recommendations for a child.

LEGAL ISSUES

Interventions: Searching for a Model

Historically, mental health professionals went relatively unchallenged in their ability to make wise and informed decisions about the treatment of institutionalized individuals (Binder, 1980).

Two landmark cases on patients' rights, *Donaldson v. O'Connor* (1974) and *Wyatt v. Stickney* (1971/1972), have led to significant reforms in the processes applied to mental health practice. These cases involved the problem of defining both minimum standards of care as well as the rights of patients to adequate treatment.

The definition of "treatment," "intrusiveness," or "intervention" has been a matter of considerable debate in the field. Several authors have sought to define criteria for "degree of intrusiveness" (Binder, 1980; Friedman, 1975; Shapiro, 1974; Spece, 1972). Spece (1972) applied a continuum model of mental health treatments from least to most intrusive. The corresponding list included: milieu therapy, psychotherapy, drug therapy, behavior modification, aversive therapy, ECT, brain stimulation, lobotomy, and stereotactic psychosurgery. Obviously, the more severe of these interventions are beyond the scope of the typical practice of most mental health professionals.

Binder (1980) presents an integration of many authors' views delineating criteria that may be used to examine intervention approaches:

> (a) the extent to which the "new mental state is foreign or unnatural" to the person in question,
>
> (b) the extent to which the effects of the therapy are reversible,
>
> (c) duration of change,
>
> (d) the rapidity with which the effects occur,
>
> (e) the extent of bodily invasion,
>
> (f) the nature of side effects,
>
> (g) the extent to which an "uncooperative" patient can avoid the effects of the treatment . . . (p. 3).

These criteria highlight the fact that mental health practice continues to function largely from a medical model perspective (Szasz, 1974) where "degree of intrusiveness" is frequently discussed in the context of medical invasion of the body (Binder, 1980). Without considering theoretical orientation or the subjective nature of defining the wide variety of therapeutic interventions, a continuum ranking, such as provided by Spece (1972), suggests that, from a legal standpoint, certain interventions should only be used after other less intrusive therapies have been tried and have failed (Binder, 1980).

As Binder proposes, there is agreement that psychological treatments cannot be easily ranked. The multitude of psychotherapies alone differ markedly in terms of definition, implementation, and general acceptance within the mental health community. Even given an agreed-upon definition, the variety of behavioral techniques such as systematic desensitization, biofeedback, and relaxation therapies would be difficult to rank order from a "degree of intrusiveness" viewpoint. It appears, however, that child mental health practitioners should consider the potential legal implications of "degree of intrusiveness" in selecting interventions. For example, the possible use of aversive techniques with school-aged children involves more complex legal and ethical principles than a more traditional counseling or consultative intervention.

Relevant Case Law

In this section three rather broad and interrelated domains of law will be discussed as they apply to interventions: confidentiality/privileged communication, informed consent, and access to records.

CONFIDENTIALITY AND PRIVILEGED COMMUNICATION. Although frequently used interchangeably, important distinctions exist between the legal concepts of "confidentiality" and "privileged communication." Confidentiality refers to a general obligation of a professional to avoid disclosing information regarding the relationship with a client to any third party. Privileged communication is narrower in scope than confidentiality. As Jagim, Wittman, and Noll (1978) note, "whereas confidentiality concerns matters of communication outside the courtroom, privilege protects clients from disclosure in judicial proceedings" (Jagim et al., 1978, p. 459). Thus, although an obligation to preserve confidentiality constitutes a broad duty owed by a professional to a client, "psychotherapist-patient privilege is a rule of evidence relevant only in court proceedings" (Hulteng & Goldman, 1987, p. 239).

The courts have generally held that mental health professionals have a common-law obligation to protect the confidentiality of the relationship with a client (Hulteng & Goldman, 1987). In *Doe v. Roe* (1977) a New York psychiatrist was held to have invaded a former client's privacy when he published a book about the plaintiff's treatment and failed to conceal personally identifiable information sufficiently. In this case the court leaned heavily on the notion that physicians implicitly agree to keep in confidence all disclosures made by the patient within the context of a contract to provide medical treatment. The court specified that these disclosures included the patient's physical and mental condition, and all matters discovered in the course of examination or treatment (*Doe v. Roe,* 1977, p. 210).

In a more recent case, *McDonald v. Clinger* (1982), a New York court held that a psychiatrist breached his "fiduciary duty" when he disclosed information to the wife of a patient under his care. A fiduciary duty is described as that duty imposed in a relationship based on professional trust. The court also ruled that damages were recoverable.

There has been spirited debate about the therapeutic necessity of absolute confidentiality. The psychiatric community has historically expressed the belief that therapy would not be successful unless the client could freely, and with security, disclose personal information. In contrast, some forms of psychotherapy are espoused that seem to quash the sentiment that there can be no therapy without complete confidentiality (Kandler, 1977; Langs, 1976). Further, as Wilson (1978) suggests, clients do not seem more reluctant to convey personal information in states that do not protect communications from legal scrutiny.

Regardless of one's therapeutic position on total versus limited confidentiality, two general reasons exist for the continued safeguard of client-counselor confidentiality. First, a confidential relationship does serve to limit clients' concerns about the social stigma often associated with participation in therapy (Denkowski & Denkowski, 1982; Sloan & Klein, 1977). A United States Department of Health, Education and Welfare (1963) survey documented the basis for the stigmatization concern. It found that 60% of those surveyed "would not act or feel normally towards a former mental patient, even though they did not learn of his illness until they had known him for some time without noticing anything about him" (1963, p. 8). Second, as discussed earlier, a central ethical obligation for professionals is the assurance that a client's right to privacy and reputation are well preserved (Denkowski & Denkowski, 1982).

The notion of a "special relationship" forms the basis of privilege as it applies to disclosures in the courtroom. The laws of various states ultimately govern the scope of privileged communication but may include husband-wife, attorney-client, clergyman-penitent, and physician-patient relationships (Fischer & Sorenson, 1985). Psychologist-client communications are privileged from disclosure in court in 41 (82%) of the 50 states (Herlihy & Sheeley, 1986). All 50 states have regulations that apply for "school counselors." Privileged communication statutes exist in 21 of these states, "providing protection from disclosure of school counselor/student communications" (Herlihy & Sheeley, 1986, p. 4); in 5 of the 21, the privilege is strictly limited to those communications relating to student drug and alcohol concerns.

Even in states which do have statutes regarding "privilege," this right is typically granted to clients of psychologists, not to psychologists themselves (McDermott, 1972). Because the right to assert or waive the privilege to prevent disclosure in courtroom proceedings is granted to the client, issues of competency are often involved. Typically the child mental health practitioner's client is a minor and is, therefore, considered legally incompetent to exercise the privilege. In this case the privilege reverts to the minor's legal guardians (McDermott, 1972). Because privileged communication for school counselors most frequently pertains to clients who are legally considered minors, some statutes include provisions for involving parents in the decision to waive counselor privilege. In fact, only two states have statutes which allow almost complete unilateral control by the student in waiving the rights of nondisclosure (Herlihy & Sheeley, 1986).

It should be noted that in states protecting the relationship between clients and psychologists, the term "psychologist" usually refers to those who have been licensed, registered, or certified by a state board of examiners or similar body for the purpose of regulating the public and private practice of psychology. This, for example, frequently excludes "school psychologists" (McDermott, 1972) or others who use similar titles but are not licensed. Privileged communication may apply, however, if a school psychologist also holds a license as a psychologist and if the licensing statute provides for privilege in that state (Knapp & VandeCreek, 1983).

The courts, although often supporting the concept of privilege, have at times insisted that a therapist divulge "confidential" client information (Denkowski & Denkowski, 1982). Judicial sentiment has found that confidential privilege for "therapists" did not apply in *State v. Bishop* (1969), *State v. Pyle* (1975), and *Stevens v. State* (1976). As Fischer and Sorenson (1985) note, even in long-recognized exemptions such as attorney-client relationships, courts have demanded that certain conditions be met:

> (a) one party in the relationship must be legally certified as a lawyer, doctor, or minister,
>
> (b) at the time of the communication in question, he or she must have been acting in a professional capacity,
>
> (c) the person making the communication, if in possession of his or her faculties, must have regarded the professional person as his or her lawyer, doctor, or minister. (pp. 16-17)

School-based professionals should note that once information is included in a school file, it cannot be considered potentially privileged communication but, in fact, falls under the provisions of the Family Educational Rights and Privacy Act (FERPA, 1974), which governs access and privacy. Privileged communication statutes, even when they do exist, do not represent absolute guarantees. Even when there is statutory support there are circumstances, including client request or clear and imminent danger to the client or others, that could prove exceptional (Herlihy & Sheeley, 1986).

It is this final exception, otherwise known as the "duty to warn principle," that has represented the "harbinger of perceived doom, gloom and tremulousness for many mental health professionals" (George, 1985, p. 291). In the well-known case of *Tarasoff v. Regents* (1976), the confidential relationship of a psychologist and his patient was the subject of a very controversial ruling.

The Tarasoff case revolved around a suit filed by the parents of Tatiana Tarasoff, who was killed in 1969 by the patient of a University of California hospital psychologist. Two months prior to her death, during his therapy sessions with the psychologist, the patient had confided his intention to kill Ms. Tarasoff. The Tarasoffs' suit claimed that there was a "duty to warn" their daughter of the impending danger. Although the psychologist did notify the campus police, the California Supreme Court ruled that the psychologist did indeed have a duty to warn a known, intended victim directly. The court held that a special relationship existed between any therapist and patient and that the duty which arose from the therapist's knowledge that his patient posed a serious threat of violence meant that reasonable care must be taken to protect a foreseeable victim of potential violence (George, 1986).

The Tarasoff case and more recent cases (e.g., *Hedlund v. Superior Court,* 1983) have caused considerable furor among mental health professionals. In tempering the "paranoia" generated by these cases, George (1986) states, "the determinative question remains whether the professional person failed to exercise that reasonable degree of skill, knowledge, and care ordinarily possessed and exercised by members of that professional specialty under similar circumstances" (p. 294). Although the controversy remains, several state legislatures have enacted laws which limit the potential liability to some degree. It is perhaps safest to assume that professionals have a duty to warn a known intended victim of his or her client's violent intent (Fischer & Sorenson, 1985).

In a more recent case, *Phyllis P. v. Clairmont Unified School District* (1986), the California Supreme Court held that a principal, teacher, and school psychologist failed to comply with their duty to warn the mother of an 8-year-old girl that her daughter was being sexually molested by another student at the school. The student, Phyllis P., stated to her teacher that another student was "playing games" with her. The teacher told the school psychologist and the school psychologist initiated counseling. The principal was also aware of the situation. The court noted that not only did the school fail to notify the mother that the assaults were taking place, it neglected to obtain informed consent for treatment and did not properly supervise the molesting student. Additionally, the court held that the mother could sue the district for this failure to warn.

To summarize, confidentiality and privileged communication are two distinct concepts and should not be used interchangeably. Though emerging case law supports a common-law obligation to preserve confidentiality, it is largely an ethical consideration. Privilege, on the other hand, deals with the admissibility of evidence into court. Although various states have enacted statutes that grant these exceptions beyond the historical relationships (e.g., lawyer-client, clergyman-penitent) to psychologist-client, some professionals may nonetheless have a legal duty to testify if ordered by a court (Fischer & Sorenson, 1985). Refusal to do so may lead to contempt citations, fines, or jail terms. Moreover, the privilege "belongs" to the client, not to the therapist.

In circumstances where a client expresses violent or harmful intentions toward another individual, a therapist has the "duty to warn" potential victims who are the targets of such threats. Further, professionals may not only have the duty to warn but may also infer a "duty to protect" third parties from violent acts (Mills, 1985). It is also clear that most professionals are "mandated reporters" for suspected cases of child abuse discovered in the course of their practice. Failure to report as required by state statute can result in both civil and criminal liability (Hulteng & Goldman, 1987).

INFORMED CONSENT. The term "informed consent" refers to the "receipt of specific permission to do something following a complete explanation of the nature, purpose and potential risks involved" (DeMers, 1986, p. 45). Informed consent is defined legally as involving three aspects: knowledge, competence/intelligence, and voluntariness (DeMers, 1986; Grisso & Vierling, 1978). Under the strictest of interpretations, the knowledge "test" requires that a professional *fully* inform the student/client/parent of all relevant information about a specific intervention approach so that the person becomes "aware" of what is being consented to (Waltz & Scheuneman, 1970). The intelligence or competence aspect of consent focuses on the ability of the child or parent to arrive at the consent rationally and independently. Within this concept are the notions of cognitive capacity and other mental health-related abilities of a client. Voluntariness refers to consent occurring in the absence of undue coercion or misrepresentation (Sadoff, 1985). The question of willful granting of permission is the typical legal standard by which this is measured (DeMers, 1986; Lidz et al., 1984).

Bray, Shepherd, and Hays (1985) suggest that the following must be included for valid consent: (a) a complete explanation of the treatment, risks, discomforts, and benefits; (b) a description of other possible treatment alternatives; (c) an offer to discuss the procedures or answer any questions; and (d) information that the client is free to withdraw consent at any time and discontinue treatment. Consent obtained pursuant to these disclosures will be "express consent." "Apparent consent" and "consent implied by law" are two other types of consent. "Apparent consent" would apply where all parties act as if consent had been given, when in actuality none was formally stated. "Consent implied by law" comes into play in questions of competency for clients most frequently seen by mental health professionals in hospital or inpatient settings (Slovenko, 1973).

One of the major controversies in this area is the age at which a person may legally consent to treatment (Bray et al., 1985; Grisso & Vierling, 1978; Sadoff, 1985). Whereas Bersoff (1982) notes that there has been a general trend for the courts to grant adolescents greater leeway in obtaining medical or psychological intervention without parental permission, there is no question that treatment of preadolescents should involve the consent of parents or legal guardians (Reynolds, Gutkin, Elliot, & Witt, 1984).

Although some state legislatures have recently sought to institute parental consent as a prerequisite, the courts have generally found that a pregnant minor may obtain an abortion and/or purchase contraceptives without parental permission (e.g., *Carey v. Population Services International, Inc.*, 1977; *Planned Parenthood of Central Missouri v. Danforth,* 1976). These decisions have been based on the belief that a requirement for parental consent might inhibit minors seeking such treatments—contrary to the individual's and society's best interest (Bray et al., 1985). To infer that adolescents thus have the right to seek the broad range of therapies without parental consent may not be prudent for the practitioner, however. Bersoff (1982), for example, reports that "it is presently very risky for school psychologists to agree to see children for any kind of therapeutic purpose without their parents' consent" (p. 1068). Unless parents are clearly endangering their children, as in the case of child abuse, the courts are decidedly "pro parents" with respect to consent (Reynolds et al., 1984). As an ethical and therapeutic consideration, the importance of parental permission for most psychological interventions is warranted. As a practical matter it must be balanced by the issue of concern, the age of the child, and the child's legal status (e.g., minor, emancipated minor, adult). The assent of the child should clearly be obtained because cooperation with any procedure affects treatment and its outcome (Schectman, Hays, Schuham, & Smith, 1982).

ACCESS TO RECORDS/RIGHT TO PRIVACY. An analogous concern to the confidentiality/privilege issue is the privacy right granted by the federal Family Educational Rights and Privacy Act (FERPA, 1974), popularly known as the Buckley Amendment. Although privilege was previously referred to as the protection of testimony or professional opinion about a client, the "data privacy" notion discussed in this section is more concerned with the release and storage of information (Lombard, 1981).

The Buckley Amendment essentially mandates the withholding of federal funds to schools or other educational agencies that fail to require parental consent or a court order for the release of records for other than defined educational purposes. With the increasing use of courts to resolve custody, child abuse/neglect, juvenile delinquency, and status offenses, the records of school-based professionals are often subpoenaed by clients, states, and adversarial parties. A subpoena may require the production of records, including notes, tape recordings, videotapes, memoranda, letters, and any other written material (Schrier, 1980). Though a detailed listing of all the provisions contained in FERPA is beyond the scope of this chapter, important requirements include that (a) parents or students 18 years or older be told the reasons for release and be given a copy of any released records, (b) parents be notified of any court order in advance of any release in order to have an opportunity to contest the contents of school records, and (c) parents be allowed to insert modifications into the record and challenge the contents. Parental consent must be obtained for release of information for children under age 18. For students 18 years of age or over or those attending postsecondary education, the rights for permission or consent shift from the parents to the student.

The Buckley Amendment does contain an exclusionary clause regarding the personal records of psychologists and counselors if these files are entirely private and not available to other individuals. This "memory aids" exception makes clear that private files of this type shall not be shared with or passed on to any other school personnel. They can be shared with a "substitute" without thereby becoming "education records" subject to FERPA (Fischer & Sorenson, 1985).

FERPA also requires that a record be kept of all parties requesting and receiving student information and that this record be made available to parents or eligible students. School districts may, however, develop policies to allow for undocumented exchanges between local district personnel by explicitly stating which school officials may have access without parental permission and noting the "legitimate educational interests" justifying the access.

With respect to the release of school records to "noncustodial parents," both FERPA and *Page v. Rotterdam-Mohanasen Central School District* (1981) clearly entitle the noncustodial parent to the same access to the child's educational records as the custodial parent (Fischer & Sorenson, 1985). This assumes that no specific court order prohibits contact between the child and the noncustodial parent. The federal law indicates that school professionals may assume a noncustodial parent's right to information unless otherwise stipulated. In cases where a child has no parent or legal guardian, educational records must also be accessible to a guardian or "an individual acting as a parent" (Fischer & Sorenson, 1985).

School-Based Interventions: Special Considerations

In this section, a variety of legal issues will be presented within the context of a range of school-based interventions, including behavior modification, the use of aversive techniques, group treatment, liability, and libel/slander.

BEHAVIOR MODIFICATION. As traditionally defined, "behavior modification" involves the application of learning principles designed to alleviate human suffering and enhance human functioning through behavior change. Behavior modification emphasizes systematic monitoring and evaluation of its techniques. Used appropriately, these techniques are intended to facilitate self-control and to expand individual skills, abilities, and independence (Stoltz, Wienckowski, & Brown, 1975).

The legal concepts that apply in this area are "due process," "equal protection," and a number of concepts from case law precedents. Constitutional due process provides that if government (e.g., school) activity affects a student in a way that deprives the student of "liberty" or "property," it must be with due process of law (Martin, 1975). Using behavioral approaches in schools could be construed as impinging on liberty. Thus, professionals in schools must be prepared to follow specific rules of due process and be able to justify therapeutic decisions in the forum of a fair hearing.

Broadly stated, "equal protection" under the Constitution suggests that a student cannot be treated in a way that differs substantially from treatment accorded others, unless there is some special justification. Therefore, any behavior change technique cannot unreasonably "single out" one group for treatment based, for example, on race or sex.

In *New York State Association for Retarded Children v. Rockefeller* (1973), the issue of inadequate or inappropriate treatment of handicapped persons was examined. In this case, the court found in favor of the plaintiff/clients whose condition was worsening after being involved in a state-run behavioral intervention program. Not only must therapy not worsen the client's condition, but persons cannot be placed in control groups for research purposes and be allowed to worsen for lack of treatment (Martin, 1975).

In the recent case of *Dickens v. Johnson County Board of Education* (1987), a time-out technique devised by a teacher and principal to isolate temporarily a disruptive sixth-grade student was ruled not in violation of procedural or substantive due process. In this case the "time-out box" had three sides and contained a school desk. The student spent as long as 4½ hours on 6 consecutive days in the box. The court noted that the judicious use of behavior modification techniques such as time-out is preferred over expulsion in disciplining disruptive students. The court also cautioned that the arbitrary "caging of students" for indeterminant lengths of time was prohibited.

USE OF AVERSIVE TECHNIQUES. Though many debate their value and the effects on the physical and mental health of students, punishment and other aversive interventions continue to be sanctioned in America's public schools (Wood & Braaten, 1983). Physical restraint, physically enforced overcorrection, and time-out procedures are among the approaches that may be employed by school-based professionals, particularly in specialized school or institutional settings.

In the last 15 years the eighth amendment prohibition against cruel and unusual punishment as it applies to behavioral interventions has been debated in the courts in a number of cases. In *Wheeler v. Glass* (1973), the court held that the restraint of two mentally retarded persons for 77.5 hours constituted cruel and unusual punishment. Restraint has similarly been viewed as cruel and unusual punishment in *Welsch v. Likins* (1974). *Wyatt v. Stickney* (1971/1972) produced a ruling which stated that whereas restraint could be used to prevent injury to others or self, it could not be used as punishment or as a substitute for habilitative programming or for the convenience of the staff.

However, in the landmark case *Ingraham v. Wright* (1977), the U.S. Supreme Court ruled that the severe paddling of two students for disciplinary reasons did not constitute a violation of the eighth amendment. In this case, the court ruled that the eighth amendment applied to the protection of criminals and was not designed to protect students in this way. Further, the court suggested that traditional common-law remedies are adequate to afford due process in a constitutionally protected liberty interest involving corporal punishment in public schools (e.g., sue for damages, assault and battery).

Time-out procedures are frequently used with exceptional children (Barton, Brulle, & Repp, 1983). The courts have distinguished between "time-out" and "solitary confinement." *Morales v. Turman* (1973) stated that seclusion was sanctioned only when it might prevent immediate physical harm to others or to the student or to prevent behavior that substantially disrupts the institutional routine. A maximum of 50 minutes in seclusion was determined in this case. *Horacek v. Exon* (1975) noted that seclusion in a locked room is forbidden.

GROUP TREATMENTS. Meyer and Smith (1977) present four interrelated axioms regarding the efficacy of group therapy. The first two are useful to the discussion of legal issues. Meyer and Smith submit that (a) confidences divulged in group therapy have the same protection under statutes of privileged communication as do those revelations made in individual therapy and (b) confidentiality is crucial to the effectiveness of group therapy (p. 638). Despite the inherent soundness of these statements, the courts have not agreed that the status of privileged communication applies to group treatments. As Fischer and Sorenson (1985) submit, this is rooted in the reluctance of courts to grant privilege or extend it to new types of relationships. Only the state of Colorado has statutes that recognize privilege for participants in group therapy. Thus, although the vast majority of group therapists and clients assume that the axiom of privilege is in effect (Meyer & Smith, 1977), there is little or no statutory or judicial assurance for this assumption.

LIABILITY. In today's litigious society, the fear many professionals may have of being sued in connection with their professional practice is a valid concern. In fact, Hendrickson (1982) argues that for counselors, liability/malpractice insurance is a must. Civil liability (when one commits a wrong against an individual) is considered in this domain. In general, civil liability for negligence occurs if one person causes damage to another through a breach of duty owed to that person. "Malpractice" refers to negligent practice in the rendering of professional services (Fischer & Sorenson, 1985).

The anxieties of many school professionals soar when they consider student issues including health matters, drug use/abuse, sexuality, and suicide. The ability to act with confidence in these areas rests not only on professional skill but on the understanding of these legal principles. Counselors legally have a "duty to use professionally accepted skills and care in working with counselees" (Fischer & Sorenson, 1985, p. 41).

In *Bogust v. Iverson* (1960), the suicide of a college-aged woman was alleged to be the result of negligence on the part of a college counselor/teacher because (a) the educator failed to secure emergency psychiatric treatment after he was aware, or should have been aware, of the young woman's incapacity; (b) he failed to advise her parents of her problems; and (c) he failed to provide proper student guidance (Fischer & Sorenson, 1985, p. 42). The Wisconsin Supreme Court ruled against the parents, finding no duty to warn, because there was no clear causal relationship between failure to alert her parents or to secure help and prevent the suicide.

Similarly, the ruling in *Bellah v. Greenson* (1978) refused to affirm the "duty to warn" principle in a case involving a suicide. In its ruling the court did not see suicide as an equivalent to impending danger of violence on members of society. The California court further noted that confidentiality is a crucial factor in the treatment of suicidal persons and that it outweighs a duty to warn the suicide victim's parents (Fischer & Sorenson, 1985).

LIBEL/SLANDER. Talbutt (1983) and Eades (1986) present brief reviews of issues relating to libel and slander in the practice of school counseling and psychology. "Libel" refers to written defamation, and "slander" refers to defamation expressed by word of mouth. Alexander, Corns, and McCann (1969) offer the necessary elements for a tort of libel or slander: (a) a false statement concerning another was published or communicated; (b) the statement brought hatred, disgrace, ridicule, or contempt on another person; and (c) damages resulted from the statement (p. 325).

Fischer and Sorenson (1985) suggest that the school-based professional is protected if he or she acted *reasonably* in carrying out the duties of his/her assigned responsibilities. The notion of what is *reasonable practice* in the field is often the legal standard applied in courtroom proceedings. "Qualified privilege" is a legal principle that protects the counselor who may communicate, in a professional manner to relevant persons, information or evaluations that may be considered negative or damaging. Mere random gossip or communication of derogatory information beyond ethical/professional guidelines may lead to successful suits for damages.

SUMMARY

Conducting psychological treatment of children's and adolescents' social-emotional problems is indeed a complex and challenging task. The clinical concerns and questions are compounded by an array of ethical and legal issues. Clinical options and plans must necessarily take these issues into consideration. At a basic level, the ethical principles of the major helping professions provide an overall guide for professional behavior. Because of age and developmental levels and the concerns of others (e.g., parents, schools), the child client presents some special ethical considerations. Similarly, there are some general legal issues that apply to persons receiving mental health services and these are made more complicated by the "minor" status of child and adolescent clients. Both statutes and relevant case law provide further guidelines for professional behavior.

The purpose of this chapter was to highlight some of the major issues present when working with children and adolescents. Although some questions in ethical and legal matters have relatively straightforward answers, there remain many grey areas. Clearly, the ethical principles, legal statutes, and case law do not completely overlap—in some cases, ethical principles may come into conflict with legal guidelines. We concur, finally, with the conclusion of Huey (1986): ethical codes do supersede the law, but legal knowledge may not always be sufficient to determine the most appropriate course of action.

REFERENCES

Alexander, K., Corns, R., & McCann, W. (1969). *Public school law.* St. Paul, MN: West Publishing.

Allen, V. B., Sampson, J. P., & Herlihy, B. (1988). Details of the 1988 AACD ethical standards. *Journal of Counseling and Development, 67,* 157-158.

American Association for Counseling and Development. (1988). *Ethical standards.* Washington, DC: Author.

American Psychological Association. (1981). *Ethical principles of psychologists.* Washington, DC: Author.

American Psychological Association. (1988). Trends in ethics cases, common pitfalls, and published resources. *American Psychologist, 43,* 564-572.

Barton, L. E., Brulle, A. R., & Repp, A. C. (1983). Aversive techniques and the doctrine of least restrictive alternative. *Exceptional Education Quarterly, 3,* 1-8.

Bellah v. Greenson, 181 Cal. App. 3d 614, 146 Cal. Rptr. 535 (Calif. App. 1978).

Bersoff, D. N. (1982). The legal regulation of school psychology. In C. Reynolds & T. Gutkin (Eds.), *The handbook of school psychology.* New York: Wiley.

Binder, V. L. (1980, May). *Legal vs. psychological aspects of intrusiveness.* Paper presented at the annual meeting of the Western Psychological Association, Honolulu, HI.

Bogust v. Iverson, 102 N.W. 2d 228 (Wisc., 1960).

Brakman, C. (1985). A human rights committee in a public school for severely and profoundly retarded students. *Education and Training of the Mentally Retarded, 20,* 139-147.

Bray, J. H., Shepherd, J. N., & Hays, J. R. (1985). Legal and ethical issues in informed consent to psychotherapy. *American Journal of Family Therapy, 13,* 50-60.

Carey v. Population Services International, Inc., 431 U.S. 678 (1977).

DeMers, S. T. (1986). Legal and ethical issues in child and adolescent personality assessment. In H. Knoff (Ed.), *The assessment of child and adolescent personality.* New York: Guilford.

Denkowski, K., & Denkowski, G. (1982). Client-counselor confidentiality: An update of rationale, legal status, and implications. *Personnel and Guidance Journal, 60,* 371-375.

Dickens v. Johnson County Board of Education. 661 F. Supp. 155 (E.D. Tenn. 1987).

Doe v. Roe, 93 Misc. 2d 201, 400 N.Y.S. 2d 668 (N.Y. Sup. Ct. 1977).

Donaldson v. O'Connor, 493 F.2d 507 (5th Cir. 1974), *vacated and remanded,* 422 U.S. 563 (1975).

Duncan, J., & Moffett, C. (1974). Abortion counseling and the school counselor. *School Counselor, 21,* 188-195.

Eades, R. W. (1986). The school counselor or psychologist and problems of defamation. *Journal of Law and Education, 15,* 117-120.

Eberlein, L. (1977). Counselors beware! Clients have rights! *Personnel and Guidance Journal, 55,* 219-223.

Ehrenreich, N. S., & Melton, G. B. (1983). Ethical and legal issues in the treatment of children. In C. E. Walker & M. C. Roberts (Eds.), *Handbook of clinical child psychology*. New York: Wiley.

Family Educational Rights and Privacy Act of 1974. 20 U.S.C.A. Sec. 123g with accompanying regulations set down in 45 C.F.R. Part 99.5.

Fischer, L., & Sorenson, G. P. (1985). *School law for counselors, psychologists, and social workers*. New York: Longman.

Friedman, P. R. (1975). Legal regulation of applied behavior analysis in mental institutions and prisons. *Arizona Law Review, 17*, 39-105.

Gelfand, D. M., & Hartman, D. P. (1975). *Child behavior analysis and therapy*. New York: Pergamon.

George, J. C. (1985). Hedlund paranoia. *Journal of Clinical Psychology, 41*, 291-294.

Grisso, T., & Vierling, L. (1978). Minors' consent to treatment: A developmental perspective. *Professional Psychology, 9*, 412-427.

Gumaer, J. (1984). *Counseling and therapy for children*. New York: Free Press.

Hedlund v. Superior Court, 34 Cal. 3d 695, 194 Cal. Rptr. 805 (1983).

Hendrickson, R. M. (1982). Counselor liability: Does the risk require insurance coverage? *Personnel and Guidance Journal, 61*, 205-207.

Herlihy, B., & Sheeley, V. L. (1986, April). *Privileged communications legal status and ethical issues*. Paper presented at the annual convention of the American Association for Counseling and Development, Los Angeles, CA.

Horacek v. Exon, CA No. 72-L-299 (1975).

Huey, W. C. (1986). Ethical concerns in school counseling. *Journal of Counseling and Development, 64*, 321-322.

Hulteng, R. J., & Goldman, E. B. (1987). Potential liability in outpatient practice: A primer for psychotherapists. In P. A. Keller & S. R. Heyman (Eds.), *Innovations in clinical practice: A source book* (Vol. 6). Sarasota, FL: Professional Resource Exchange.

Ingraham v. Wright, 430 U.S. 651, 97 S. Ct. 1401, 51 L.ED.2d 711 (1977).

Jagim, R. D., Wittman, W. D., & Noll, J. O. (1978). Mental health professionals' attitudes toward confidentiality, privilege, and third-party disclosure. *Professional Psychology, 9*, 456-466.

Johnson, J. H., Rasbury, W. C., & Siegel, L. J. (1986). *Approaches to child treatment: Introduction to theory, research, and practice*. New York: Pergamon.

Kandler, H. O. (1977). *Issues of confidentiality in psychiatry*. Newsletter, Society of Adolescent Psychiatry, New York.

Knapp, S., & VandeCreek, L. (1983). Privileged communications and the counselor. *Personnel and Guidance Journal, 62*, 83-85.

Koocher, G. P. (Ed.). (1976). *Children's rights and the mental health professions*. New York: Wiley.

Langs, R. (1976). *The therapeutic interaction* (Vol. 2). New York: Aronson.

Lidz, C. W., Meisel, A., Zerubavel, E., Carter, M., Sestak, R. M., & Roth, L. H. (1984). *Informed consent: A study of decision making in psychiatry*. New York: Guilford.

Lombard, T. J. (1981, August). *Current legislative and policy issues related to school psychological services.* Paper presented at the annual meeting of the American Psychological Association, Los Angeles, CA.

MacDonald v. Clinger, 84 A.D. 2d 482, 446 N.Y.S. 2d 801 (N.Y. App. Div. 1982).

Martin, R. (1975). *Legal challenges to behavior modification.* Champaign, IL: Research Press.

McDermott, P. A. (1972). Law, liability, and the school psychologist: System of law, privileged communication, and access to records. *Journal of School Psychology, 10,* 299-305.

Meyer, R. S., & Smith, S. R. (1977). A crisis in group therapy. *American Psychologist, 32,* 638-662.

Mills, M. J. (1985). Expanding the duties to protect third parties from violent acts. In S. Rachlin (Ed.), *Legal encroachment on psychiatric practice.* San Francisco: Jossey-Bass.

Morales v. Turman, 364 F.Supp. 166 (1973).

National Association of School Psychologists. (1985). *Professional conduct manual.* Washington, DC: Author.

New York State Association for Retarded Children v. Rockefeller, 357 F.Supp. 752 (1973).

Page v. Rotterdam-Mohanasen Central School District, 441, N.Y.S.2d 323 (Sup. Ct. 1982).

Phyllis P. v. Clairmont Unified School District (86 Daily Journal D.A.R. 2795, July 30, 1986).

Planned Parenthood of Central Missouri v. Danforth, 428 U.S. 52 (1976).

Prasse, D. P. (1986). Litigation and special education: An introduction. *Exceptional Children, 52,* 311-312.

Rachlin, S. (Ed.). (1985). *Legal encroachment on psychiatric practice.* San Francisco: Jossey-Bass.

Reynolds, C. R., Gutkin, T. B., Elliot, S. N., & Witt, J. C. (1984). *School psychology: Essentials of theory and practice.* New York: John Wiley.

Ross, A. O. (1980). *Psychological disorders of children: A behavioral approach to theory, research, and therapy* (2nd ed.). New York: McGraw-Hill.

Sadoff, R. L. (1985). Competence and informed consent. In S. Rachlin (Ed.), *Legal encroachment on psychiatric practice.* San Francisco: Jossey-Bass.

Sales, B. D., & Grisso, T. (1978). Law and professional psychology: An introduction. *Professional Psychology, 9,* 363-366.

Schectman, F., Hays, J. R., Schuham, A., & Smith, R. (1982). Accountability and confidentiality in psychotherapy, with special reference to child treatment. *Clinical Psychology Review, 2,* 201-211.

Schrier, C. J. (1980). Guidelines for record-keeping under privacy and open-access laws. *Social Work, 25,* 452-457.

Shapiro, M. H. (1974). Legislating the control of behavior control: Autonomy and the coercive use of organic therapies. *Southern California Law Review, 47,* 237-356.

Simmonds, D. W. (1976). Children's rights and family dysfunction: Daddy, why do I have to be the crazy one. In G. P. Koocher (Ed.), *Children's rights and the mental health professions.* New York: Wiley.

Sloan, S., & Klein, C. (1977). Psychotherapeutic disclosure: A conflict between right and duty. *University of Toledo Law Review, 6,* 55-85.

Slovenko, R. (1973). *Psychiatry and law.* Boston: Little, Brown.

Spece, R. G. (1972). Conditioning and other technologies used to "treat?" "rehabilitate?" "demolish?" prisoners and mental patients. *Southern California Law Review, 45,* 616-681.

State v. Bishop, 128 Vt., 227-228, 260, A. 2d, 393, 398 (1969).

State v. Pyle, Kan. 423, 442, 531, P.2d, 1309, 1323 (1975).

Stevens v. State, 354 N.E. 2d 727 (Ind. 1976).

Stoltz, S. B., Wienckowski, L. A., & Brown, B. S. (1975). Behavior modification: A perspective on critical issues. *American Psychologist, 30,* 1027-1048.

Szasz, T. S. (1974). *The myth of mental illness* (rev. ed.). New York: Harper & Row.

Talbutt, L. C. (1983). Libel and slander: A potential problem for the 1980's. *The School Counselor, 30,* 164-168.

Tarasoff v. Regents of the University of California, 13 Cal. 3d 177, 529 P.2d 553 (1974), *vacated,* 17 Cal. 3d 425, 551, P.2d. 334 (1976).

Thomas, S. B. (1985). *Legal issues in special education.* Topeka, KS: National Organization on Legal Problems of Education.

United States Department of Health, Education and Welfare. (1963). *Public opinions and attitudes about mental health.* Washington, DC: U.S. Government Printing Office.

Wagner, C. A. (1981). Confidentiality and the school counselor. *Personnel and Guidance Journal, 59,* 305-310.

Waltz, J., & Scheuneman, T. (1970). Informed consent to therapy. *Northwestern University Law Review, 64,* 628-650.

Welsch v. Likins, 373 F. Supp. 487, *affirmed* 525 F. 2d 987 (1974).

Wheeler v. Glass, 473 F. 2d 983 (1973).

Wilson, J. P. (1978). *The rights of adolescents in the mental health system.* Lexington, MA: Lexington Books.

Wood, F. H., & Braaten, S. (1983). Developing guidelines for the use of punishing interventions in the schools. *Exceptional Education Quarterly, 3,* 68-75.

Wyatt v. Stickney, 325 F.Supp. 781 (1971); 334 F.Supp. 1341 (1971); 344 F.Supp. 373 (1972); 344 F.Supp. 387 (1972).

Chapter 3

Psycholanalytic Approaches

Frederick Weisz, Ph.D.
Constance Benoit, M.S.W.

INTRODUCTION

Psycholanalysis owes its origin to Sigmund Freud. Freud (1955a, 1955b) defined psychoanalysis as (1) the procedure by which mental processes are investigated, (2) the method by which neurotic disorders may be treated, and (3) a body of information which describes human behavior.

All psychoanalytic therapies stem from classical Freudian psychoanalysis and apply psychodynamic understanding of human development in an effort to alter maladaptive behavior. The term *psychodynamic* implies that behavior is the product of mental forces, motives, or impulses as well as certain psychological processes that serve to regulate or control them. Psychoanalysis is based on the premise that the antecedents of daily behavior are largely beyond the realm of conscious awareness. It espouses a deterministic point of view wherein behavior is seen as neither haphazard nor random but as having determinable causes and as being goal directed, although on the surface it may appear irrational.

Psychoanalytic theory originally followed a hydraulic model of tension reduction in which intrapsychic conflict was viewed as originating from the repression of disturbing childhood material. Early theory placed great emphasis upon instinctual drives although later modifications have shifted to a focus on the organism's capacity to adapt to the realities of the environment.

History and Status

Interest in psychoanalysis in the United States first appeared in the lectures of William James at Harvard University in 1894. In 1900 a group of American psychiatrists went to study in Europe, and upon their return they formed a psychoanalytic society. In 1909 the Department of Psychology at Clark University invited Freud to give a series of lectures. Two years later the American Psychoanalytic Association was organized in Washington.

The first reference to child psychoanalysis appeared in 1909 with Freud's report of "Little Hans" in which he treated a case of infantile neurosis, specifically a phobia, through information and material provided by the boy's father.

As a subspecialty of psychoanalysis, child psychoanalysis has been in existence for almost 60 years. An early contributor was Hermine von Hug-Hellmuth (1921) who introduced the concept of play as a specific child analysis technique. Hug-Hellmuth visited the homes of young children, conducting her work in these settings through sharing in the child's play. Siegfried Bernfeld (1929) and August Aichorn (1935) were among the first individuals to study adolescents and delinquent phenomena. Sigmund Freud's daughter, Anna Freud (1965), credits Berta Bornstein with the discovery of the analysis of defenses in child psychoanalysis.

In 1926 and 1927 Anna Freud delivered a series of four lectures at the Vienna Institute of Psychoanalysis on the technique of child analysis, thereby opening wide the door to child psychoanalysis. Subsequent seminars quickly followed, and case studies were reported that are still considered relevant. The early period of the twentieth century was in general a time of great interest and rapid growth in child development, especially among psychologists and educators.

From the outset, the new movement in child psychoanalysis was conducted cautiously in order to avoid the phenomenon of "wild analysis" which had already occurred in the treatment of adults. These analysts tended to experimentation and often deviated from "orthodox" theory, itself still in a state of transition. Still, in the late 1940s, child psychoanalysis witnessed a split, and there exists today an ongoing controversy between two schools of thought: Melanie Klein and her followers, known as the *English School,* and Anna Freud and her followers, known as the *Vienna School.* Basic differences separate these schools both in theory and in technique. Klein proposed that the structure of personality is intact at birth, and she emphasized the treatment of children from even the earliest periods of life. She equated children's play with free association and interpreted play as an attempt to mitigate against the superego, which is viewed as extremely harsh. She suggested that the superego is present from early infancy. Anna Freud believed that children develop a superego only at the resolution of the oedipal complex (3 to 5 years old). Her focus was on the child's ego development, and she emphasized the importance of working with teachers and parents. Although Kleinian technique is well developed (Klein, 1932; MacKay, 1981) and accepted in some psychoanalytic circles, Kessler (1966) questions the method in the light of known developmental and maturational information about childhood.

Work with childhood depression and borderline adolescents reflects areas of current interest among child psychoanalysts such as Peter Giovacchini and Peter Blos. Other analysts who have contributed significantly to our knowledge of ego development, depression, and separation-individuation include Edith Jacobson, Rene Spitz, and Margaret Mahler.

Psychoanalysis has broadened its original scope beyond the early, often narrow, traditional focus. Psychoanalytic theory has permeated many forms of psychotherapy, and it is now fair to refer to psychoanalytically based psychotherapy as a distinct technique for psychoanalysis. Psychoanalytic psychotherapy encompasses a broad spectrum of therapies which utilize psychodynamic principles to comprehend unconscious processes operating in the individual. For the purposes of this chapter, we will confine ourselves primarily to basic principles of classical psychoanalysis, which are often incorporated in even the less intensive psychotherapeutic procedures.

The formal teaching of psychoanalysis began in Berlin in 1920. The New York Psychoanalytic Training Institute, the oldest in North America, was founded in 1929, the Chicago Institute in 1932. Today there are numerous institutes in the United States and Canada as well as throughout the world. The foremost center for training in child psychoanalysis is the Hampstead Child-Therapy Clinic in London, formerly under the direction of Anna Freud.

All training for psychoanalytic psychotherapy takes place in psychoanalytic institutes. The formation of a child psychoanalyst is a long and arduous process. In addition to undergoing a personal analysis, the candidate is expected first to acquire skill and training as an adult analyst and subsequently to take additional training, specifically in child psychoanalysis. The program entails the successful completion of several "control" cases, which are closely scrutinized by a supervising analyst. Anna Freud (1970/1971) argued for the separate and independent training of child and adult psychoanalysts, and the Hampstead Clinic offers a course directed to the primary goal of training child psychoanalysts. As a subspecialty, child psychoanalysis gained increased status through the formation of the American Association for Child Psychoanalysis. Controversy still exists regarding the acceptability of so-called lay (nonmedically trained) analysts. American institutes have been historically less willing than the European centers to accept candidates who are not first trained as physicians. In those centers where nonmedically trained applicants are accepted, prior professional experience—for example, in social work, psychology, and counseling—is highly valued.

The institutes provide not only the training ground for would-be psychoanalysts; they are also the forum for the professional exchange of current theory and practice of psychoanalysis. One of the major publications in the child subspecialty is the annual volume of the *Psychoanalytic Study of the Child,* first published in 1945.

OVERVIEW OF THEORY

Basic Theory and Assumptions

Freud initially proposed a topographical model of the mind in which he delineated an unconscious, a conscious, and a preconscious. The *unconscious* is made up of desires, fantasies, and wishes of which the person is unaware and which are mostly of a sexual or an aggressive nature. The *conscious* contains those thoughts and feelings of which the person is aware, and the *preconscious* consists of ideas which, though not conscious, can be readily made conscious through the effort of attention. Later, Freud superimposed on this model a structural theory of the mind that included the id, the ego, and superego. The *id* forms the unconscious basis of the psyche and is dominated by primary urges or instinctual drives. The id is governed by the pleasure principle, which seeks constantly to reduce tension. The id is characterized by primary process functioning, which means simply that images of objects are formed not on the basis of reality but rather to reduce tension and thus provide pleasure. The *ego* is a higher order structure which guides and controls. Conscious perceptions are a function of the ego; it mediates between the organism and the environment and assists in adaptation. When the ego performs an inhibitory function, it usually does so through its defense mechanisms, which are largely unconscious. The ego is governed by the reality principle, which seeks to procure objects in the real world for the safe gratification of the id. The ego is characterized by secondary process functioning which is logical, rational, and realistic. The *superego* is the final structure. It is concerned with right and wrong and is believed to develop from the oedipal wishes of the young child. The superego is the introjected parental authority. The interplay of these three structures constitutes intrapsychic functioning and provides the basis for normal and abnormal psychological functioning.

Freud proposed that individuals are born with a basic sex drive or instinctual energy. He called this force *libido* and described it as the energy of the life instincts with its source in the id. Libido is fluid and can be invested in a wide variety of objects and activities beyond those narrowly considered sexual. Mental energy is accumulated around an idea, activity, or object, and this is called *cathexis*. To his libido theory Freud later added a second basic instinctual drive: *aggression*. He viewed aggression as a derivative of the death instinct. The death instinct is not supported by any known biological principle.

Freudian metapsychology is built upon six basic constructs or core areas:

1. *topographical*—the assumption of three "areas" of the mind: unconscious, preconscious, and conscious.
2. *economic*—the assumption that a quantitative relationship exists between drives and resistances.
3. *genetic*—the assumption that psychological phenomena proceed according to an epigenetic plan, building upon earlier forms, and that the past exists into the present.
4. *structural*—the assumption that mental structures (id, ego, and superego) mediate conflicts, implicit in all behavior.
5. *dynamic*—the assumption that all behavior is motivated, purposeful, and meaningful and that there is interplay between drive discharge and regulatory forces.
6. *adaptive*—the assumption that the environment or real world is a determining factor of behavior and that the organism has the capacity of relating to and fitting in with the environment.

The cornerstone of psychopathology rests upon the model of intrapsychic conflict arising out of an imbalance among id, ego, and superego forces. Freud assumed that an unconscious force or resistance which he called *repression* was used to control the direct expression of id impulses. In the formulation of the structural model, he viewed repression as a defensive function of the ego. Later he introduced the key concepts of *anxiety* and *symptom* as a means of elaborating the process of intrapsychic conflict. Freud believed that anxiety is disturbing to the organism and that defense mechanisms develop in response to the danger signal of anxiety.

Anna Freud provided greater elaboration of the various defenses in *The Ego and the Mechanisms of Defense* (1937). Among the most frequently acknowledged are:

1. *repression*—the most generic defense mechanism in which threatening feelings or impulses are forced out of consciousness.
2. *denial*—the process whereby the individual refuses to acknowledge external reality.
3. *projection*—the process whereby the individual defends against an unwanted feeling by attributing the feeling to someone other than himself or herself.
4. *negation*—the form of denial in which an individual acknowledges the existence of an unwanted idea or feeling by stating that it doesn't exist.
5. *displacement*—the expressing of an impulse by changing its object and disguising its real intent from the ego.
6. *introjection*—a form of identification involving taking on characteristics of a formerly significant object and internalizing them into self structure.
7. *reaction formation*—an alarming desire or wish is replaced in consciousness by its opposite.
8. *isolation*—the intrapsychic separation of idea and affect resulting in repression or displacement of the content or affect.
9. *undoing*—the individual employs a specific action or symbolic act in a magical fashion in order to dismiss or cancel out another.
10. *rationalization*—the unconscious justification of an individual's actions to avoid or ward off negative affect.
11. *intellectualization*—the individual engages in systematic and rational thinking in order to avoid or control affect rather than experiencing it.
12. *sublimation*—the individual attempts to gratify an impulse or wish that is basically socially unacceptable by channeling the energy into a socially acceptable activity.

The function of defense mechanisms is to avoid or to terminate anxiety. Defense mechanisms per se are not pathological. They are a necessary means of control, and some (for example, sublimation) are characteristic of the mature adult. The extensive use of defense mechanisms to control inadequate psychosexual adjustment, however, can result in psychological disturbance. In the psychoanalytic treatment process, defenses are analyzed in order to uncover the conflict arising from sexual and aggressive drives.

Freud observed two key phenomena in the process of psychoanalysis: *transference* and *resistance*. Transference refers to the repetition during therapy of earlier feelings or patterns of responding. The patterns are directed toward the therapist. In analysis the transference phenomenon is a form of resistance in which the individual attempts to avoid remembering or verbalizing earlier infantile conflicts by repeating old patterns of behavior. This natural phenomenon allows the therapist to observe directly the derivatives of the past conflict. Transference and transference resistance are central to psychoanalysis; the treatment situation is designed to promote transference and its development into a transference neurosis. Transference neurosis represents the intensified feelings of the patient toward the psychoanalyst, who becomes the central figure in a dramatization of the emotional conflicts that began in the patient's childhood. Whereas transference involves fragmentary repetitions of attitudes from the past, transference neurosis is a pervasive theme wherein the patient's fantasies and dreams center on the therapist. Transference neurosis is analyzed back to infantile roots in an attempt to resolve the original unconscious conflict.

Resistance refers to all attempts by the patient to ward off unconscious material. The analytic situation promotes the expression of unconscious repressed material through free association, a technique in which the patient expresses everything that comes to mind. Resistance represents an effort to distort the source of the actual connections. It is the interpretation of resistance which ultimately uncovers the repressed childhood memories. Finally, Freud considered "working through" transference and resistance to be the very essence of psychoanalytic treatment.

The patient is not the only individual with emotional reactions to therapy. When the psychoanalyst expresses emotional responses based on his or her inner needs, he or she produces countertransference. The therapist maintains constant awareness of countertransference which, if unchecked, may reinforce the patient's early psychic conflict. One reason for the lengthy training of psychoanalysts is that it provides the time for analysts to develop this awareness of possible countertransference of feelings.

Freud proposed a theory of human development consisting of stages through which the child passes on his or her way from birth to adulthood. The point of distinction of each stage is the locus of the child's pleasurable activities, which correspond to an erogenous zone. Hence, Freud referred to these stages as pyschosexual.

Oral. The earliest psychosexual stage, lasting approximately from birth to 18 months, is characterized by a focus on the mouth as a primary source of pleasure. The infant attempts to gratify sexual and aggressive impulses through such behavior as sucking, swallowing, chewing, and biting.

Anal. The second stage extends from 18 months to around 3 years and is defined by the concentration of erotogenic pleasure in the anal region of the body. Sphincter control develops during this stage, and gratification focuses on the sensations associated with retaining and expelling feces. The anal stage is marked by ambivalence and a struggle for control.

Phallic. Between 3 and 6 years of age the child passes through the phallic stage, during which time the primary source of libidinal pleasure lies in the genital organs. Erections, masturbation, and voyeurism are common occurrences, and the child may engage in sex play with other children. There is recognition of anatomical differences between the sexes which fosters penis envy in girls and castration anxiety in boys. The major occurrence, however, is the emergence of the *oedipal complex.* The superego develops during this stage, completing the structural components of personality.

Latency. The period between approximately 6 years and puberty marks a time in which sexual interest is dormant. The earlier infantile stages are closed as the child represses and forgets the intense strivings that characterized the oedipal conflict. Latency is a period of relative quiescence with respect to libidinal urges. Maturation and elaboration of ego functions is paramount.

Genital. The onset of puberty marks the end of latency. The genital organs again become the major erotogenic zone, but the shift in sexual interest is toward outside objects. The adolescent re-experiences many of the repressed earlier sexual urges as the libidinal energy associated with each of the erogenous zones is fused and synthesized. Much of the libidinal energy of the genital stage becomes sublimated into socially accepted outlets as the adolescent moves closer to normal adulthood.

In the psychoanalytic framework, child development can be examined in terms of three phases: *prelatency, latency,* and *adolescence.* In the *prelatency* phase the development of object constancy is paramount. Object constancy refers to the individual's ability to recognize differences among objects and to maintain a relationship to one specific object even in its absence. Object constancy implies that the relationship goes beyond simple need satisfaction and that the individual has an emotional investment in the relationship. Psychoanalysis was expanded to include object relations when Freud proposed the structural model in *The Ego and the Id* (1961). The early view held that objects were important as the basis of need gratification and drive discharge. Later, as the emphasis on the external world developed, the importance of the fit between the infant and its primary object, the mother, became the focal point of all psychological development.

Ronald Fairbairn was a leading proponent of the British School of Object Relations. Winnicott (1965) further emphasized the importance of primary objects when he described the "good enough mother." The transitional object, a term also coined by Winnicott, reflects the idea that a familiar object such as a toy or blanket helps replace the absent mother as a source of comfort and thereby acts as a bridge to autonomous functioning.

With the prelatency phase the major developmental occurrence is the formation and resolution of the oedipal conflict. The oedipal conflict refers to the intense love of the child for the opposite-sex parent and the attendant rivalry, hostility, and identification that ensues with the same-sex parent. The resolution of the oedipal conflict is believed to result in the establishment of the superego. Because of the nature of the intense, complicated strivings of the oedipal triangular situation, Freud viewed this event as the nucleus for the later development of neurosis and symptoms.

The *latency* phase of development is divided into two periods, corresponding roughly to 6 to 8 years of age and 8 to 10 or 12, depending upon the age of onset of puberty. The early phase is characterized by the child's preoccupation with himself or herself along with a demise of impulse gratification. With the resolution of the oedipal conflict there is a reduction of sexual preoccupation. Real objects are denied and fantasy becomes an important method of adjusting to emotional stresses. The newly emerging superego is harsh and punitive. The second phase of latency is accompanied by an increased interest in the outside world as the source of objects. Object fantasies contain more realistic representations. The superego becomes less punitive as the child develops better reality testing.

The final phase of child development is *adolescence,* which Freud (1953) described as the time for the establishment of a final sexual orientation. Adolescence can be divided into four periods. *Preadolescence* from age 9 to 13 marks the resurgence of libidinal and aggressive drives. There is a general striving toward strengthening the sexual identification. Regression at this stage is often reflected in an increase in fighting, gang activity, temper outbursts, and depression. *Early adolescence,* which corresponds roughly to the 12- to 15-year age range, is associated with the emergence of a definite genital drive orientation. The adolescent experiences a more varied emotional life with slightly less regression. There is an increase in peer relationships with the same sex and concurrent dissolution of family ties which accompanies the cathexis to peers and work interests. The adolescent will oscillate between regression and forward movement often reflected in extreme behavior such as rebelliousness or submission. Acting out, depression, feelings of isolation, and running away are common reactions during this period. *Middle adolescence,* approximately 14 to 18 years of age, is accompanied by greater attempts to attain mastery of object relationships. There is greater ease in developing heterosexual relationships, superficial attachments, and, in general, an increase in the desire for objects. Hero worship and social group identification are common at this time. The later phase of middle adolescence also witnesses an increased concern on the part of the adolescent for world and sociopolitical issues. Finally, *late adolescence,* which encompasses approximately 17 to 20 years of age, is marked by a resolution of the separation-individuation conflict. Character formation as a result of identification is complete, and the young person accepts parental ideas and attitudes previously rejected.

In adolescence, there is a general resurgence in interest of gratification of id impulses marked by heightened sexual or aggressive activity and a conjoint struggle for ego integration. Adolescence, therefore, reflects both a second chance for resolving the struggle among the intrapsychic forces as well as a period of greater clarification of sexual identity. If there has been adequate resolution of the oedipal conflict, adolescence is likely to pave the way for normal development into adult sexual relationships.

VIEW OF PSYCHOPATHOLOGY

Originally, Freud viewed the development of psychopathology as a consequence of early sexual trauma. Based largely on his work with hysterics, he was impressed by the significant sexual content of their complaints. He proposed that psychic events, especially early sexual experiences, develop into pathogenic behavior when they become repugnant to the individual's conscious self. Freud assumed that mental illness is the psychic consequence of early sexual seduction which is repressed from consciousness. The belief that psychological disturbance lies in early sexual development remains a cornerstone of psychoanalytic theory, and infantile sexuality is viewed as a normal developmental phenomenon. However, Freud realized that the theory of actual sexual trauma was itself incomplete. He subsequently postulated that infantile sexual impulses, arising in the unconscious, create conflict, which thus forms a second explanation of psychopathology. The conflict which arises from oedipal strivings reflects one of the most important issues in Freudian theory. Recall that in the oedipal phase the child experiences a strong desire for union with the opposite-sex parent while at the same time there exists a wish to exclude or eliminate the same-sex parent. The child's fear of retaliation usually thwarts the direct expression of the sexual drive. Failure to resolve the oedipal conflict invariably leads to later problems with adjustment.

The conflict theory assumes that sexual and aggressive drives are blocked through fear, and the urge toward drive discharge is expelled from consciousness, usually through repression. Repression does not reduce drive discharge; it merely renders the drives unconscious. Neurotic symptoms develop as a result of repressed tendencies which press toward conscious expression. Inner conflicts stem from childhood experiences, and the emergence of neurosis in later life presupposes earlier neurotic patterns.

Psychoneuroses orginate from conflict between the id (drive discharge) and the ego (defense mechanism). In psychoanalytic theory *symptoms* develop as a result of an imbalance of forces within the personality as earlier conflicts are reactivated and as the ego's mechanisms of defense are threatened with disintegration. Neurotic symptoms, which are well-delineated patterns of behavior, reflect a compromise between unacceptable wishes and an unconscious fear. Symptoms are not chosen haphazardly but are purposeful, and meaningful. They are defenses against unconscious desires and serve to gratify the unconscious wishes symbolically. Because symptom formation reflects underlying conflict which is inadequately resolved, attempts to alleviate the symptom will prove ineffectual if the underlying conflict remains. Accordingly, symptom substitution will result. By analyzing the symptom it is possible to uncover the hidden meaning of the conflict. Psychoanalysis is less concerned with symptom removal than with the exposure and mastery of underlying conflict. To summarize, a neurotic symptom reflects an imbalance in the intrapsychic forces; represents a reactivation of infantile conflict; and signifies an effort at "spontaneous cure" or adaptation.

Anxiety develops from the fear of an unconsciously imagined danger and is one of the most common symptoms of psychopathology. Anxiety is an unpleasant affect with psychological and physiological manifestations. It is considered normal when it is appropriate in intensity to a given situation and when it does not result in disorganization of the personality or in maladaptive coping behavior. Because anxiety implies danger, even the threat or anticipation of anxiety, which is called signal anxiety, can lead to symptom formation. A crucial aspect of mental development is the ego's capacity to experience, tolerate, and master internal conflict and to marshal defenses in response to the signal of danger. Defenses allow the ego to achieve adaptation and to channel the basic drives. In the course of normal development each psychosexual stage evokes feelings of danger that are related to the specific developmental tasks. A fundamental issue in psychic development, then, is learning to tolerate phase-related anxiety and to marshal defenses in an adaptive fashion. In this sense anxiety is not always negative but reflects an integral part of successful maturation.

In Freud's view the severe forms of psychological disturbance, that is, the psychoses, reflect serious conflict in the individual's ability to adapt to environmental stresses. The lack of successful adaptation to the real world stems from a primary deficit in the synthetic function of the ego which is basic to the integration of all other mental functions. As in the neuroses, psychotic symptoms are meaningful in content and reflect an attempt toward adaptation. However, the psychotic state is one of total personality decompensation and severe impairment of reality testing. Freud had little actual experience with psychotic patients, and he cites only a few clinical cases. He believed that psychotic individuals could not benefit from psychoanalysis.

General Therapeutic Goals and Techniques

As a treatment form psychoanalysis is still more concerned with the psychoneuroses, although recent advances have included its application to borderline and psychotic conditions. Minimal importance is attached to symptom relief; rather, the goal remains to break down early boundaries of id, ego, and superego, bringing repressed or warded-off unconscious material to the surface so that it may be reintegrated in the context of reality. Thus, the goal is to make the ego face what it had repressed from the id, or, as Freud (1964a) explained, "where id was, ego shall be." This process takes place within the emotional context of the transference in which the unconscious, repressed conflict is interpreted. Through the therapeutic alliance in which the analyst allies himself or herself with the patient's ego to join in the struggle against the neurotic conflict, the technique of interpretation demonstrates to the patient the anachronistic nature of his or her transference feelings and their inappropriateness for adaptation to his or her contemporary object relationships.

The analytic process utilizes several components which serve to induce regression in the therapeutic situation, resulting in the development of a transference neurosis, which then becomes the central axis of the interpretive work. These components are the well-known features of free association, the couch position with the analyst out of the patient's eyesight, frequency of sessions (usually four or five times a week), and an objective passivity on the part of the therapist. They serve to create an atmosphere in which the patient feels inferior or childlike in relation to the analyst; and the patient's dependent needs are aroused, propelling him or her to earlier regression points, with the consequent projection of attitudes, demands, and impulses characteristic of his or her past conflictual relationship onto the therapist. The work of the analyst is then to demonstrate to the analysand the irrational and unrealistic component of his or her projections. Interpretation of the patient-therapist axis thereby becomes the central focus, with insight into the neurotic repetitive pattern and the working through of the conflicts involved the supreme curative agent. Fenichel (1945) describes this as "a process of working through which shows the patient again and again the same conflicts and his usual way of reacting to them, but from new angles and in new connections" (p. 31). Length of treatment may vary, although it is generally accepted to be long-term therapy.

INDIVIDUAL PSYCHOTHERAPY WITH CHILDREN

Psychoanalysis as a therapeutic technique has been applied to children for well over 50 years (A. Freud, 1974). Natural evolution of the theory has resulted in a broadening of the parameters of child psychoanalysis, and consensus regarding the appropriate use of the technique is not uniform. All analysts can agree that psychoanalysis is the preferred mode of treatment with certain types of psychoneuroses. Controversy remains lively, however, when the discussion turns to the universal applicability of such therapy or to the psychoanalytic treatment of the more severe forms of childhood psychopathology.

Anna Freud outlined a number of critical factors in the evaluation of a child for therapy. In general, it is the opinion of the Freudian child analysts that psychoanalysis should be restricted to the severe forms of infantile neurosis. The most frequent manifestations of neurosis in children include phobias, anxiety states, conversion hysteria, traumatic experiences, and obsessional behaviors. Unlike adult cases wherein the decision for treatment can be made as a function of the amount of suffering from neurotic symptoms, children do not usually present the same degree of neurotic suffering. Moreover, the problem is often divided equally between parent and child. Frequently, it is the reaction of the parents to the symptom, e.g., feeding disturbances or enuresis, that results in treatment being sought. The child, if left untreated, would remain indifferent to the symptom. The anxiety that accompanies such symptoms in the child may be warded off by phobic or obsessional mechanisms. The reactions which these mechanisms create in the environment often become the deciding factor in whether or not treatment is initiated. When the symptoms are highly disturbing to the environment—for example, in the case of aggressive or destructive behavior—treatment is usually sought. A second consideration is the degree of disturbance of the child's normal capacities, specifically the capacity for object love and for play. The direction of libidinal urges either inward or outward becomes the measure for assessing object love. In general, the excessive and prolonged manifestation of narcissistic behavior implies that autoerotic gratification is of greater importance to the child than are the objects in the environment. Similarly, disturbances in the child's capacity for constructive play, often manifested in the excessive and repetitive use of imaginary play, are an indication of neurotic conflict. *Such factors must always be measured against the backdrop of normal development, which is the final and most critical variable in the treatment decision.* The structure of the child's personality evolves slowly and becomes crystallized as he or she moves through the psychosexual stages. During these periods all children show clinical signs of conflict between instinctual drives and antagonistic forces of the ego. Such transitory disturbances actually facilitate development; when the conflict is resolved, the symptoms disappear and the integration of the various structures is strengthened. The seriousness of an infantile neurosis rests ultimately upon the prolonged display of symptoms and the degree to which they restrict the developmental processes.

Neurotic manifestations are an indication for therapy primarily when (1) the conflict has been internalized and the hope of recovery is slight, (2) the conflict has resulted in fixation at some stage of development, or (3) the conflict has resulted in regression to an earlier stage of development. In such instances where interference with the maturational process has occurred, treatment is always warranted.

Within the aforementioned framework, let us now turn briefly to some specific examples of the appropriate use of psychoanalysis with children. Pearson (1968) advocates psychoanalysis as the desirable form of therapy for the following types of situations:

1. With children who, despite satisfactory intellectual levels, display marked inhibitions or restrictions in ego functions. These children are frequently loners, with poor adjustment to social life. Their interests are very narrowly focused, often upon an activity which requires little participation from other children of the same age.
2. Occasionally a child who has been completely toilet trained will suddenly become enuretic or encopretic, and there is no identifiable organic basis. This circumstance reflects a regression in psychosocial development and is another situtation in which psychoanalysis can be employed. In these cases the regression reflects a defense against an unconscious conflict.
3. Sexual perversions when they occur without other marked delinquent symptoms are suitable for psychoanalysis as are cases in which a child expresses conscious wishes to be a member of the opposite sex.
4. Some conversion syndromes, such as tics and stuttering, reflect disturbances of physiological function due to repressed instinctual wishes and are treatable through psychoanalysis.
5. Finally, some forms of antisocial behavior, notable when the behavior is caused by an unconscious need for punishment brought about through excessive guilt, are appropriate cases for child psychoanalysis.

Techniques and Considerations

Psychoanalytic techniques vary as a function of the age of the child, the nature of the child's symptoms, and his or her ability to respond to therapy. The technical situation differs from that with adults in that the child experiences an ongoing "developmental pull" to replace primary process functioning with secondary process thinking as part of the gradual maturation process. Psychoanalysis is an intensive form of therapy, requiring three, four, or even five sessions a week on a weekly basis. The emphasis upon frequency of visits insures a continuity of flow of material while at the same time it promotes an intensification of feelings toward the therapist that is crucial for the development of a transference.

Frequently, children, especially the preschool child, the latency child, and the prepubescent child, are incapable of free association, the technique by which adults are analyzed. It is important, therefore, to employ some other method by which the therapist can make contact with the child's unconscious. One such approach is through the child's play. Recall that repetitive and stereotyped play patterns are often an indication of an underlying unconscious conflict. Work with children almost always involves play although child psychoanalysts make different uses of it. Kleinian analysts, for example, interpret the symbolic significance of play as a *direct* expression of unconscious conflict. Freudian child therapists invoke play although the interpretation tends to be conservative. Interrupting a child's play for an interpretation or otherwise setting limits on the play, aside from the realistic curtailment of actual destructive behavior, is counterproductive to the goal of understanding the meaning of the play. Play is thus a source of information about the child which lays the groundwork for interpretation. The conservative view toward interpretation is based on the assumption that free play has an inherent therapeutic effect by allowing the discharge of instinctual impulses, thereby relieving intrapsychic tension. However, play by itself will not resolve the neurosis.

Interpretation is the basis of all psychoanalytic techniques. The essence of interpretation lies in uncovering a connection for the child where the child sees none. Such connections may be between past and present events, between defenses and impulses, or between fantasy and reality (Kessler, 1966). The use of interpretation in working with children requires skill and training because timing is an all-important factor.

The manner in which transference develops in child psychoanalysis is affected by the fact that the child experiences an ongoing relationship with his or her parents. In analysis, transference is composed of the patient's feelings about his early object relations, and this is expressed in intense feelings and behavior toward the therapist. There is little doubt that children are capable of transference. However, the nature and shape of the transference are affected by the dependency relationship of the child to his or her parents. Based on this, Anna Freud (1974) believed that the child is incapable of developing a transference neurosis. Transference in child psychoanalysis reflects both the *current* relationship of the child to the parents as well as the earlier feelings and past experiences. Transference may appear temporary and less intense. For some children, transference emerges quickly as the child reenacts conflicts which may be of only recent origin. On the other hand, resistance may be equally strong for the same reason. Resistance in child psychoanalysis may stem from the parents who direct and control much of what the child thinks and says. In this sense resistance as a phenomenon of psychotherapy is viewed more broadly by the therapist in working with children.

Finally, let us comment briefly on the selection of play material. The objective is always to provide a setting in which the child may express fantasies and unconscious conflicts. Some analysts advocate a sparsely furnished room consisting only of a sink, toilet, small table, and a cot or bed. To this setting the child will bring a special collection of toys and materials which he or she alone will use. Other analysts work in a well-equipped playroom, consisting of some of the following materials: dolls, puppets, and toy furniture with which the child can act out his or her relationship with different members of the family in the home; drawing and painting materials and a blackboard for the free expression of ideas; clay or plasticene, sand, water, and rubber animals as primitive elements for the expression of preoedipal conflicts; toy soldiers and policemen, plastic guns, and various games for the expression of aggressive material. A controversial point is the controlled use of fire in the playroom. Some analysts include the availability of matches, particularly with children whose problems have an enuretic component. Nearly all psychoanalysts allow the child to bring to the playroom any desired toy or object from home since such material is always chosen because of its significance to the child.

The case study which concludes this chapter provides a specific example of the use of play techniques in the psychoanalytic treatment of a child.

INDIVIDUAL PSYCHOTHERAPY WITH ADOLESCENTS

With adolescence there occurs a resurgence of instinctual drives brought about in part by the biological and physical changes of puberty. Because adolescence reflects the transition period from childhood to adulthood, it is not surprising that the behavioral manifestations include elements of both of these stages. Psychoanalytic technique likewise must combine the methods of child and adult analysis. In general, adolescence is *not* a favorable period for initiating analytic treatment. There is little stability as the adolescent moves from crisis to crisis brought about by the various libidinal drives. Moreover, there is increased resistance to cooperation in treatment, especially if the treatment has been imposed by an outside force. However, psychoanalysis is indicated in those cases where the symptoms are long-standing and have their origins in the *earlier* stages of psychosexual development. In particular are those cases where the oedipal and pre-oedipal psychopathology has resulted in neurotic symptoms or rigid ego structure. As with children, the symptoms for which psychoanalysis is advocated in adolescence are largely psychoneurotic. Some types of impulsive behaviors are also amenable to psychoanalysis: delinquent tendencies which are not a function of a generally impoverished environment but rather which stem from early unconscious conflicts; eating disorders, including obesity which is tied to an actual greed for food, and its counterpart, anorexia; and impulsive sexual behavior when it is clearly an expression of pregenital sexuality. Truancy as a phobic reaction is considered appropriate for analysis as are excessive needs for order and cleanliness. Certain forms of learning problems, when it can be demonstrated that the difficulty is a function of an inability to take in information despite otherwise normal intelligence, are inappropriate for psychoanalysis. These cases are not equivalent to specific learning disabilities. In all adolescent cases it is desirable that the patient have relatively cohesive self-structure, resistant to fragmentation, and a capacity for developing transference neurosis. In terms of personality structure which admittedly is in a state of flux, one looks for a relatively strong ego and an overly severe superego.

The all-important rule of thumb of child psychoanalysis applies equally to adolescents: It is necessary to assess the symptoms always in the context of the interference they pose to normal development. Of significance in adolescence are the following developmental tasks: separation and individuation from the family structure; promotion of significant peer relations; development of a positive self-esteem and sexual identity; control of sexual drives and adaptation to sexual norms. Laufer (1981) emphasizes the importance of sexuality, concluding that adolescent pathology must be understood developmentally as a breakdown in the formation of a final sexual organization. However, neither a diagnostic label nor severity of symptoms per se is a clear indication for the ability of an adolescent to benefit from psychoanalysis. One has to assess further the phase of development with special regard for the individual's level of object relations and the ego's ability to relinquish old object ties. The quality of object relations can be assessed from both dependency expectations and reactions to actual disappointments. Relinquishing old object ties is commonly seen in the adolescent development of "crushes" and hero worship which reflect reinvestment of libidinal energy into outside objects. Adolescents frequently retreat from family involvement in an exaggerated manner reflecting ambivalent feelings and attachment to parental figures. The major defense mechanisms utilized to counteract strong attachment to objects include regression, a preoccupation with the self in the form of grandiose fantasies, displacement, and withdrawal. Ultimately, the therapist's most useful reference point in the determination of an adolescent's appropriateness for psychoanalysis is the normal or usual rather than the pathological. The most valuable guidelines continue to be the impact of puberty on the youngster coupled with his or her reactions to it, the emotional tasks he or she must accomplish in becoming an adult, and the degree to which his or her adolescent experiences make a positive contribution to the process of adulthood.

Techniques and Considerations

Because adolescence spans a broad period of time, commencing with puberty and terminating with adulthood, the techniques of psychoanalysis are varied. With younger and generally immature adolescents it may be necessary to continue employing the technique of play although understandably the nature of the older child's play becomes increasingly sophisticated. In fact, the nature of play and its relationship to fantasies and feelings is actually useful knowledge for analysts who treat adolescents. It serves the same purpose as in the treatment of children, namely as an insight into the unconscious material. Although adolescents are quite capable of free association, they may feel too unstable to risk the amount of regression that accompanies the free association of thoughts. Therapy with young adolescents must focus on creating a dependency relationship toward the therapist. A central assumption is that the neurotic conflict will emerge in the context of the developing closeness of therapist and patient. The environment of the therapy sessions must become comfortable and provide an actual relief from the outside world, which is often perceived as critical and unsupportive. The analyst, if he or she is to be successful at all, will offer himself or herself to a far greater extent to the adolescent; he or she will be both friend and role model, albeit in a reserved and restrained fashion. The therapist must be objective but understanding, and especially firm when necessary. Still, it is difficult to create a positive transference because the adolescent is usually mistrustful of adult values and is actually attempting to assert his or her independence.

Most psychoanalysts agree that treating adolescents requires modification from classical lines because transference in the case of adults presupposes a significant degree of identity closure. Transference in adolescence is rather a mixture of a reality-based relationship with a new adult authority, paired with demands based on neurotic conflicts, the patterns of which are repeated on the therapist. Although ever cognizant of the influence of early experience, the analyst directs his or her efforts toward the here-and-now, increasing the adolescent's ego tolerance to pathogenic conflicts. Laufer (1980) divides the analytic material of adolescents into two categories: the immediate past, which reflects the crises of puberty, and the preadolescent past, which reaches back to the oedipal and pre-oedipal stages of development. He stresses that both need to be understood and interpreted, but unless the adolescent understands the immediate past, interpretation of oedipal and pre-oedipal material will be of limited value. Additional emphasis must be placed on helping the adolescent learn to test reality accurately. In-depth and comprehensive analysis of the defensive structure is less important in adolescent psychoanalysis, and in some cases it becomes counterproductive to the goals of treatment. The rationale, as most analysts agree, is that the process of "working through" is still limited in adolescence.

The adolescent's view of the mechanics of psychotherapy is from time to time distorted, and he or she can be expected as a matter of course of action to say and do things which will embarrass not only himself or herself, but in some cases the therapist. The analyst working with middle-phase adolescents can assume that he or she will be the target of manipulative efforts as the adolescent tests the limits of the new relationship and compares it with previous adult contacts. The nature of the therapeutic alliance between the analyst and the adolescent is so delicate and vulnerable that Meeks (1971) has characterized it as the "fragile alliance."

Striking differences occur around countertransference issues which arise from the amount of aggressivity among adolescents and the lack of positive feedback which characterizes adolescents in turmoil. Special demands are placed upon the therapist as the patient expresses an intensity and an urgency for immediate symptom relief but feels no obligation to return that which he or she is receiving. The repetitive nature of the demands is often so great as to lead the therapist to question the vicissitudes of the approach.

The analytic setting itself is frequently viewed with suspicion and anxiety by the adolescent. Whereas the setting for psychoanalytic treatment of the child is normally the playroom and for the adult it becomes the couch, there is no easy solution for the adolescent. Particularly in middle and late adolescence there is clear rejection of play as "babyish" and immature. The couch is threatening, and it undermines the adolescent's need for a direct relationship. Face-to-face contact, four or five sessions a week, is maintained as in all forms of psychoanalysis.

Selma Fraiberg (1955) sums up the issues in the treatment of adolescents in the following manner:

> What the child in puberty fears is loss of control, surrender to the demands of drives. What he fears in therapy is the further disturbance of his precarious equilibrium. What he longs for most of all is the restoration of harmony. If our treatment is to have meaning for him, if we can hold out to him a concrete goal, we need to help him see therapy as a means of reestablishing equilibrium, of helping him to become master of himself. (p. 280)

Many of the therapeutic issues relevant to child therapy are equally germane in adolescence. Transference and resistance provide the central axes for which interpretation is the major technique. However, in late adolescence when physical appearance corresponds more closely to the adult, there is a tendency for greater expectations which are sometimes unwarranted. Usually, the therapist who is comfortable in the treatment of children finds greater ease in the world of adolescence than does the therapist whose work has been largely adult oriented.

GROUP PROCEDURES WITH CHILDREN AND ADOLESCENTS

Psychoanalytic techniques were applied to group treatment only after their initial use in individual treatment. In the literature there appear to be no universally accepted criteria nor clear diagnostic categories by which to judge the appropriateness of candidates for group therapy. Normally, psychoneurotic problems that indicate a need for individual therapy can also be treated through a group experience.

Freud's theories concerning the organization of groups evolved from his study of transference. Freud (1921/1955a) commented that the major dynamic process occurring in a group is the projection and giving up of the individual's superego and ego ideal to that of the group and/or the group leader. It follows then that individuals with weak ego structure become vulnerable in the group process. The ego is threatened in the face of regression. Additionally, narcissistic individuals frequently react adversely to the group therapy situation and there is a tendency to withdraw object interest in other members of the group. These individuals become preoccupied with their own concerns reflected in demanding and dominating behavior.

The use of psychoanalytic technique in group treatment places considerable emphasis on developmental issues. It appears more appropriate to organize children into groups based first on developmental competency and second on diagnostic category. Mullin and Rosenbaum (1962) argue that psychoanalytic group therapy is appropriate for all age levels but the process and mode of communication will vary as a function of maturational level and overall psychosexual development.

Anna Freud stressed the importance of observation of young children in nursery group play periods in order to provide more information upon which to base individual treatment. Group intervention is also an important modality for promoting developmental tasks in latency and adolescence as well and can be an important adjunct to individual treatment.

With preschool and early school-age children, psychoanalytic group treatment appears contraindicated when the child has not developed the necessary primary object relationships. Sociopathic children and children with perverted sexual experiences generally do not respond favorably to psychoanalytic group treatment. Psychoanalytic group therapy has successfully been employed for such problems as phobic reactions, effeminacy in boys, and shy and withdrawn types of behavior.

The importance of peer relationships for latency-age children facilitates the use of group therapy at this age. Selection for group therapy during latency is in part based on obtaining a variety of personality types and intellectual levels. Contraindications again include psychopathological children, homicidal types, and overt sexually deviant children.

The selection of adolescents who may be appropriate for psychoanalytic group treatment is a more difficult matter. Sociopathic individuals, homosexuals, drug offenders, and psychotics are usually considered unresponsive to psychoanalytic group treatment. However, as is occurring in individual treatment, recent literature reports that psychoanalytic group work has been successful in the treatment of borderline adolescents.

Techniques and Considerations

Bion's (1961) work in analytic group therapy contains three basic assumptions: (1) the assumption that the leader provides satisfaction of dependency needs; (2) the assumption that the group will promote aggression as a means of flight or resistance; and (3) the assumption of hope and expectation unrelated to reality arising from pairing behavior among group members.

These basic assumptions complement psychoanalytic theory with its emphasis on a dynamic unconscious, intrapsychic conflict, and the existence of ego-defensive forces. Resistance and transference also occur in group therapy and must be worked through in order to achieve improvement. In psychoanalytic group therapy the focus remains on the individual, and attention to the group as a separate entity is limited. Regression to earlier stages is fostered in an effort to undo repression and work through conflict. A transference neurosis is evoked and analyzed along with interpretations about unconscious conflict in order to promote personality reconstruction.

Generally, group therapy is viewed as supporting and assisting the patient through peer group interaction with a goal of intrapsychic change and an increase in capacity for reality testing. Identification as a coping mechanism provides a major element for therapeutic change; it fosters a split in the ego that allows the patient to experience as well as to observe intrapsychic processes. Identifications are thought to develop in the group as a result of the transference of love or hate feelings which group members secretly maintain for the group. The network of potentially positive forces operating in a group includes identification, transference, and object ties. Group cohesion is based on these positive factors.

Age and developmental considerations provide guidelines for techniques in group therapy. With younger children psychoanalytic group therapy is conducted in a permissive play atmosphere. In play group therapy, materials are similar to those used in individual therapy. Toys such as plastic guns and rubber animals can be employed to act out aggressive impulses. Doll houses and puppets help to re-create with group members and the therapist some of the problems experienced in the home. The other group members act as stimulants in producing ego-freeing cathartic play. Therapists' interventions include interpreting the child's transference to the therapist and to the other children. For younger age groups Slavson (1950) advocates the use of female therapists to promote maternal fantasies.

Latency-age groups usually focus on specific activities. Children in this phase of development are experiencing greater synthesis of ego functions in an attempt to master and adapt to the environment. Mastery of the environment is often facilitated through direct accomplishments. The aim of latency groups is to channel the developing ego structure into socially approved modes. After about 9 years of age, the focus shifts to greater verbal communication.

Adolescent psychoanalytic groups employ verbal communication techniques with a goal toward insight. Special consideration is directed toward similarity and homogeneity regarding the phase of adolescent development. Psychoanalytic group treatment in adolescence promotes peer reliance and decision making. The open sharing of feelings with peers helps to resolve conflict about dependency and guilt. Transference and authority issues are explored as a means of helping adolescents to see adults as allies, thereby producing greater self-confidence. Group treatment assists the adolescent in dealing with ambivalence and hostility toward authority figures and adults in general. It utilizes the adolescent's natural tendency to form into groups, allowing him or her to feel less anxious and isolated. As an adjunct to individual treatment, group therapy can dilute the transference in the adolescent with intense dependency strivings and allow him or her to make progress by establishing peer relationships.

In psychoanalytic group treatment the analyst must be ever aware of potentially adverse developments. He or she maintains a vigilance against overtly and covertly destructive behavior. Aside from this restriction the therapist remains open and accessible and refuses to censor any of the group members' verbalizations.

In group therapy several members are available as objects for transference, and the analyst is a more real person in contrast to the "blank screen" which characterizes his or her approach in individual analysis. Multiple transference reactions, multiple siblinglike reactions, and multiple identifications make this a complicated method of treatment, and the therapist may feel he or she is falling behind in understanding the process, particularly with older children. However, the real advantage to group work is in providing for greater object cathexis, thereby reducing narcissistic cathexis; this leads to ego strengthening as a result of the multiple transference.

Gender balance is also an important consideration. Although it was originally thought that groups should contain only same-sex children, particularly in the phases where instinctual drives are paramount, it is now recognized as highly desirable to provide the reality context of both sexes in order to enhance the capacity for resolving sexual problems and conflicts.

Child and adolescent groups are generally smaller in size than adult groups. With young children the optimal size of the group is three to five members. The number of children that a group can include increases with age up to about eight members as the ideal size for adolescent groups.

Psychoanalytic group therapy sessions are usually an hour to an hour and a half long and occur from one to five times a week. It is generally considered to be a long-term form of treatment, usually 1 to 3 years, but length varies with the age of the child and the severity of the problem.

CLASSROOM AND EDUCATIONAL APPLICATIONS

Anna Freud stressed the importance of natural observation of children; it was, therefore, a logical next step for psychoanalysis to direct its attention to the role of education in the 1920s and 1930s. Because the atmosphere of education in the early 20th century was still very punitive, the early analysts addressed issues of control in the classroom. The disappointing state of affairs at that time suggested that the therapist whose work consisted of resolving inhibitions and developmental disturbances could see education only from its worst point. Anna Freud (1974) criticized education for its restrictive characteristics and claimed that psychoanalysis advocated limiting the punitive effects of education. Psychoanalytic theory stresses normal development in which education can play a key role.

On a more positive note, Anna Freud proposed that psychoanalysis could offer education qualified criticism and awareness of the complex nature of the relationship between children and adults. Finally, she recommended psychoanalysis as a treatment for actual injuries sustained by the child through punitive educational methods.

Anna Freud was concerned with the relationship between the child's personality structure and his or her behavior in the classroom. In several papers (A. Freud, 1968b, 1968c), she described the teacher's changing role in child development. She promoted the idea that teachers be exposed to children of different ages, teaching at different levels, so that they might have a better grasp of the child's emotional and cognitive development. In a lecture delivered at the Harvard Graduate School of Education in 1952, she responded to teachers' questions on how to handle the so-called problem child, and she discussed the role of teachers' emotional attachment to the children they taught.

Certain misconceptions of psychoanalytic theory have detracted from its successful application to education. For example, the notions that frustration is bad because it can lead to neurosis and that all defense mechanisms are bad because they can lead to repression of unconscious conflicts were popular ideas in educational reform. Total permissiveness per se has never been feasible nor desirable in the classroom. Fenichel (1945) addressed this issue directly in discussing the application of psychoanalytic theory to education. Could education avoid or diminish children's conflicts? He concluded that psychoanalysis is helpful in individual cases, but it faces real limitations when applied to the broad spectrum of the whole population. He viewed education in its historical and social context and proposed that the repression of drives is not only a by-product of education but that it is part of an inevitable fact of social life. Somewhat pessimistically, he concluded that for psychoanalysis to have an impact on education, the whole structure of society might have to change. Waelder (1960) also addressed this point, concluding that a psychoanalytic approach in the classroom does not mean that children should be pampered or allowed total freedom. Rather, one must strive for the optimal balance between gratification and frustration in order to promote each child's potential for learning.

Concern today focuses on the relative importance of the various structural components of personality. Controversy exists regarding the emphasis in education. Are ego functions the focus to the exclusion of id or instinctual needs? There is danger that teachers may be so oriented toward promoting ego functions that they will disregard instinctual life, conflict, and their impact on the child's object relationships. Certainly, education has been concerned with inducing guilt in an effort to repress aggressive or sexual impulses. As such, education has fostered inhibition with the rationale that these restrictions are in the service of adaptation.

Psychoanalysis has acknowledged the teacher's role as an important object for the child. Kris (1975a) stressed the importance of psychoanalytic understanding of interpersonal relationships in the education process. The influence of the educator and his or her own conflicts can be crucial in the child's process of identification with significant objects. At times in the child's life the teacher can be a replacement for parental influence.

Psychoanalysis has also contributed to the introduction of mental hygiene within the context of the normal curriculum. As early as 1941, interest was directed toward progressive education within the total education scene (Zachary, 1941), and certain changes were inevitable. Greater emphasis was directed toward psychological causes for poor schoolwork. Guidance counselors, social workers, psychologists, and nurses were employed by school districts as one means of promoting mental hygiene. In some cases, consultants were engaged with the specific recognition that some children have difficulty learning as a result of emotional problems.

Many schools today provide mental health services with active mental health team consultants. Psychoanalytic theory offers the consultant a knowledge of psychic structure, providing greater understanding of what a child's behavior may be expressing. Consultation is highly effective when there is continuous dialogue between school personnel and the consultation team. In this atmosphere a consultant can provide education for students, parents, and staff on specific emotional issues. In this model, as well as providing assessment and limited individual and group treatment, the consultant can apply his or her knowledge of group and individual psychodynamics to make the classroom an environment in which to facilitate learning and growth.

In order to achieve these goals, consultants *use the backdrop of normal development to describe dynamic conflicts.* The resolution of psychosexual conflict at each stage is crucial for optimal learning to occur and for the child to develop a sense of competence. Successful conflict resolution frees energy for learning. In turn, the child with conflicts can benefit from positive classroom experiences that promote his or her self-esteem and peer relationships. Teachers can provide good models of authority and can promote adult relationships in cases where the child's parents are inadequate.

Teacher Techniques

Psychoanalytic theory assumes that the school can provide a restorative-supportive environment. The school provides a miniculture, and its psychological potential is, therefore, endless. A teacher employs therapeutic teaching techniques when he or she deals with the affective-cognitive mix. That is, teaching is effective when there is recognition of the child's intellectual and emotional makeup.

Certain goals in teaching can serve to facilitate psychological development (Rhodes & Tracy, 1972). From a psychoanalytic perspective these goals would include (1) minimization of stress in the school environment, (2) minimization of undesirable interactional gains, and (3) employment of curricular approaches as specific interventions.

Stresses in the school environment are frequent and often serious. They result in insecurity, feelings of failure, and sometimes open rebelliousness even in normal children. The teacher attempts to minimize stress by providing an atmosphere that is warm and caring and by promoting participation from students in decision making. The mutual working through of issues is, therefore, both adaptive and therapeutic. To be truly successful, the school should be viewed as a place of pleasure and satisfaction.

Historically, teachers have failed to recognize underlying unconscious motivational structures. One frequently catches glimpses of transference-like phenomena in the classroom that are for the most part unrecognized and simply ignored. These behaviors may reflect earlier beliefs which have been distinctly maladaptive. These occurrences provide the opportunity for a corrective influence which can be readily incorporated through the student's relationship with his or her teacher.

Rhodes (1963) suggests specific educational interventions which can be incorporated in the curricular approach. For example, he recommends that the child be exposed to new opportunities which will emphasize positive motives, such as adventure or discovery. Other curricular materials, though not specifically psychoanalytic, reflect similar emphasis on motivational and affective issues (Jones, 1968; Weinstein & Fantini, 1970).

Structured Educational Programs

To date, the psychoanalytic model has been most frequently employed in certain private schools, such as the Orthogenic School in Chicago, and in day-treatment programs based within hospital settings. Special classes do exist for emotionally disturbed children (Cruickshank & Johnson, 1975), but there has been less direct application of psychoanalytic theory to curriculum development in these settings. There is even less evidence that psychoanalytic theory has permeated program development in normal classrooms.

The Cornerstone Method (Lopez & Kliman, 1980) is one example in which psychoanalytic techniques are integrated into the therapeutic nursery education of preschool children. This program is based in a community clinic. A child psychoanalyst works simultaneously in the classroom with teachers 4 to 5 days each week. The psychoanalyst treats the children individually in brief sessions within the classroom, and each child receives three or more weekly sessions. The aim is to modify drive behavior and to divert it into play, learning, and work. The therapist and teacher engage in complex interactions while maintaining separate roles wherein the former provides the interpretive stance and the latter is the therapeutic educator.

The application of psychoanalytic concepts to the process of education holds great promise. Psychoanalysis contributes specifically to the knowledge and awareness of child development. Psychoanalytic theory can be applied in the classroom both in teaching technique and basic teaching materials. Yet its real potential remains largely unrealized. This gap presents a real challenge to psychoanalysis and to the field of education.

PARENTING SKILLS

Contemporary parent education programs are based on recognition of the importance of the relationship between parent and child. Psychoanalytic theory emphasizes the importance of early object relations, especially between mother and child. Parental attitudes and feelings obviously affect the development of the child's psychology. Kris (1975a) stressed both adaptive capacity and empathic response to changes, noting: "Adaptability of the parent . . . may prove a factor which may throw light on some neglected aspects of [the] parent-child relationship, and its impairment may possibly gain importance in early diagnosis of expected difficulties" (p. 156). Psychoanalysis has contributed greatly to an increase in awareness of parental influences on child development.

The application of psychoanalytic theory was extended to child-rearing techniques in the 1930s and 1940s. Parents attempted to reduce the fears and anxieties within their children through increased permissiveness as a result of Freudian theory. Unfortunately, they met with some disappointment because one of the common side effects was an increase in their own guilt feelings. Through misunderstanding and misapplication of psychoanalytic principles, some parents attempted to reduce the severity of their children's superegos only to witness the deepest of all anxieties, "that is, the fear of human beings who feel unprotected against the pressure of their drives" (A. Freud, 1965, p. 8).

Anna Freud (1965) pointed out that, in retrospect, children whose development was influenced by the application of psychoanalytic principles were in some respects different, although they did not necessarily escape exposure to neurotic conflicts. On a slightly more positive note, she admitted that there are occasions when "an analytic upbringing promotes better health."

There appears to be no simple parental solution of facilitating healthy development in children, and great care must be exercised in assessing the impact of the parents on the child's development. For example, some parents maintain such strong attachment to their child that they represent in him or her an ideal of themselves. The child in turn is shaped into an image that promotes these fantasies. Other parents may extend their own pathology to the child, relating to the child on this basis rather than on the basis of the child's real needs. In the most severe cases there can be a fusion of the symptomatology between mother and child. Parents may also unwittingly maintain a child's disturbance because of the anxiety that is created both in the parents and in the child. All of these point to the need for careful assessment of the interaction between parent and child.

Sometimes a discrepancy exists between the parent and the child that is a function of the psychological meaning of specific experiences. Parents may assess demands placed on the child with logic and practical necessity while failing to realize that the child interprets in the light of his or her own stage of psychic reality. Thus one aspect of education for parents is to recognize discrepancies that exist as a function of the child's incomplete assessment of reality.

Anna Freud (1968b) discussed the role of knowledge for the average mother. Historically, mothers were assumed to be competent and informed on the complexities of child-rearing; popular belief attributed such wisdom to "mother instinct," a notion comparable to maternal behavioral patterns in animals. Recognizing the incompleteness of such an analogy, she pointed out that young parents frequently feel inexperienced and incapable of dealing with problems in child development. Parents express the desire that their children develop into free, unrestrained individuals, and this necessitates greater information on normal psychological development. Several specific points have been discussed in the context of psychoanalytic theory: aggression and negativism in young children, importance of sexual development, and early object attachments.

Psychoanalysis stresses the importance of recognizing that aggression and negativism are a reflection of instinctual forces which demand immediate gratification. Parents' responsibility, then, is not to eradicate aggression but to guide the child to channel aggression into an acceptable form of expression. Greater understanding of early sexuality results in further acceptance of the normality of such behavior as masturbation and mutual sex play. Parents who accept the significance of such behavior for healthy undisturbed development will not attempt to eliminate sexual expression. Rather, they will assist the child in determining its appropriate context. The child's early relationship to his or her parents stems from the dependency upon them for need satisfaction. In normal development the relationship of comfort and satisfaction, in particular to the mother, is offset by developing rivalry of the child in the oedipal phase. Every child's fantasy of replacing either a mother or a father must be recognized by parents as a deadly serious matter for the child. It becomes, then, the responsibility for the parents to assist the child through the disappointment of such unmet wishes in order to minimize harm to his or her self-esteem and confidence.

Techniques in Parent Education and Counseling

Child guidance clinics with their focus on parent-child interaction have been a primary resource for parent education. When it is a question of a disturbed child, the role of the parents assumes greater importance and the intervention technique may of necessity be intensified with the parents. Such techniques are likely to include individual counseling and in other cases individual psychoanalysis.

Direct observation of children also serves to enhance parents' knowledge of child development and needs. Anna Freud utilized this method at the Hampstead Child-Therapy Clinic. Direct observation is promoted in those areas where the mother and/or father have themselves experienced deprivation in their early object relations.

In working with parents, Kessler (1966) stresses the need to provide educational explanations of behavior. At the same time she cautions that such explanations require good general knowledge both of the specific dynamics of the case and of child psychology and psychopathology. She describes three types of explanation centering on normality, symptom, and defense. Explanations of normality include couching the behavior within the guidelines of what is normal and phase-appropriate behavior. Examining the behavior for its symptomatic component helps the parent to understand the underlying meaning of the behavior. Similarly, an explanation of a defense provides parents with a clearer understanding of the source of conflict, for example, in a case where a child is using aggression as a defense against his or her own fears of aggression.

There are no "packaged" programs stemming from psychoanalytic techniques. However, information that stresses the importance of such issues as sexual education and early emotional development is available through various health and social welfare pamphlets, and this literature has been influenced by psychoanalytic theory. Guidelines are available, for example, on the methods that parents can employ to answer children's questions regarding sex. Critical developmental events, such as toilet training, are frequently discussed in such pamphlets. One of the more widely read works in the 1940s was Dr. Spock's *Common Sense Book of Baby and Child Care* (1946), which provided parents with concrete developmental guidelines. Spock's early work contained a strong undercurrent of psychoanalytic theory.

FAMILY THERAPY

The prime focus of psychoanalysis remains the individual. Yet in working with children and adolescents, it is impossible to ignore the impact of the family and its influence as the singularly most important environment in the child's development. Interest in the psychoanalytic treatment of families stemmed from a multitude of problems associated with the individual treatment of children and adolescents. Early indications of the importance of the family were inferred from the transference reactions of children rather than from direct observation of family interaction. Specific concern arose over impasses and treatment failures. Freud (1963) maintained that the individual failures in treatment are always due to external circumstances and that the internal resistances can always be overcome. Psychoanalysts also observed gradually that improvements due to therapy with children often resulted in actual deterioration of the family system. The initial focus on the family was largely limited to the mother-child dyad because there existed an underlying assumption that the mother was the earliest and most important object in the child's environment. Anthony (1980) reports that much of the psychoanalytic literature still fails to consider the family as the unit of focus but rather continues to report on parent-child relations or on the child's fantasy of the family during treatment. Psychoanalysts have been tempted to view problems in terms of two distinct spheres: the child or adolescent as the individual patient on the one hand and the parents and/or family on the other. This artificial division has frequently resulted in a further division of responsibility in which a second mental health professional, often a social worker, works with the family while the child undergoes individual psychoanalytic treatment. Some psychoanalysts believe this provides a protective barrier that shields the analyst from directing too much attention to the environment.

There is wide variation in analytic technique with parents and family. On the one end of the continuum are analysts who exclude the family completely from treatment, focusing only on the child's neurotic conflicts. More frequently, parents are kept informed, sometimes actually participating in sessions with young children. In other instances, parents and family are treated, even analyzed, simultaneously but separately. At the other extreme the family may be treated for the child's pathology rather than the child (Bowen, 1978).

The impact of the environment should not be underestimated. Anna Freud (1965) proposed a classification system of childhood disorders in which conflicts are viewed as either primarily external or primarily internal. In those cases where the environment has failed to provide adequately for the child, management becomes an integral aspect of the therapeutic work, and this necessitates work with the parents and sometimes the entire family. Kramer (1968) reports that child psychoanalysis is less successful when there is a high degree of external conflict and family pathology. In these cases he advocates family therapy as a first step until the child can be sufficiently freed up for analysis. As interest in ego development assumes greater prominence, it is likely that more attention will be paid to the child's extrapsychic world in which the entire family plays a critical role.

Psychoanalytic family treatment developed as an extension of individual psychoanalysis and later as a treatment form for more severe disorders which resisted adequate resolution in individual treatment. In this sense it can be viewed as an alternative in those cases in which psychoanalysis is ineffective. Yet in treating the entire family, the emphasis remains closely tied to traditional psychoanalytic theory.

Conditions in which the child's psychopathology reflects unconscious conflicts of other members of the family are usually accompanied by either parental or family treatment. In these cases it is hypothesized that the child serves to gratify unconscious impulses of the collective family, and the whole system operates in a dynamic fashion which forces all of the problems onto one member. Frequently there is a history of emotional deprivation in the backgrounds of the individual parents. Neurotic conflicts are revisited on the family as the cycles are repeated from generation to generation. One indication that the child is responding to family conflicts or pressures is found in the transference development, especially in the child's unconscious attempts to replicate the parent's behavior in the analyst.

Conditions in adolescence which are frequently treated by a family approach and which may or may not include additional individual treatment include borderline problems, narcissistic difficulties, and antisocial acting-out behavior. Indeed, one of the problems associated with individual treatment of adolescents is that the unconscious assumptions in the family are often very powerful at this stage and can lead to resistances which interfere with the individual therapy more than do the adolescent's own internal resistances. For example, in one family the unconscious wish of the collective family is that the adolescent male replace the father and thereby become the mother's partner. Such dynamics present serious obstacles to normal adolescent development and introduce external conflict which may be dealt with in family treatment. Family separation-individuation, interpersonal conflict, and communication breakdown result in enmeshment and thereby maintain a predominantly gratifying neurotic family homeostasis. The family is literally in no position to allow the adolescent to mature and emancipate himself or herself. A clinical example often associated with this type of family constellation is adolescent school refusal.

Techniques and Considerations in Family Therapy

Psychoanalytic family therapy employs analytic theory in the treatment of families. There is an assumption that the family operates in ways of which they are not fully aware. As a collective unit they promote certain unconscious wishes just as does the individual. Freud (1913/1918) first described these ongoing processes in *Totem and Taboo.* He referred to the *family psyche,* which corresponds closely to the individual psyche. The family psyche maintains a continuity of emotional life that is passed on from generation to generation. The existence of a collective psychological life serves to provide an unconscious understanding of psychic conflict within members and this too can be transmitted across generations.

One technique in family work, then, is to look at the family organization in order to understand the child and to infer from the collective defenses the underlying unconscious meanings. Frequently, the process is one of identification just as it occurs in group work. Identification is, of course, a method of introjection by the ego. For example, a father will dismiss his son's aggressive and destructive behavior on the playground at school with the offhand remark, "I was just like that when I was his age." Treatment consists of understanding and working through the transferences of the parental introjections in order for the parents to see and experience how the problems in the present family have arisen from unconscious efforts to master or repeat old conflicts stemming from their families of origin. Projective identification occurs in families as well when there is a blurring of ownership of personal characteristics which become attributed to other family members. In the extreme cases, Bowen (1978) describes the "undifferentiated family ego mass" as the situation in which all members are totally enmeshed in the systemic functioning and are incapable of maintaining separate identities. In these cases individual psychoanalytic treatment frequently results in an impasse, and family treatment is the preferred mode of intervention.

Despite an orientation that demands constant awareness of the past and unconscious processes of each of the family members, psychoanalytic family work also strives to interpret transferences and resistances of the family as a collective unit. The neurotic family interaction is then reinterpreted in terms of the individual's neurosis which is rooted in the family structure.

Although family techniques are undergoing rapid changes and revisions with the introduction of systems theory (e.g., Haley, 1977; Papp, 1977), psychoanalytically based intervention remains reconstructive in focus. That is to say, the same need exists in family work as in individual work: to pull apart the structural aspects of personality and to rebuild them through insight and interpretation. Therapy is, therefore, considered long-term although this time period can vary from several months to several years. Despite variations in style, the techniques maintain (1) a focus on the individual in treatment, (2) reinforcement of the individual in the minds of the other family members, (3) a recognition of the unconscious components of the family dynamics, (4) acknowledgment that the family will often impede the separation and individuation of its members, and (5) acceptance of the fact that core components of each family member's personality are difficult to modify and that change occurs only over a long period of time.

EFFICACY

In one of Freud's last published papers, *Analysis Terminable and Interminable* (1964b), there is a general impression of pessimism with respect to the therapeutic efficacy of psychoanalysis. Freud was always conscious of the limitations of his theory, and consequently he frequently revised his formulations. One of the early attempts to examine outcome of patients treated at the Berlin Psychoanalytic Institute was based on 10 years of collated statistics and was published by Fenichel in 1930. The results indicated that psychoanalysis was often only partially successful yet still remained the foundation for reconstructive therapy. In general, one of the problems in evaluating psychoanalysis as a technique is the fact that it rests more on clinical knowledge than on quantitative evaluation. Freud's findings were deduced from numerous hours of direct patient contact and as such describe specific details of human personality that are assumed to apply to all human behavior. Moreover, the details of this theory and technique are frequently expressed in a language that is not operational and, therefore, not easy to test. Psychoanalysis thus presents great difficulty when viewed from an empirical basis. The psychoanalyst focuses on conscious thought and feelings as the raw data, and within the psychoanalytic method there is less emphasis upon observing behavior to determine the consistency of thought and feelings with action. Psychoanalytic theory has unfortunately paid little attention to the processes by which a conscious thought is manifested in behavior. The other data that are most frequently used in psychoanalytic research are the analyst's observations of the patient's remarks, and these are highly susceptible to individual bias (Lustman, 1963; Schlessinger, Pollock, Sabshin, Sadow, & Gedo, 1966). Furthermore, such data are the result of extrapolation from abnormal subjects with the fundamental assumption that they apply equally to normal behavior. At the theoretical level criticism has been leveled against psychoanalysis for its lack of precision as to the specific nature of the structural aspects of id, ego, and superego at each stage of development.

Still, some outcome studies have been mildly encouraging (Feldman, 1968; Luborsky, 1971). More detailed investigations such as the Psychotherapeutic Research Project of the Menninger Foundation (Wallerstein, 1975) and the Research Project of the Hampstead Child-Therapy Clinic (A. Freud, 1958) can shed additional light on this difficult question. The Menninger Foundation Research Project has attempted long-term prediction of outcome based on assessment of the structure of personality and the type of pathology. The major shortcoming of psychoanalysis efficacy evaluation has been the fact that, with few exceptions, those most skilled in the technique are least skilled in the methods of research investigation.

Psychoanalysis does not attempt to eliminate all of the personality defects and neurotic factors in patients. It does attempt to mitigate the rigors of a punitive superego, and this is a significant criterion of the effectiveness of treatment. Symptom alleviation is less significant than the patient's overall feeling of adjustment or need for continued psychotherapy. The chief basis of evaluation, then, is the patient's capacity for attaining reasonable happiness and his or her ability to contribute to the happiness of others. This achievement is measured in the patient's willingness to deal with normal life stresses and to enter into and sustain mutually gratifying relationships. On the theoretical level, successful treatment involves the reduction of unconscious and neurotic inhibition, accompanied by a decrease of infantile dependency needs and a release of the individual's normal potential previously blocked by neurotic conflicts. Ideally, these changes pave the way for internal growth and mature personality functioning.

The proliferation of psychoanalytically based forms of psychotherapy has made it extremely difficult to evaluate the efficacy of psychoanalysis. Marmour (1973) argues that psychoanalysis has never been a fixed entity at any time in its history. Such expansion has been useful, however, in specifying more refined techniques for treating a wider segment of the disturbed population. In fact, there appears to be somewhat of a blurring of therapeutic technique among child psychotherapists (Koocher & Pedulla, 1977). Psychoanalytic theory, although still a very powerful force in child psychotherapy, is not rated among the most frequently used techniques despite the fact that its principles are often employed in interventions in the child and adolescent area. One obvious reason for its limitation is the lack of adequately trained child psychoanalysts. A second, equally important, reason is the intensity of the intervention. Clearly, only a very small percentage of children and adolescents actually undergo psychoanalysis in the traditional Freudian sense.

With respect to child and adolescent psychoanalysis, a particular problem emerges when one attempts to determine successful outcome. Glover (1953) questions whether analysis of young children is ever completed because the standards are quite different from those used to evaluate adult cases. For example, persistence of symptoms in children, albeit in a modified form, may not be interpreted as failure when evidence exists of strengthened character formation. Fenichel (1945) argues that the advantage to treating young children and adolescents lies in the relatively short period of time in which the inhibition has been maintained. The most traditional analysts maintain that the success of child analysis cannot be satisfactorily assessed until at least 15 years have elapsed. Estimating the therapeutic efficacy of psychoanalysis thus excludes entirely children under the age of puberty. Glover concludes that the real test of child psychoanalysis remains in the patient's capacity in later life to withstand stresses and frustrations without resorting to symptom formation.

The superiority of psychoanalysis over any other form of treatment is an unsettled issue, but it is evident that neither psychoanalysis nor any other form of psychotherapy provides the solution to all emotional problems of childhood and adolescence. Psychoanalysis remains, above all, a form of education rather than a cure. In this sense it provides a great hope in the treatment of children and adolescents.

CONCLUSIONS

The importance of psychoanalytic theory to the practicing clinician lies in its depth of understanding of the nature of human development and in its exploration of the unconscious. The survival of psychoanalysis may ultimately rest upon its flexibility with respect to such technical issues as length and intensity of treatment. The specific challenge to psychoanalysis is to make it more readily accessible to a wider spectrum of the population in terms of both presenting problems and economic feasibility. One means of achieving this goal is to develop a more direct application to education—for example, in curriculum materials that recognize the developmental tasks inherent in each of the psychosexual stages. Psychoanalysis must also expand its horizons beyond its narrow parameters as a subspecialty of psychiatry. For psychoanalytic treatment to flourish, it will be increasingly important to demonstrate its relevance to the broader spectrum of professionals within the mental health field. Finally, it is recognized that additional research is needed that will operationalize the theoretical constructs inherent in psychoanalytic technique. Psychoanalysis bears the responsibility for developing an adequate research strategy that takes into consideration the psychoanalyst's insistence that treatment can be validated only through the actual process of psychoanalysis.

CASE STUDY

The Case Study of the Leopard Boy[1]

The clinical example describes the psychoanalytic treatment of a young boy whose development was normal until he experienced a terrifying event, resulting in a traumatic neurosis. The follow-up report emphasizes the need for awareness of both the intrapsychic structure of the child and the dynamics of family life.

HISTORY AND ASSESSMENT. At the time of assessment, the patient was a 3½-year-old boy, the only child of an upper middle class family. He was referred by his father, who reported that 5 months prior to the assessment the boy had been bitten on the neck by a leopard. Since the time of the attack, he had experienced numerous problems—he would awaken two to four times each night and would have frequent nightmares involving "animals and monsters," and he exhibited a reluctance to

---

[1]From "Psychic Trauma and Traumatic Neurosis," by G. MacLean, (1977). *Canadian Psychiatric Association Journal, 22,* 71-76, and "Addendum to a Case of Traumatic Neurosis," by G. MacLean, (1980). *Canadian Journal of Psychiatry, 25,* 506-508.

be apart from his mother. The onset of these symptoms began with the bite of the leopard and represented a marked change from his behavior prior to the event. In addition, over the 5 months that had elapsed from the time of the attack to the time of the assessment, little amelioration of the symptoms had occurred.

On review of the history, it was related that a week following the boy's discharge from the hospital after having his tonsils removed, he and his father went to their local pet store. The store kept a leopard on display, enclosed in a peculiar cage that was made up of bars and a protective glass shield, with a gap between the top of the cage and the ceiling of the display room. While the boy was watching, the leopard leaped up, managed to get through the gap and bit the boy and his father on the neck and head. Bleeding and finding no help available, the father managed to keep the leopard away to permit their retreat out of the store. They were taken to their local hospital where the lacerations were repaired.

The attack by the leopard marked the onset of the boy's symptoms. Immediately after the attack, he acted terrified. He cried and screamed, "Why did the leopard bite?" "He bit Daddy!" "Daddy has blood all over him!" On his return home from the hospital emergency department, he began to experience problems with sleeping. Two or three or perhaps four times a night, he would awaken and come into his parents' room and climb into bed with them. He would be crying and complaining about "bad dreams" and about "animals and monsters."

Prior to the meeting with the leopard, the boy had been content to play outside by himself, and he was always happy to stay with a baby-sitter. However, with the accident, he began to show a reluctance and concern about being separated from his mother and father. His mother described this concern as being "more clinging." Whenever she went out, he would be full of questions as to where she was going, for how long, and when she was coming back. In addition, he showed an interest in where his father was going. Whether it was to work or out in the evening, he would constantly ask where his father was, and he would demand to be told repeatedly about his father's exact whereabouts.

The boy was an appealing child who was quite talkative, warm, and interested. On the initial meeting, he played freely with the toys and he showed a good ability to fantasize. In this initial meeting, he loudly announced that he had been bitten by a mosquito on the way to the assessment; however, this wasn't too bad because mosquitos could "never eat you up," because "Mummy would help." Members of a toy family then began to "get hurt." They would fall and "hurt their legs." Members of the family "couldn't help" for they "got hurt too." Doctors were called but "they got hurt" and "no one would help anyone!"

The parents were both industrious, successful people with a good relationship, interested and able to parent. They presented no evidence of neurotic or characterological problems. In particular, no parental contribution to the development of the symptoms could be discovered.

The problem was diagnosed as a traumatic neurosis, and an offer of individual psychotherapy for the boy was made and accepted. Subsequently, over a period of 8 months, 24 sessions were held at a frequency of about one session a week. Scattered throughout this period and at infrequent times there were a number of conjoint interviews with the parents—never less than once a month, never more than twice a month.

TREATMENT. One major theme that progressed throughout all of the sessions was the re-enactment in play of the traumatic event. In myriad ways, the actual attack of the leopard was re-enacted. Every detail—the trip with father, the interior of the pet store, the attack of the leopard, what was said, where the scratches and cuts occurred, the police ambulance, and so on—was reviewed over and over again. This re-enactment might consist of a detailed verbal description of the traumatic encounter, or a simple, small part of the entire adventure might be symbolically or directly present in play. For example, in play, a toy rubber tiger might be contained in a small cage, only to escape over the toys, "like the leopard in the pet store." Similarly, a great cage might be built of the toy furniture and blocks to contain the rubber animal but to no avail for he "always gets out." The playroom frequently became the pet store or the leopard's cage, and the play centered about that. When this would be interpreted, it often prompted a verbal description of the actual traumatic event.

For the first few sessions, the boy stayed in the playroom and played. The theme of re-enactment was the major emphasis. However, with the re-enactment and the emotions of fear and anger involved, it was noted that the sessions quickly became shorter and shorter. Whereas the first two lasted the complete 45 minutes, the next several sessions quickly decreased in length, until he was spending only about 10 minutes in the playroom before asking to leave to see his mother. It was conceptualized, at that time, that a number of reasons existed for the brevity of the sessions. In producing the frightening material in his re-enactment of the traumatic encounter, the boy had on a number of occasions adopted the appearance and manner of a leopard and attacked the therapist. One reason, therefore, for the brevity of the sessions was thought to be the feared retaliation for his attacks on the therapist. In addition, it was thought the playroom itself was becoming a frightening place because of the "monsters" existing in the toy box and the boy's associations. The feared retaliation was thought to be of particular significance because it most probably was linked to the child's anger at his father and the subsequent fear of retaliation from him. With the partial interpretation of this anger and fear, the boy immediately began to spend entire sessions in the playroom.

The child's anger at his parents, especially his father for allowing the leopard attack, became a major issue in the transference. The expression of anger was followed by his fears of retaliation. A typical situation in therapy would be described as follows. The boy would come into the playroom and play quietly with a number of toy figures. Then rather quickly, the entire population of his toy drawer sought refuge and were safe in the toy house, safe from the attack of a rather vicious rubber leopard. Then the house proved not to be safe as he knocked it from the table and smashed it to the floor, at which time the boy would shout, "Look what 'you' did! Now everybody in the house has been hurt!" The interpretation would be made at this juncture, "you are angry at 'me' for letting that happen, and you are angry at 'me-daddy' for letting the leopard bite you." Perhaps, he would respond with a quick "yes," as then he escalated in his anger to throw all the toys, the blocks, and a great quantity of water all over the playroom. The interpretation would be repeated, and he would be interpreted in terms of his need to make a recompense for his angry attack, because of his fear of retaliation.

The range and type of affect expressed in the sessions varied tremendously—love, anger, fear, and hate were expressed, rapidly and quickly in succession. Ambivalence was marked. Facing his emotions and the consequent conflicts, the boy employed a variety of defenses in the context of his therapy.

For example, frequently and suddenly in the play, the therapist would find himself attacked by the boy who would be growling and scratching out "like a leopard." We could see that the boy was attempting to deal with his fear and his anger by identifying with the aggressive animal and by showing the therapist what it was like to be suddenly attacked. The defense of identification, however, not only occurred in the identification with the leopard, but it was also exhibited when the boy would act like a father or mother or therapist. In play, often his voice would lower and he would assume the role of father in the re-enactment of the traumatic event. Even the detail of bringing a small toy police ambulance to the sessions and playing the part of the policemen "taking the little boy and his father to the hospital" occurred.

In addition, not only because of his identification with the leopard but also because the world had proven to be a dangerous place, he began to project his own anger onto the environment and, in particular, to fear retaliation from the therapist. In play, the therapist became the leopard, and the boy dealt with the leopard as best he could, by constructing cages or by actively running away, out of the playroom.

Over the sessions the therapist was confronted with another subtlety of defense that constituted more of a characterological trait. As previously described, the boy was a bright, verbal, creative child and in his pressure to activity, which in itself was a defense, he became quite beguiling. If in play, for example, the boy identified with the leopard and swatted the therapist across the neck, as he had been swatted by the leopard, he would frequently, immediately become a changed person. For example, he would begin to be very creative and with talent imitate a rock singer, or entertain the therapist in some other manner. He would imitate a baby, facing the therapist with the apparent question as to "how can you get mad at me—I'm just a little boy?"

Over the 8 months of therapy, the child's symptoms decreased and at the time of termination, they had disappeared.

FOLLOW-UP. The boy came for reassessment when he was 7½ years of age. The father related that after good experiences in kindergarten and Grade 1, a problem had been encountered by the boy in Grade 2. He began to express a newfound dislike of school, and his parents began to receive reports from his teacher that his schoolwork had deteriorated. All of this was in marked contrast to his previous good performance and his former enjoyment of school. In addition, the boy had become sad and morose, and his mood had concerned the parents. The parents described the boy's teacher as an angry woman who they felt was the major cause of the boy's dislike of school and his poor performance. However, they were more concerned about how upset and affected the boy was with this identifiably difficult relationship. On certain days he appeared to be a happy child who played well with his friends and who performed well in his tasks. On other days, his sadness and what was described as a "complaintive pessimism" appeared to intrude and "nothing was right, nothing went right." He would not play with his friends, and his schoolwork would not get done.

A thorough educational assessment was made which included both comprehensive testing and classroom observation. This revealed the boy to be above level in reading and mathematics. There were no deficits found in the testing of perceptual modalities. The educational consultant concluded with certainty that the boy should have no difficulty in achieving and maintaining a good school performance.

The classroom observation, however, was extremely valuable because it revealed that the boy's teacher was a very angry woman who, for some reason that remained unknown, openly disliked the boy and who treated him within the classroom with marked disfavor. This teacher's attitude was in arresting contrast to the general reaction to the boy as an appealing child whom everyone liked. When in the actual presence of the school teacher, it was observed that he became withdrawn and that his performance became impaired.

The parents were interviewed. Of significant occurrence over the intervening 3 years was the birth of another child, a girl, one and one-half years earlier. The pregnancy had been difficult and with complications resulting in the mother having spent much of this period in hospital. In addition, the father's mother had died one year previously. The parents noted the complaints about the school performance and about the boy's mood. In addition, they observed that another problem existed, which they described as a "fear of water." The boy refused to go swimming or even to go near swimming pools or the ocean. He told them that he was afraid of drowning. He refused even to go to Boy Cubs as he heard that they went swimming. The parents stated that in all other areas their son appeared to be functioning well.

The boy was assessed. He had grown considerably over the 3 years since he had last been seen. He was a tall 7½-year-old who was friendly and interested, and who immediately described a vague memory of having been seen before. He commented that he remembered the playroom, but that he remembered it as being much larger then. The play began slowly. He played with the clay, and snakes began to appear. "Boa Constrictors, King Cobras, rattlesnakes, flying snakes, and snakes that spit their venom 20 yards to kill people" were created. People were variously killed. He drew a picture of a storm with black clouds and lightning. The world was seen to be a "dangerous place, full of dangerous things." There were good things, helpful things in the world, but there were mostly bad things and dangerous things. Dangerous things had the characteristic of surprising you, of following you, of suddenly coming upon you and threatening you. He provided a list of dangerous animals, of dangerous objects, and a list of potential natural disasters. Soon all this led back to the leopard. He recounted the attack of the leopard as he had 4 years previously when he was first seen. In this play, accidents happened, people fell, cars overturned, lightning struck, monsters appeared, and people died. The boy recounted how he was frightened of his teacher, who in play became the "wicked witch." A hospital appeared in the play where "some were lucky enough to go and get fixed," but "some people weren't so lucky and died."

On assessment, the boy was seen to be capable of excellent performance in all spheres of emotional and cognitive functioning and in relationships with peers and adults. However, symptoms based on neurotic conflict appeared to interfere with such ability. These neurotic symptoms again appeared to have been precipitated by an environmental stressor—the harsh school teacher. This was related to the original overwhelming stressor—the leopard. However, concern was felt about the regression under stress. Although this was felt to represent neurotic "inner" conflict linked symbolically to the original trauma; the tendency to regression had the potential of being, or becoming, a characterological fault.

In addition, on this occasion, it appeared that a parental contribution to the development and maintenance of the boy's symptoms was present. In retrospect, this contribution was seen to have been an important, unrecognized factor in the original traumatic neurosis. It was seen in the assessment interview that the boy was especially preoccupied with death. When this was taken back into the second conjoint interview with the parents, their anxieties about death became obvious. They were concerned about the loss, through death, of loved ones. Of most recent note was the death of the paternal grandmother, and the threatened loss of the last pregnancy. This loss and threatened loss were described by the parents as being difficult topics for them to consider.

Over a 6-month period, 26 individual sessions were held with the boy and four conjoint sessions were held with the parents. In these two situations, two parallel themes were dealt with. The boy expressed his fear of death and his fears of the "dangers of the world." The world was a dangerous place where people were hurt and died. This was seen to be intimately linked with the attack of the leopard. At that time, his ego had been overwhelmed when he had it demonstrated to him in an overwhelming way that the world was dangerous, where he could be destroyed.

The parents revealed that the attack of the leopard had also been overwhelming to them. They had been frightened by the prospect of suddenly losing their son. They could talk of experiencing this fear at the time of the attack only in retrospect. They felt they could not admit it to themselves at the actual time of the attack. The boy's mother discussed the loss of her mother when she was 13, and the loss of her father when she was 16. With such losses she was convinced at that time that she would never be loved or love anyone again. When she married, she had been surprised to experience love, and when she had a son she could scarcely believe it to be true. The boy wanted to talk about death, but the parents could not. They were aware of the boy's fears in general outline, but they could not talk with him about them. The boy had mentioned his concern about his mother's health and about the baby's chances of living. His disapproval of his father's smoking and of his father's flying on business trips was known. The parents could not help their son deal with his fears of this dangerous world and of the mortality of men, because they could not deal with their own fears.

Over the course of therapy, a change in the boy occurred: He became more optimistic and enthusiastic in his relations with the world. Gradually, his fears disappeared. In addition, the school year was coming to an end and he looked forward to the advent of a new teacher in the coming year. The brief therapy of the parents had as a focus their fears of loss. They quickly became insightful and they could understand the parallel nature of the family problem. With such insight they were able to contain their fears and with their lessened anxiety and increased confidence they were able to help their son contain his fears.

ANNOTATED BIBLIOGRAPHY

Blos, P. (1962). *On adolescence.* New York: The Free Press.

Blos' work provides a comprehensive psychoanalytic framework upon which to view adolescence. With emphasis on theory, he describes five phases of the adolescent process. Little reference is made to either psychopathology or treatment.

Brenner, C. (1973). *An elementary textbook of psychoanalysis* (rev. ed.). New York: International Universities Press.

Available in a paperback edition, this work provides a comprehensive, concise overview of psychoanalytic theory and technique. It provides greater detail and refinement of basic concepts, including intrapsychic conflict, resistance, and transference.

Erikson, E. H. (1963). *Childhood and society.* New York: W. W. Norton.
This text originated from Erikson's work in psychoanalysis. Consistent with current interest and emphasis on the study of the ego, it stresses the concept of man's capacity to organize his experience and his action in an adaptive fashion. With references to culture, religions, and revolution, the work deals with the understanding of neurosis in the wider perspective. Erikson discusses the eight stages of man's development from basic trust to ego integrity.

Freud, A. (1968). *The writings of Anna Freud* (7 vols.). New York: International Universities Press.
These volumes contain the major writings of Anna Freud, stemming directly from her clinical work, teaching activities, and lectures. Of special interest are Volume II, dealing with the ego and the mechanisms of defense; Volume IV, which discusses the indications of child psychoanalysis; and Volume VI, in which she provides a guide to assessment of psychopathology.

Pearson, G. H. (Ed.). (1968). *A handbook of child psychoanalysis.* New York: Basic Books.
Intended as an introductory handbook on the psychoanalysis of children and adolescents, this work offers guidelines and indications for treatment, gives a description of initial interviews with both the child and the parents, and discusses issues of transference, resistance, and termination. A case is described in detail in an attempt to present a picture of the day-to-day interaction between the analyst and the child.

The psychoanalytic study of the child. Published in annual volume form. New York: International Universities Press.
These annual volumes, first published in 1945, provide a collection of current topics of interest to child and adolescent psychoanalysts and reflect perhaps the most recent findings on etiology, treatment, and theoretical understanding from a psychoanalytic perspective. The articles vary in emphasis, including research, theory, and practice.

Winnicott, D. W. (1977). *The piggle.* New York: International Universities Press.
This classic work describes a case study of a young girl in psychoanalytic treatment. Delightfully written in an easy-to-understand format, it provides a running account of the actual treatment process, including comments and notes by the analyst, which give the reader an understanding of theory and technique.

REFERENCES

Aichorn, A. (1935). *Wayward youth.* New York: Viking Press. (Original work published 1925)

Anthony, E. (1980). The family and the psychoanalytic process in children. *Psychoanalytic Study of the Child, 35,* 3-40.

Bernfeld, S. (1929). *The psychology of the infant.* London: K. Paul. (Original work published in 1925)

Bion, W. (1961). *Experiences in groups.* London: Tavistock.

Blos, P. (1962). *On adolescence.* New York: The Free Press.

Bowen, M. (1978). *Family therapy in clinical practice.* New York: Jason Aronson.

Brenner, C. (1973). *An elementary textbook of psychoanalysis* (rev. ed.). New York: International Universities Press.

Cruickshank, W., & Johnson, G. (Eds.). (1975). *Education of exceptional children and youth* (3rd ed.). Englewood Cliffs, NJ: Prentice-Hall.

Erikson, E. H. (1963). *Childhood and society.* New York: W. W. Norton.

Feldman, F. (1968). Results of psychoanalysis in clinic case assignments. *Journal of the American Psychoanalytic Association, 16,* 274-300.

Fenichel, O. (1930). *Zehn jahre Berliner psychoanalytischer institut.* Vienna: International Psychoanalytischer Verlag.

Fenichel, O. (1945). *The psychoanalytic theory of neurosis.* New York: W. W. Norton.

Fraiberg, S. (1955). Some considerations in the introduction to therapy in puberty. *Psychoanalytic Study of the Child, 10,* 264-288.

Freud, A. (1937). *The ego and the mechanisms of defense.* London: Hogarth Press.

Freud, A. (1958). Clinical studies in psychoanalysis (research project of the Hampstead Child-Therapy Clinic). *Proceedings of the Royal Society of Medicine, 51,* 938-942.

Freud, A. (1965). The psychoanalytic view of childhood: Long-distance and close-up. *The writings of Anna Freud* (Vol. 6). New York: International Universities Press.

Freud, A. (1968a). *The writings of Anna Freud* (7 vols.). New York: International Universities Press.

Freud, A. (1968b). Nursery school education: Its uses and dangers. *The writings of Anna Freud* (Vol. 4). New York: International Universities Press. (Original work published in 1949)

Freud, A. (1968c). Answering teachers' questions. *The writings of Anna Freud* (Vol. 4). New York: International Universities Press. (Original work published in 1952)

Freud, A. (1971). Child analysis as a sub-specialty of psychoanalysis. *The writings of Anna Freud* (Vol. 7). New York: International Universities Press. (Original work published in 1970)

Freud, A. (1974). The role of transference in the analysis of children. *The writings of Anna Freud* (Vol. 1). New York: International Universities Press. (Original work published 1926-1927)

Freud, S. (1918). *Totem and taboo* (A. A. Brill, Trans.). New York: Vintage Books. (Original work published in 1913)

Freud, S. (1953). Three essays on the theory of sexuality. In J. Strachey (Ed. and Trans.), *The standard edition of the complete psychological works of Sigmund Freud* (Vol. 7). London: Hogarth Press. (Original work published in 1905)

Freud, S. (1955a). Group psychology and the analysis of the ego. In J. Strachey (Ed. and Trans.), *The standard edition of the complete psychological works of Sigmund Freud* (Vol. 18). London: Hogarth Press. (Original work published in 1921)

Freud, S. (1955b). Two encyclopedia articles. In J. Strachey (Ed. and Trans.), *The standard edition of the complete psychological works of Sigmund Freud* (Vol. 18). London: Hogarth Press. (Original work published in 1923)

Freud, S. (1961). The ego and the id. In J. Strachey (Ed. and Trans.), *The standard edition of the complete psychological works of Sigmund Freud* (Vol. 19). London: Hogarth Press. (Original work published in 1923)

Freud, S. (1963). Introductory lectures to psychoanalysis. In J. Strachey (Ed. and Trans.), *The standard edition of the complete psychological works of Sigmund Freud* (Vol. 16). London: Hogarth Press. (Original work published in 1917)

Freud, S. (1964a). New introductory lectures on psychoanalysis. In J. Strachey (Ed. and Trans.), *The standard edition of the complete psychological works of Sigmund Freud* (Vol. 22). London: Hogarth Press. (Original work published in 1933)

Freud, S. (1964b). Analysis terminable and interminable. In J. Strachey (Ed. and Trans.), *The standard edition of the complete psychological works of Sigmund Freud* (Vol. 23). London: Hogarth Press. (Original work published in 1937)

Glover, E. (1953). *Psycho-analysis and child psychiatry.* London: Imago.

Haley, J. (1977). *Problem-solving therapy.* San Francisco: Jossey-Bass.

Hug-Hellmuth, H. von. (1921). On the technique of child analysis. *International Journal of Psychoanalysis, 2,* 287-305. (Original work published in 1920)

Jones, R. (1968). *Fantasy and feeling in education.* New York: New York University Press.

Kessler, J. (1966). *Psychopathology of childhood.* Englewood Cliffs, NJ: Prentice-Hall.

Klein, M. (1932). *The psycho-analysis of children.* London: Hogarth Press.

Koocher, G., & Pedulla, B. (1977). Current practice in child psychotherapy. *Professional Psychology, 8,* 275-287.

Kramer, C. (1968). *The relationships between child and family psychopathology.* Chicago: Kramer Foundation.

Kramer, E. (1975a). On psychoanalysis and education. *Selected papers of Ernst Kris.* New Haven: Yale University Press. (Original work published in 1948)

Kris, E. (1975b). The study of variations of early parental attitudes. *Selected papers of Ernst Kris.* New Haven: Yale University Press. (Original work published in 1953)

Laufer, M. (1980). On reconstruction in adolescent analysis. In S. Feinstein, P. Giovacchini, J. Looney, A. Schwartzberg, & A. Sorosky (Eds.), *Adolescent psychiatry* (Vol. 8). Chicago: University of Chicago Press.

Laufer, M. (1981). Adolescent breakdown and the transference neurosis. *International Journal of Psychoanalysis, 62,* 51-59.

Lopez, T., & Kliman, G. (1980). The cornerstone treatment of a preschool boy from an extremely impoverished environment. *Psychoanalytic Study of the Child, 35,* 341-375.

Luborsky, L. (1971). Quantitative research on psychoanalytic therapy. In A. Bergin & S. Garfield (Eds.), *Handbook of psychotherapy and behavior change.* New York: John Wiley and Sons.

Lustman, S. (1963). Some issues in contemporary psychoanalytic research. *Psychoanalytic Study of the Child, 18,* 51-74.

MacKay, N. (1981). Melanie Klein's metapsychology: Phenomenological and mechanistic perspective. *International Journal of Psychoanalysis, 62,* 187-198.

MacLean, G. (1977). Psychic trauma and traumatic neurosis. *Canadian Psychiatric Association Journal, 22,* 71-76.

MacLean, G. (1980). Addendum to a case of traumatic neurosis. *Canadian Journal of Psychiatry, 25,* 506-508.

Marmour, J. (1973). The future of psychoanalytic therapy. *American Journal of Psychiatry, 130,* 1197-1202.

Meeks, J. E. (1971). *The fragile alliance: An orientation to the outpatient psychotherapy of the adolescent.* Baltimore: Williams and Wilkins.

Mullin, H., & Rosenbaum, M. (1962). *Group psychotherapy.* New York: Free Press of Glencoe.

Papp, P. (Ed.). (1977). *Family therapy: Full length case studies.* New York: Gardner Press.

Pearson, G. H. (Ed.). (1968). *A handbook of child psychoanalysis.* New York: Basic Books.

Rhodes, W. (1963). Curriculum and disordered behaviour. *Exceptional Children, 30,* 61-66.

Rhodes, W., & Tracy, M. (Eds.). (1972). *A study of child variance* (Vol. 2). Ann Arbor: The University of Michigan.

Schlessinger, N., Pollock, G., Sabshin, M., Sadow, L., & Gedo, J. (1966). Psychoanalytic contributions to psychotherapy research. In L. Gottschall & A. Auerbach (Eds.), *Methods of research in psychotherapy.* New York: Appleton-Century-Crofts.

Slavson, S. (1950). *Analytic group psychotherapy with children, adolescents, and adults.* New York: Columbia University Press.

Spock, B. (1946). *The common sense book of baby and child care.* New York: Duell, Sloan and Pearce.

Waelder, R. (1960). *Basic theory of psychoanalysis.* New York: International Universities Press.

Wallerstein, R. (1975). *Psychotherapy and psychoanalysis.* New York: International Universities Press.

Weinstein, G., & Fantini, M. (1970). *Toward humanistic education: A curriculum of affect.* New York: Praeger.

Winnicott, D. (1965). *The maturational process and the facilitating environment.* London: Hogarth Press.

Winnicott, D. W. (1977). *The piggle.* New York: International Universities Press.

Zachray, C. (1941). The influence of psychoanalysis in education. *Psychoanalytic Quarterly, 10,* 431-444.

Chapter 4

Adlerian Approaches

Don Dinkmeyer, Jr., Ph.D.
Don Dinkmeyer, Sr., Ph.D.

INTRODUCTION

Adlerian psychologists believe that all behavior is purposeful and goal directed. The behavior of children and adolescents is influenced by their search for significance and social acceptance. Adlerian psychology observes "psychological movement" to understand the purpose and the pattern of behavior. By understanding a child's goal, one can understand the meaning of the child's behavior.

A primary purpose of Adlerian counseling and therapy is goal reorientation. This approach has practical and far-reaching implications for the professional working with children and adolescents.

Adlerians view the child or adolescent as a social being. The family is the first group in which each child must find a significant place. The child's place within the family constellation influences his or her personality and sibling relationships.

In the child's search for belonging, the child's behavior is sometimes misbehavior, actions which are not acceptable to others. A clear understanding of the child's belief behind the misbehavior allows the therapist to move toward corrective action.

History and Status

Adlerian psychology was founded by Alfred Adler (1870-1937), a Viennese physician. Today, Adlerian psychology is a recognized precursor to many current schools of psychological thought, including Albert Ellis' Rational-Emotive Therapy and William Glasser's Reality Therapy, as well as Transactional Analysis.

Adler was invited to join Freud's Vienna discussion groups and became president of the Psychoanalytic Society in 1910. He resigned from the Society one year later, taking with him many members of the Society who were not comfortable with the direction of Freud's emerging psychology. Two years later, in 1912, Adler founded the Society for Individual Psychology.

Alfred Adler published more than 300 articles and books and was the first to demonstrate techniques of working with parents, teachers, and children through public demonstration. At that time, it was a controversial method as many professionals felt the mystique of "mind-healing" should not be disclosed in such a public and educational setting.

One of Adler's major contributions was the establishment of dozens of Child Guidance Clinics across Vienna. The Clinics were the basic unit for an educational and counseling approach, which was made available to social workers, teachers, medical doctors, and parents. As a result of the establishment of these clinics, Adlerian psychology became a resource to both professionals and laymen.

Adler made his first lecture tour of the United States in 1926, and soon settled in the United States after an escape from the conflicts of World War II, which destroyed much of his work in Vienna and throughout Europe.

Subsequently, Rudolph Dreikurs became the standard-bearer for this school of psychology, which became known as *Individual Psychology*. Despite extreme resistance to Adler's ideas by professionals and strong pressures to conform to Freudian psychology, Dreikurs nourished Individual Psychology's growth in the United States. This period of heavily psychoanalytic dominance in psychology was not equal to the forceful persistence of Dreikurs. His writings and demonstrations encouraged the development of the Adlerian movement in the United States and abroad.

Dreikurs made many contributions to Adlerian theory. One of the most perceptive and widely used was his understanding of children's misbehavior. Commonly referred to as the *four goals of misbehavior,* this understanding is today the cornerstone for Adlerian parent education and child counseling and psychotherapy.

Family Education Centers throughout the United States and Canada offer education and counseling resources, including parent education. Each summer an international summer school teaches Adlerian concepts and is attended by individuals from around the world. In the United States, the Alfred Adler Institute of Chicago, also founded by Dreikurs, is the largest Adlerian training institute.

Individual Psychology's central organization in the United States and Canada is the North Amerian Society for Adlerian Psychology (NASAP), located in Chicago, Illinois. Founded by Dreikurs in 1952, NASAP has more than one thousand members representing all helping professions. NASAP holds an annual convention, and the Society publishes a quarterly journal, the *Journal of Individual Psychology,* devoted to research and applications of Adlerian psychology. The Society recently created five Interest Sections: Clinical, Education, Family Education, Theory and Research, and Business and Organizations. This movement reflects the renewed and diverse interest in individual psychology across the continent.

OVERVIEW OF THEORY

Basic Theory and Assumptions

Adlerian psychology is based on an explicit theory of human behavior. This theory, applied to the counseling process, provides a concrete understanding of an effective counseling relationship.

Each person, even the youngest child, is seen as an individual, with the creative capacities to decide and choose. The actions of each person are purposeful, indivisible, and socially based. Adlerian psychology makes the following basic assumptions:

1. *All behavior has social meaning.* Each child is always faced with opportunities for interactions with other children

and adults. Questions such as, "Does she get along with her classmates?" and "How does he get along with siblings and parents?" are concerned with the social context or meaning of a child's behaviors.

2. *All children and adolescents seek to belong.* The goal of behavior is to belong, to be accepted as part of a group. Experiences within the first group, the family, often shape the way in which children approach the opportunities for belonging in other groups such as school classes and groups based on friendship and mutual interests. The goal of belonging transcends most definitions of right and wrong; gangs and groups of delinquents are conforming to their own mutual goals.

3. *Personality has unity and pattern.* The unity and purpose of an individual's behavior are often misunderstood. Questions like the following are thus asked: If a child has a high IQ, why is he or she doing poorly in school? Why does the affluent adolescent shoplift?

   A person moves through life in identifiable patterns of behavior which conform to the goals the person is seeking. Dreikurs (1953) stated: "The doctrine of the unity of the personality gave Individual Psychology its name. This name, which is so often misunderstood, is derived from the Latin word 'individuum,' which literally means 'undivided,' 'indivisible' (*individere)*" (p. 56).

4. *Behavior has a purpose.* Goal-directedness (purposiveness) is perhaps the most important explanation in our understanding of behavior and misbehavior. Instead of looking backward for a causative or historical explanation of a current situation, Adlerians seek to understand the current purpose (goal) of behavior.

   Each individual exercises a creative capacity to choose goals. The goal-directedness of behavior explains, rather than explaining away, the current conditions, pleasant or unpleasant, which children or adolescents find themselves creating.

Within each of us is a *private logic*. For example, while the common logic may be that alcohol and driving do not mix, an adolescent's private logic may be, "I don't care what they say; I can handle driving and drinking." Holding this belief, the adolescent acts on that basis, not on the basis of the common logic.

If a counselor does not understand the private logic of the client, counseling will not produce change. Adlerians have developed procedures and techniques to identify the entire set of beliefs and logic which a person holds. These beliefs are reflected in the person's *life-style.*

5. *Motivation is a striving for significance.* At birth, an infant is dependent upon others for survival. Infants accurately perceive that they are, in many ways, less significant than adults and older children. Life thus becomes a constant struggle for us to become more significant than those around us. Equality and superiority are universal goals for children and adolescents.

   This striving for significance first takes place within the family. The concept of sibling rivalry is simply the competition for unique and significant places within the family group.

To summarize, Adlerian psychology believes that man is an indivisible, social, decision-making being whose psychological movement and behavior are purposive. It teaches the therapist to understand psychological movement and purpose as the final cause of patterns of behavior.

BEHAVIOR AND MISBEHAVIOR. All behavior is the result of a person's beliefs and goals. The four goals of misbehavior are the cornerstones of the Adlerian understanding of child misbehavior. Formulated by Dr. Rudolph Dreikurs, the four goals are a basic part of a pragmatic, systematic theory of child behavior.

The four goals of misbehavior are: to get attention, to achieve power, to get revenge (to get even), and to display inadequacy (to give up). The goals are on a continuum which displays increasing discouragement. If, for example, recognition or being noticed is a belief of the child, then the goal of the behavior will be to seek attention. But not all attention-seeking behaviors are acceptable to the adults in a child's life. This fact, however, does not alter the attention-seeking goal. For example, a young child may do something annoying or even dangerous to attract the attention of the mother. These inappropriate behaviors may make the mother feel annoyed, but she still will pay attention to these behaviors. Even saying, "Stop it!" is paying attention to the child. Thus, the goals of attention-seeking misbehavior are to get the parent to respond and to make the parent feel annoyed while responding to the misbehavior.

By identifying the adult's feelings and actions in response to the misbehavior, the adult can take corrective action. Attention-getting misbehavior can be ignored, and the goal of attention can instead be recognition for appropriate behaviors. Each of the four goals of misbehavior has a corresponding mistaken child's belief, adult's feeling, and adult behavior in response to the misbehavior (Dinkmeyer & McKay, 1989).

Parents and teachers frequently use the Adlerian concept in their homes and classrooms. Counselors and therapists also use it for diagnosis and corrective action. The four goals constitute one of the most basic and useful Adlerian contributions to child psychology.

MISTAKEN BELIEFS. Relatively mild discouragement about being accepted and belonging in the family and classroom groups is demonstrated in the four goals of misbehavior. Children, in their search for belonging, may mistakenly believe that any form of behavior is acceptable so long as it meets their goals. For adolescents, common mistaken beliefs often center around their need to conform to their chosen peer group which brings with it a uniform rejection of their family values or family atmosphere.

Neurotic behaviors are characterized by a pessimistic attitude and a lack of the courage to be imperfect. A neurotic child or teenager may fear the worst, refuse to try, and withdraw from interaction with others. These actions are all characterized by the discouragement the child feels about his or her place in the world.

A common childhood neurosis is school phobia, a problem which can be more easily treated when the counselor recognizes the purpose of the behavior, as seen through the eyes of the child or adolescent. The school-phobic child is often extremely discouraged about his or her abilities and has given up. If the child is allowed to remain at home, the adults have agreed with the child's mistaken self-assessment.

HEREDITY AND ENVIRONMENT. The role of heredity in the development of personality is recognized but not emphasized. The child's biological inheritance may account for physical traits, but implicating heredity as a rationale for behavior reflects an ineffective understanding of genetic endowment. Little can be done if the counselor believes that genetics are responsible for current and past behavior; it is a convenient rationale from which there is little hope of escape and represents a pessimistic approach to the situation.

The human infant comes into the world with a specific set of inherited endowments and into a specific social environment in which the siblings, parents, and grandparents create a continuous set of trial-and-error learning experiences.

Children have biological and social needs for food, comfort, attention, and other priorities. Interaction at first may be limited, but children are well equipped to make their needs known to those who care for them. Behaviors that meet their needs are repeated. Those that are not successful are soon abandoned.

The early ability to perceive and make choices is demonstrated in the normal-hearing children of deaf-mute parents. When crying, screaming, or other vocal noises do not attract attention from the parent, nonverbal actions such as making facial grimaces or kicking the feet are used. Though we are shaped by our environment, we are also capable of shaping it.

FAMILY ATMOSPHERE. Adlerians use the term *family atmosphere* to describe the climate in the home. This climate includes the relationship between the parents and their relationship with the children.

Within each family atmosphere there exist identifiable family values. For example, families frequently value, and thus hold expectations for athletic excellence, academic excellence, or musical or artistic abilities. Other attitudes such as conformity, submissiveness, competitiveness, or economic success may be interpreted correctly by the children as family values. A family value can also be defined as something which is important to both parents whether they agree or disagree about the issue. For example, a family value may be education, yet not all of the family members may have the same goals.

Each child must respond in some way to the family values. These values are the rules of the first group—the family. The child decides whether or not to accept each element of the family atmosphere. Whatever the stand taken on a particular family value becomes part of that child's developing personality and this influences the behaviors chosen to attain that goal. Thus the importance of the family atmosphere in the child's decisions and perceptions and emerging personality cannot be overstated.

FAMILY CONSTELLATION AND BIRTH ORDER. The interaction of the family members is the most important influence on the child's personality development. Many studies of the influence of birth order on personality development do not take into account each child's subjective perceptions and the subsequent interpretations of his or her place in the family.

Family constellation is the Adlerian concept which describes the all-significant family members. Stepparents, grandparents living within the home, and even stillborn children can all be part of the psychological basis for the family constellation. Greatest emphasis, however, is placed on siblings and parents.

Each child is born into a different family situation within the same family. A family composed of three children, for example, will include a child who initially is the only child, then later the oldest; a child who initially is the younger child, and then the middle child; and a child who will always be the youngest. Each child is also influenced by parents who are changing and behaving differently than they did with their previous children. Parents are influenced by the preceding children and, therefore, will treat younger children in different ways. For example, parents may be less protective of a second or third child, having gained confidence in their experiences with the first.

The birth order positions are: the only child, first child, second child, youngest child, and middle child. The generalized characteristics of these positions in the birth order are most useful to the counselor when it is realized that each child creatively interprets his or her chronological position.

The so-called only child may be in an extremely advantageous or disadvantageous position depending upon his or her perceptions. Being an only child in a world of adults, he or she may, if encouraged by the parents, become highly responsible and adultlike in behaviors and attitudes. In contrast, the only child may choose to resent the lack of siblings. Opportunities to learn how to get along with others, to stand up for themselves, and to learn how to settle differences with others may be limited.

The first child always experiences a dethronement when he or she is moved from the only child position with the birth of a second child. The first child decides whether to continue to compete for the number one position or to relinquish this position to a highly competitive second child. Competition for parental attention and approval is a frequent cause of sibling rivalry.

The second child often feels that he or she has been placed in an unfair race throughout life. The "competition," i.e., the older child, has been given a head start. The second child, in seeking ways to find a unique place within the family, will often excel in areas in which the first child can easily be overtaken. Among all the siblings, the first and second children may have the most pronounced differences in interests and traits. For example, if the first child excels in academics, the second child may seek to be known for musical, athletic, or other capabilities.

The youngest child may never leave the baby position within the family. The position has many advantages, as little is expected of a baby and babies are taken care of by others. Yet, as in all other birth positions, youngest children may decide to move in an opposite direction and surpass all older siblings in one or more areas. This turn will often occur when the family atmosphere and values emphasize the importance of achievement, competition, or excellence.

The middle child has neither the privileges of the older child nor the special attentions of the younger child. Often feeling squeezed from both sides, middle children may act on the perception by attempting to treat others unfairly. From their subjective point of view, life is unfair.

These general characteristics of birth order positions outline the potential family group dynamics from each of the five positions. There may be several family constellations within the same family as a result of death, divorce, remarriage, or large age differences between children. If two children are more than 8 years apart, they generally do not have as strong an influence on each other and are part of separate constellations and birth orders.

VIEW OF PSYCHOPATHOLOGY

The Adlerian view of psychopathology may initially present problems for counselors unfamiliar with Adlerian psychology. With the exception of organic dysfunction, mental illness is understood as a combination of mistaken beliefs, extreme discouragement, and a faulty private logic. Symptoms often associated with what is commonly called neurosis result from the condition of failure and discouragement. Neurotics are essentially aware and accepting of common sense and know what they should do. However, they manage to arrange to avoid certain tasks of life through various creative symptom complexes. They know the correct path to follow but are not happy with the obvious required direction and fail to act correctly. Neurotics may present lofty ambitions, lack of courage, and a pessimistic attitude. They may present an image and engage in behaviors which convince themselves and others that they are really trying, yet still avoid the basic responsibilities of life. The presenting symptoms are chosen by chance occurrence when the individual discovers that a certain symptom can relieve responsibility or provide unusual control over other people. The base of neurosis may include past life experiences, family values, genetic tendencies, and chance alone when a symptom gives the unexpected excuse.

With children, psychopathology is best understood in terms of the goals of their behavior. As described above, school phobia, for example, is usually directed against the parents. Children may avoid school in various ways to gain attention, to show their power, to get even, or to demonstrate their "disability." Parents, as well as teachers and school administrators, must learn to withdraw from the unreasonable demands of the child. With any failure to function, one must observe the psychological movement and, except in strictly organic cases, ask "For what purpose?" One will see the purpose then as the final, ultimate cause for the failure to function.

Adolescents face a complex, value-orienting process, and the task of value formation may dominate the adolescent's life. The problems presented are often tied to one of the many life tasks currently being encountered by the adolescent. The adolescent is more aware of the variety of factors, sometimes seemingly unchangeable, and the result may be a defeated and pessimistic outlook on life.

In contrast to psychopathology in adults, disturbances in adolescents and children are relatively responsive to counseling and psychotherapy. The patterns of behavior and supporting beliefs are usually not as long-standing, and, as a result, intervention may take weeks or months, not years.

General Therapeutic Goals and Techniques

Adlerian counseling and psychotherapy have four main goals which correspond to four phases of the counseling process.

1. *Developing an empathic relationship between client and counselor in which the client feels accepted and understood by the counselor.* Adlerian counselors seek to establish an equal, collaborative relationship with their clients, in which both are active partners in moving toward mutually agreed-upon goals. This relationship may be spelled out in a contract, specifying client goals and responsibilities that each partner will undertake. Goals are made explicit so that both client and counselor can monitor progress. The counselor, recognizing the power of encouragement, offers continued support and helps the client become aware of and accepting of his or her assets and how to use these assets. Analysis of deficits and liabilities is minimized.

2. *Assisting the client in understanding the beliefs, feelings, motives, and goals that determine his or her life-style.* This represents the analysis and assessment phase. An active listening approach that pays attention to both verbal and nonverbal communication enables the counselor to assess the person's life-style, i.e., a personal construct built on the person's beliefs, perceptions, and feelings about himself or herself and others. The counselor looks at the meaning of the pattern and total psychological movement, focusing on the client's purpose as revealed through the counseling communication. Once a thorough understanding of the client's life-style is reached, the counselor is in the position to help the client reach the same understanding and see how the basic beliefs and perceptions influence the client's life-style.

3. *Assisting the client in developing insight into his or her self-defeating behaviors and mistaken goals.* The counselor's primary function in this phase is to help clients recognize their mistaken ideas and to understand why they act the way they do. It is necessary that clients understand the purpose of their behavior and how that behavior helps them achieve their often unconscious goals. Confrontation and interpretation are based on the client's present behavior, his or her position in the family constellation, and the various challenges of living (social contracts, work, spiritual concerns, self-image, etc.). The interpretation is always done with regard to life-style, which is the central theme, and will deal with the purpose and consequences of behavior, with little attention being paid to the cause. Interpretation may be offered to the client in a tentative, open-ended, hypothesis-sharing manner or in a more direct confrontational approach where the counselor points out discrepancies between verbalized intent and actual beliefs.

4. *Assisting the client in considering alternative ways of dealing with problematic behaviors and situations and making a*

commitment to change. This is the action-oriented phase of counseling, also known as the reorientation stage. Recognizing in the client the mistaken and self-defeating beliefs and goals, the counselor offers alternative ideas and beliefs for the client's consideration. Establishing realistic goals is a beginning step in the reorientation process. The counselor offers encouragement to promote confidence and thus to promote change. Adlerians, in this phase, are oriented toward modifying motivation, rather than behavior, and focus on changing the client's attitudes, beliefs, perceptions, and goals. These changes will result in behavior change.

INDIVIDUAL COUNSELING WITH CHILDREN

Counseling children younger than 5 or 6 years of age requires the involvement of the parents. This counseling is actually a form of family counseling. The purpose of the counseling is to change the beliefs and behaviors in all of the family relationships while working within the context of the family system.

At age 5 or 6, children are ready for individual counseling or group counseling, as well as family counseling. Their language and cognitive abilities have progressed to a point which makes the verbal interaction in a counselor-client relationship a meaningful process for them.

Young children's misbehaviors are usually so easily diagnosed that a formal life-style assessment is not necessary. The four goals of misbehavior are often sufficient diagnostic tools for both the counselor and parents.

We do not suggest that the very young child is unable to participate in the counseling. In fact, one of the most useful Adlerian contributions is the significance of the *recognition reflex.* It is a spontaneous facial reaction (a smile or grin as a response) to verbal statements, a reaction which cannot be suppressed. The recognition reflex confirms the verbal statements of adults which are made as tentative hypotheses. Children at the pre-verbal level are capable of listening to the discussion between parents and counselor, and their recognition reflexes, or lack of them, are a continuous assessment of the empathy and progress occurring in the counseling.

Techniques

Although it is important for the counselor to empathize with a client, it is also important not to belittle him or her. Counselors sometimes fall into the habit of speaking down to children. It is ultimately confusing for a child to hear an adult try to talk like a child. Counselors can use their own words and tone of voice, taking into consideration the restricted vocabulary of children. Of course, experience helps in developing empathy and rapport with younger children.

Nonverbal modes such as dance, art, or puppetry are all fertile avenues of communication with children as an adjunct to the counseling process. Play therapy may be most useful as a diagnostic tool. It allows the counselor to observe the child's interaction skills and physical capabilities in addition to providing insight into the child's perception of family relationships.

Counselors must recognize the importance of working with the child's entire world. A child's world includes siblings, parents, grandparents, teachers, and sometimes others. Children are not yet independent of these people. Changes in the child often come about when the adults around them change first.

To influence a child's attitudes and behavior effectively, the counselor needs to understand the child's perceptions. Table 1 presents the *Children's Life-Style Guide* (CLSG) (Dinkmeyer & Dinkmeyer, 1977a), which is a modification of the adult assessment technique. CLSG is a structured questionnaire that allows children to respond in their own language. The counselor uses the CLSG to elicit information to make a life-style assessment. Adlerian child counseling usually includes the CLSG assessment.

The CLSG provides unique direction for the early interviews, and the assessment is used in establishing specific goals for the counseling. First, the CLSG asks the child to make comparisons between himself or herself and the other siblings. The questions, "Who is most different from you? Why?" lead to an understanding of how the child perceives himself or herself. It provides immediate insight for the counselor into the child's self-image.

The section on functioning at life tasks gives a clear picture of the child's psychological movement, revealing goals and beliefs. A knowledge of the child's attitudes about school, future plans, and social relationships allows the counselor to investigate the child's approach to the challenges of living.

The information on the family atmosphere details the child's perception of each parent and the way in which the child perceives his or her treatment at home.

The rating of the child and the siblings in the family again gives a picture of how the child perceives himself or herself with regard to various basic traits and in relation to his or her siblings. It can be used by the counselor to identify areas of strength or places where the child perceives strength. This provides the counselor with the unique opportunity to inventory the individual's "claim to fame." At the same time, the counselor can note where there are feelings of inadequacy.

Early recollections identify an area that is relatively new as a technique in child counseling. Some psychologists feel that this technique is an inappropriate one to use with children. However, it is our experience that children do have recollections, and these recollections can be used diagnostically to get at the child's basic perceptions of life. The counselor collects the recollections by saying to the child,"Think back as far as you can remember to something that happened when you were very young. It can be anything, but it should be something you can describe as a one-time incident."

The three wishes section is designed to generate projective data on the child's perception of self (self-concept).

The life-style assessment develops a summary that includes:

1. Beliefs about self, the world, and others.

2. Motivations (goals and intentions).

3. The choice of behaviors to reach life's goals.

Although children find it difficult to pay attention to the goals and objectives throughout the entire counseling period, they will respond to a session that is structured and has purpose. The major reason for lack of effective child counseling often resides in the counselor's belief that the child is not ready to be counseled and instead is ready only to play.

Counseling is conversation with a purpose. It is very important to have the goals of the counselor and counselee aligned and moving in the same direction. This task is obviously much more challenging when the counselor is working with young

TABLE 1
CHILDREN'S LIFE-STYLE GUIDE (CLSG)

1. *Family Constellation:*

Name	Age	Educational Level

Who is most different from you? Why?
Who is most like you? Why?
Tell about your life before you went to school.

2. *Functioning at Life Tasks:*
If you had the choice to go to school or stay home, which would you do? Why?
What do you like about school? Why?
What do you dislike about school? Why?
What is your favorite subject? Why?
What is your least favorite subject? Why?
What would you like to be when you grow up? Why?
Who is your best friend? Who is your best friend at school?
Are you a leader or a follower?
What do you usually do when you are with your friends?
When you play a game, are you usually picked first or last or in the middle?

3. *Family Atmosphere:*
What kind of person is your father?
What kind of person is your mother?
How do your mother and father get along?
Which child acts most like your father?
Which child acts most like your mother?
When you misbehave, who disciplines you? Why?
What do your parents expect of you at home? In school? At play? During special activities?
What do you like to do best with your mother or father? Why?
What do like to do least with your mother or father? Why?
What jobs do you have at home?

4. *Rating* (List highest & lowest sibling for each attribute; include yourself):

Intelligent	Critical	Materialistic
Hardest Worker	Considerate	Most Friends
Best School Grades	Shares	Most Spoiled
Conforming; Obedient	Selfish	Athletic

TABLE 1 (Continued)

Rebellious	Responsible	Strongest
Helps Around House	Temper	Prettiest
Tries to Please	Bossiest	Most Punished
Cares About Other's Feelings	Sensitive; Feelings Easily Hurt	High Standards of Achievement; Wants to be Best

5. *Early Recollections:* (Think back as far as you can remember to something that happened when you were very young.)

6. *Three Wishes:*
   If you were going to pretend to be an animal, which would you choose? Why?

   Which animal would you not want to be? Why?

   What is your favorite fairy tale or story? Why?

   List of Mistaken Self-Defeating Perceptions
   Assets

children. It is important not only to understand and empathize with feelings but to establish boundaries and limits.

Children will respond to and learn much from confrontation and tentative interpretation. When a goal or a purpose is alluded to in a tentative format (e.g., "Could it be . . . ?" or "Is it possible . . . ?" and then alluding to one of the four goals of misbehavior), the child often gains insight.

With children it is very important to go beyond insight to "outsight." This involves having the child put the concepts he or she has learned into action.

Effective child counseling also involves contact with the other major forces in the child's experiences. When parents and teachers are involved, a greater impact is made upon the behavior of the child.

INDIVIDUAL COUNSELING WITH ADOLESCENTS

Counseling with adolescents usually provides an opportunity to utilize almost all the techniques available in working with adults. It is particularly important for the counselor to listen and be empathic. The adolescent has not been accustomed to being heard. This in itself can be therapeutic.

Frequently adolescents come into counseling because they are sent by someone else. It is essential in any case to clarify what the adolescent wants to learn and to gain from the relationship. The adolescent responds well to a clearly defined and commonly accepted goal, benefiting more from being a partner in an equal relationship.

Adolescents also prefer "straight talk" to analytical language. When their behavior is out of line and in conflict with society, they will respond to confrontation by the counselor.

Adolescence is a period of time in which teens are confronted with challenges in all the major arenas of life. Adolescents are expected to do well in school, perhaps to hold down a job, and to be planning a career. Their social contacts and male and female friends are often under close surveillance. They are often still exploring the meaning and purpose of life. Because a large number of external values appear to be imposed upon them, it is important to help adolescents develop their own values in order to increase their self-esteem and their ability to cooperate with others.

Adolescents respond well to an active approach to therapy and can be excellent candidates for group psychotherapy, as will be discussed later.

Adolescents present a unique challenge to the counselor. Counseling is directed toward seemingly opposite goals: to stimulate more autonomy and self-reliance, and to create a greater ability to function within the system. These goals, however, are not mutually exclusive, and both reflect the position adolescents hold in our society.

Adolescents may seek counseling because they are deeply discouraged. Adolescent suicide and depression are increasingly frequent occurrences. An effective relationship with a counselor or therapist may be the only aspect of their lives which provides hope and encouragement for the adolescent.

The other extreme finds adolescents whose delinquency, promiscuity, drug use, or other forms of rebellion point to an active and intense movement away from societal group norms. The counselor may be perceived as just another intruding element of the unwanted set of values. These adolescents are also extremely discouraged about finding an adequate and fulfilling place to belong within the society, town, school, peer group, and family.

Techniques

The counselor must have a high degree of awareness of the adolescent's subjective perception of the counselor's role. Some may see a counselor as a spokesperson for the values they are rebelling against, regardless of the intentions of the counselor. Adolescents frequently feel that the age difference represents an insurmountable obstacle in establishing rapport with a counselor. Many adolescent pressures along with parental or sibling problems represent interpersonal problems at the core. It is for these reasons that group therapy is often recommended.

Adolescence may be characterized by several universal concerns. Drug use and sexual experimentation are so widespread that counselors must be prepared to become a resource for accurate information. In addition, counselors can facilitate the acquisition of the interpersonal skills such as dating which can be taught effectively in groups.

GROUP PROCEDURES WITH CHILDREN AND ADOLESCENTS/CLASSROOM AND EDUCATIONAL APPLICATIONS

Adlerian psychological principles have been extensively applied to child and adolescent groups. The concepts of belonging, social interest, and humans as social beings are basic to Adlerian group counseling. Because Adlerians recognize the significance of groups and belonging in everyday life, they also recognize the group as an effective vehicle for counseling and therapy.

Inherent in the Adlerian approach to classroom and educational settings is the advantage of early educational intervention. Behaviors of children ages 6 to 10 have been found to be moderately good predictors of similar behaviors in early adulthood (Kagan & Moss, 1962). There has been a paradox in American education relating to the mental health of children and their subsequent adult years. If reading is an accepted priority but we do not teach it in the schools, should we be surprised that we have a nation of illiterates? Similarly, we have not attended to the mental health education of our children. Yet we are constantly faced with the effects of this situation.

Groups have advantages at many age levels. For younger children, shyness or unwillingness to talk with adults can be lessened in a group. With adolescents, groups can become a valuable place for sharing feedback and peer group perceptions. The groups are structured to take advantage of group forces such as universalization, linking of similar ideas and concerns, and awareness of the purposive nature of behavior and misbehavior (Dinkmeyer & Muro, 1979).

Children and adolescents are always part of a group during their schooling. Their behavior is goal directed and influenced by their search for significance and social acceptance in the group. This points to the importance of training teachers in group dynamics and practical activities.

Counselors in elementary schools use groups for both therapeutic and educational purposes. This technique provides an effective and efficient method for working with students. Problem-solving groups in elementary schools focus on areas such as friendship, weight loss, divorce, and discipline. The experiences of divorce and child abuse can result in the failure to develop successful interpersonal skills. As discussed later in this section, counselors working with special groups should be aware of specific structuring procedures for successful group experiences.

Another type of elementary group focuses on the developmental concerns of children and can be conducted by both counselors and teachers. The purpose of such a group is to teach systematically affective and problem-solving skills, which should be a basic part of each child's education.

Group Techniques

Educational groups can be conducted with entire classrooms. Whenever possible, smaller group activities in which the group is divided into dyads, triads, or minigroups of six should be used to maximize each child's participation in the activities. Large group discussions can become dominated by more talkative children unless the teacher or counselor deliberately seeks to involve all children in the discussion.

Counseling groups have much smaller group sizes. Experience in working with elementary school children indicates that groups of four to six children are ideal. Adolescent groups should not exceed ten to twelve members. The relatively small size of these groups is intended to encourage each student to participate.

There are five steps in developing special topic groups. First, the adult leader should be able to define clearly the group's purpose. Group-building activities and experiences within the purpose of the group should be identified prior to the first group meeting. The group is developed in a systematic fashion in the early stages to maximize cohesion, interaction, and involvement.

In the second step, pre-interviews with the prospective group members can be conducted. This allows the leader to assess each student's prospective readiness for the group as the purpose and rules of the group are outlined. The pre-interview enables the leader to ascertain the student's goals. These goals become the guidelines for monitoring the individual's progress.

The third step involves the balancing of the group composition. The ratio of male to female members (and the possible exclusion of one sex) must be considered. The balance of the group should also reflect its purpose. For example, an adolescent group on dating would include males and females, with varying degrees of dating skills and interpersonal skills represented by the participants.

The fourth step is the use of opening activities for the groups which should be structured regardless of the purpose of the group. Group-building activities help accelerate the group's cohesion and promote mutual trust. The leader also uses techniques which structure the group, such as asking each member to share verbally a summarizing statement at the close of each group session.

The fifth step involves the classroom teacher in promoting group development. We have observed that classroom teachers frequently do not take advantage of group-building opportunities within their classes. It has been demonstrated that discipline and motivation problems can be alleviated through systematic group activities. For example, the classroom meeting can become an ongoing problem-solving and goal-setting experience for students.

Teacher Techniques

Adlerian psychology has much to offer even the most challenging situations in the contemporary classroom. Today's teachers frequently report that discipline is their number one problem in the classroom, almost regardless of the grade level. Traditional discipline methods, which rely on control and unquestioning respect for authority, no longer seem to work.

Classroom teachers are frequently untrained in the ability to work with groups, the most basic teaching skill. It appears that classroom teachers are functioning without a practical understanding of human behavior.

Developing an understanding of self and others is central to the educational process. Emphasizing a return to the basics of education is understandable, but it is inconsistent when these basics do not include the nurturing of the child's feelings of self-worth. Studies have indicated that the educational process is a significant contributing factor in the development of a child's attitudes, values, and involvement with others (Dinkmeyer & Dinkmeyer, 1982; Kagan & Moss, 1962).

Adlerian psychology is applied to the educational process in three major areas:

1. Building awareness of self and enhancing feelings of self-worth. Academic achievement, including the mastery of basic reading, writing, and math skills in the early primary grades, is severely handicapped when the

child feels he or she is incapable or less able than other students. The educational opportunities in our classrooms must include developing an understanding of self and others. Affective education must be seen as a partner with cognitive education in the classroom.

2. Taking advantage of positive group forces. Each classroom has its own set of classroom dynamics. Through Adlerian principles, the teacher becomes aware of these interrelationships among the children and the teacher and the children (Dinkmeyer, McKay, & Dinkmeyer, 1980). For example, the classroom meeting is one technique which recognizes the value of the group and gives a democratic outlet for problem solving and growth (Dreikurs, Grunwald, & Pepper, 1971).
3. Dealing with discipline in a logical and nonpunitive way. Discipline that allows for a mutual sharing of power is more efficient and less wearing on both teachers and students. It removes the teacher from the enforcer role and removes many of the common power struggles from teacher-child relationships. Each child is given an opportunity to learn from his or her choices, within the acceptable bounds of the classroom. This approach, using logical consequences, is part of the Adlerian approach to classroom discipline.

Structured Programs

One of the most widespread applications of Adlerian psychology in classrooms is the *Developing Understanding of Self and Others* (DUSO) (Dinkmeyer & Dinkmeyer, 1982) program. Published in 1970 and revised in 1982, DUSO-1 and DUSO-2 are planned for use in the prekindergarten through fourth grades as part of the elementary school curriculum. The affective education emphasis of the DUSO program does not preclude its relevance to other academic skills. Communication activities, songs, and fantasy relaxation activities are some of the media through which the 42 DUSO goals in each kit are achieved.

Individual Education (IE) is an alternative to the traditional educational system. Developed by Dr. Raymond Corsini, IE has been implemented in schools since 1972. The basic premise of IE is that children are responsible for their own education (Corsini, 1977). The Individual Education approach was renamed the Corsini 4R system (C4R) in 1986. The program is now implemented in more than a dozen schools across the world. Significant developments have occurred in the United States and Israel, as well as in the Netherlands.

All partners in the educational process are affected by the Adlerian principles inherent in an IE school. Students are taught not only traditional academic learning but practical life skills and socialization skills. Teachers are given comprehensive training in Adlerian discipline and encouragement skills. Parents are oriented to the IE system through workshops, are required to participate in parent education classes, and are encouraged to allow their children to become responsible for their own education.

Systematic Training for Effective Teaching (STET) is a 14-session teacher in-service program that presents classroom applications of Adlerian concepts. Participants in the program receive materials which give them not only numerous classroom activities based on Adlerian principles but a new understanding of elements such as misbehavior, encouragement, discipline, group dynamics, working with special students, and the role of parents. STET is similar to STEP (a parent program discussed below) in that it recognizes the power of the peer group to stimulate change, in contrast to individual consultation with a professional, such as the school counselor.

PARENTING SKILLS

Adlerians have made a special contribution to the field of parent education. The lack of parenting skills in our society has resulted in many broken homes and marriages, and it has affected children in countless instances. Counselors and therapists now recognize the need for parent education in both educational and therapeutic settings.

The Adlerian commitment to parent education began in Vienna in Alfred Adler's Child Guidance Clinics, which served as resource centers for therapy and education. The public demonstration of counseling, which was opened to parents, teachers, and other professionals, showed the applicability of Adlerian ideas to the family. Today, in the United States and Canada, parent education classes are frequently the cornerstone of the Adlerian Family Education Center.

Parenting is a very complex responsibility yet few people acquire the formal skills necessary to carry it out. A basic shift in our society, from autocracy to democracy, has made traditional parenting roles and skills ineffective. To learn to be a parent on the basis of observing other parents, trial and error, or experience as a child is often discouraging (Dinkmeyer & McKay, 1973).

We believe that parents may be one of the last minorities to be liberated. Children today function on the assumption that they are equal to their parents—not in age or skill but on the basis of an open relationship. When parents have been raised to obey their own parents and their children do not respond to commands and demands, it is the parent who suffers in the relationship.

New parenting skills must be taught to parents. The therapist or counselor who works with children and adolescents often sees a child who is, in part, the product of parental mistaken beliefs and behaviors. These can create in a child problems such as resistance and neurosis, which require counseling and therapy. Far greater are the numbers of children who do not receive counseling, yet are raised in a relationship which reduces their feelings of self-worth and their desire to be a cooperative member of society. Finally, the frustration and suffering of parents who are not yet capable of effective parenting are equally devastating to the parents' self-esteem.

We believe that all parents can benefit from parent education. Increasing their skills can help to reduce the number of children who lack self-esteem, feel resentment, or seek to escape their homes. Parenting skills can be taught as an adjunct to therapeutic interventions with children or adults. The vast majority of parents have no need for therapy but want increased satisfaction in their parenting role through learning ideas and skills.

School counselors have become a major resource for the teaching of parents. But parent education is not limited to the schools. Agency counselors, psychologists, clergy, and others in the helping professions are finding that educating parents is an important preventive step.

Techniques in Parent Education

The goal of parent education is to expose parents to new ideas and techniques. Professionals can call on a wide variety of books and programs which effectively present these new ideas. Effective implementation of parent education does not require that the leader be a parenting expert, or even a parent.

Instead of one-to-one parent counseling, the use of groups is strongly recommended. This approach is a more effective use of time. It brings into use the force of universalization which is often ignored in counseling and therapy. Groups are places where people learn that they have common problems and can learn from one another.

Group parent education does not consist of lecturing by a leader. Instead, parent experiences and insights into the ideas presented are the basis of the skill-building experiences within the group. For example, parents of a 3-year-old may believe it is their "fault" that they are unable to get their child to bed without protests. Until the parent education group, these parents had no understanding of the nature of the problem and no indication as to whether the bedtime problem was "normal" or "abnormal." In the parent education group, however, the parents then learn a way to meet the child's need for attention effectively and also learn that other parents of 3-year-olds experience similar attention-seeking behaviors in their children.

Leaders of parent education groups utilize group forces such as universalization, linking, and feedback. Sharing of experiences allows parents to realize that there is a universality in child behavior. It is the leader's responsibility to link parents to their similar concerns and ideas with one another. At the start of parent education groups, parents are so concerned with their own children that they do not realize that other parents have similar concerns.

Leaders limit their verbal involvement in the group. For example, when a parent presents a problem or the results of the use of a new parenting idea, feedback from other parents allows him or her to understand how he or she is being perceived by the other parents. If the leader were to provide feedback, it is more likely that the same comment would be viewed as a critical evaluation instead of an honest reaction from a peer.

Parent education groups must be highly structured, so that several separate educational experiences can occur. If parent involvement were limited to group meetings, there would be little chance that any real change in their homes would occur. Thus, it is important that parents leave each session with a specific activity assignment—a new skill to be utilized—which will be reviewed during the following week's session.

New parenting techniques and ideas can be presented through assigned reading, minilectures, charts, or other effective presentation means. After each concept has been presented and discussed, an application of the skill occurs within the group. Parents literally practice the new skill, such as reflective listening or applying logical consequences, with other parents in the group.

Structured Programs

Adlerians have been conducting parent education book discussion groups for more than a quarter of a century. *Children: The Challenge* (Dreikurs & Soltz, 1964), *The Practical Parent* (Corsini & Painter, 1975), and *Raising a Responsible Child* (Dinkmeyer & McKay, 1982)—all written by Adlerians—can be used in the book study format. It is the responsibility of the group leader to structure the group time into discussion and application segments.

Perhaps the most widely used, standardized Adlerian parent education program is *Systematic Training for Effective Parenting* (STEP). The program, written by Don Dinkmeyer and Gary D. McKay (1976), consists of nine sessions, each devoted to a specific parenting skill. Parents begin by learning that all child behavior, including misbehavior, has a purpose. This purpose is ascertained by becoming aware of the parent's reactions to and feelings about the child's misbehavior. The link between misbehavior and parental reaction is then clarified to the parents.

STEP has become a widely used parent education program, used by school counselors, mental health agency professionals, and others. It has now reached more than two million parents and has been translated into Spanish, Greek, and Japanese. A study showed that more than 93% of the participants recommended the STEP course for other parents, citing elements such as the group atmosphere and the increase in parenting knowledge as reasons for their satisfaction with this Adlerian approach to parent education (Dinkmeyer, Jr., 1981).

The STEP was revised to include video-based training incidents (Dinkmeyer & McKay, 1989). A survey of parent educators showed overall satisfaction with the program content, scope, and teaching method. However, the section concerning motivation through praise and encouragement was revised to further clarify the differences between these approaches.

FAMILY THERAPY

Alfred Adler was the first to publicly demonstrate family counseling techniques (Dinkmeyer & Dinkmeyer, 1977b). The Adlerian approach to family counseling emphasizes family dynamics, and interrelationships among all members of the family are studied. Other therapies sometimes neglect the importance of the sibling relationships. They concentrate primarily on the parent-child relationship. The importance of the children's need to belong within the family unit makes family interventions, in the Adlerian mode, a group approach.

Frequently a parent or teacher will refer a child to a family counselor as the "problem" child of the family. Individual treatment of this child will not solve the family's problem. The child's problem, to no small degree, is often his or her current inability to find an acceptable place within the family. Poor grades at school, delinquency, or problems with siblings and parents all point to a failure in the entire family.

Family intervention, therefore, must be guided by working with the family system and not be simply dealing with the symptom or original reason for referral. The goal of family therapy is to improve the abilities of the group members to live together. This goal is frequently accomplished by teaching communication and encouragement skills, while reorienting family members away from destructive communication patterns and faulty beliefs. Family therapy is a specialized form of group therapy (Dinkmeyer & Dinkmeyer, 1977b).

The great need for therapeutic intervention in many families has tempted some helping professionals to engage in family therapy with little background or experience. Family counseling is perhaps the most demanding type of counseling, one which quickly saps the unprepared counselor of initiative or techniques. Counselors might assess a family situation to see if the family can benefit from less difficult forms of intervention. Parent education, for example, may be appropriate if it appears that a family lacks education and information to meet so-called typical problems or concerns.

Techniques in Family Therapy/Counseling

This section will briefly present Adlerian techniques in family interventions.

USING MULTIPLE THERAPISTS. It is extremely difficult for a single therapist to deal effectively with a family. The multiple therapist approach allows the family to benefit from multiple perceptions. In addition, the multiple therapist approach is an excellent training procedure.

GIVING ENCOURAGEMENT. The importance of encouragement in producing change cannot be overemphasized. Numerous articles and books now allow the therapist to understand fully the applications of encouragement (Dinkmeyer & Dreikurs, 1963; Dinkmeyer & Losoncy, 1980; McKay, 1976). Unlike praise, encouragement can be effective with family members who are the so-called problem. Encouragement is the process of instilling confidence to do something different; it is not the reward after the change. Therapists must find ways to encourage all family members, beginning with the first session. The "problem" family member usually needs the most encouragement.

STOPPING ARGUMENTS. Family members often engage one another in verbal fist fights. Through "antisuggestion" the counselor can deflate the benefits of these random arguments. For example, when it is clear that a father and daughter argue frequently, the therapist can ask them to make a daily commitment to fight. At the close of the session, the therapist asks the father and daughter to argue diligently, at a specific time, for one half-hour each day. They may feel that this recommendation is absurd, but the counselor earnestly asks them to make this commitment. At the following session, the father and daughter frequently report that they are unable to argue on schedule and have more awareness of the purpose of their fighting behavior.

HOLDING FAMILY MEETINGS. The purpose of the family meeting is to provide a structured time for the family to deal with relationships and plans. Many typical concerns can be legitimate discussion items at the family meetings held with the therapist. This simple concept, when overlooked, accounts for many repetitive, unresolved disagreements within a family. In the family meeting, usually held weekly, new approaches can be brainstormed, reviewed, and modified. Feelings can be ventilated. The meeting becomes a guaranteed time at which problems can be resolved and positive family issues discussed or planned.

RECOGNIZING PROGRESS. The therapist must be aware of the slightest progress in the family, because the family is so caught up in their problems that they often do not see any positive change. The model for encouragement must come from the therapist.

EFFICACY

Empirical evidence does indicate that Adlerian psychology has been successful with children and adolescents. In fact, much of the research has been conducted with these populations in educational settings and family education centers. This research reflects the commitment Adlerians have maintained toward preventive mental health programs.

Kern, Matheny, and Patterson (1978) have compiled a comprehensive review of Adlerian research. Their investigation covered a 26-year period, producing one of the most thorough investigations of the Adlerian approach. They concluded that most of the research focused on the schools and parent education.

For example, research has been conducted for more than 10 years on the DUSO program. The research into this affective education program generally supports the effectiveness of the DUSO activities. The research also indicates that affective education, like cognitive learning, is best taught on a regular basis within the classroom like other basic skills (Dinkmeyer & Dinkmeyer, 1982).

Another major area of Adlerian research is parent education. Book discussion groups studying Adlerian-approach texts (Corsini & Painter, 1975; Dinkmeyer & McKay, 1976; Dreikurs & Soltz, 1964) have been studied in both clinical and educational settings. Adlerian parent education has been successfully conducted in both of these settings. Dinkmeyer, Jr. (1981) indicates that Adlerian parent education has reached more than one million parents.

Adlerian research with the child and adolescent populations is one of the largest and most successful areas of research:

> Clients most positively affected by the [Adlerian] approach were preadolescent and adolescent youth experiencing difficulty with classroom behavior, school achievement, or interpersonal relationships. (Kern et al. 1978, p. 89).

A large body of research on the STEP and STEP/Teen programs has been conducted (Dinkmeyer & McKay, 1976, 1983). More than 50 studies have measured parent, child, and teen perceptions and behaviors. Instruments to measure parent perceptions and behaviors have been developed.

Although Adlerian psychology may not be researched as extensively as some other approaches, there is a substantial body of empirical evidence which indicates that it is successful. These successes result in changed beliefs and behaviors based on the education clients received in Adlerian ideas.

CONCLUSIONS

Adlerian psychology provides a sound theory and pragmatic techniques for working with children and adolescents. It understands children and adolescents as goal-directed, decision-making, social beings whose behaviors always have a purpose. This theory provides guidance for the many varied interactions of counseling and therapy.

The Adlerian movement has been very much involved with Family Education Centers, parent education, teacher consultation, and family therapy. There is an abundance of articles, books, and materials for use with these populations.

Counseling children and counseling adolescents are distinctly different approaches. When working with young children in counseling or therapy, it is important that the counselor include the parents and teachers in the process. The focus is on the family system and on consulting with teachers. Counseling adolescents also often involves the entire family. However, it may be that the therapist, instead of working against adults, will encourage the teen to establish active-constructive goals. Adolescent counseling encourages development of conflict resolution skills, self-esteem, and an increased ability to get along with others.

Education is an equal partner to therapy in the Adlerian approach to counseling children and adolescents. The school years are an opportunity to teach lifelong affective and coping skills. Group dynamics are an effective approach in teaching these skills, as well as in counseling and therapy.

CASE STUDY

Mr. and Mrs. L. came to counseling because of their problems in dealing with their oldest daughter, Mary, age 12.

The parents—father and stepmother—were seen alone at the first counseling session to get their perception of the conflict. Mary's father and mother were divorced a year ago, and Mr. L. remarried. Mr. L. obtained custody of the children, and Mary still feels deeply the loss of her mother. Because they moved about 150 miles from their former residence, Mary seldom sees her mother. Mary has internalized her grief; she has few friends and has a hard time showing love and positive emotions to her father. She has refused to accept the divorce. She has also not accepted her stepmother, and Mr. L. feels trapped in the middle of Mary's conflicts.

The therapist suggested that the L.'s be patient and willing to listen with empathy to Mary's feelings. An appointment was scheduled to meet with Mary, who, according to Mr. L., was very willing to come for counseling.

The first interview with Mary focused on listening to Mary's feelings and indicating empathically that her feelings were being heard accurately. The therapist recognized the difficulty Mary was having in still loving her mother, yet trying to adjust to and accept her stepmother. Mary stated that she did not accept her stepmother as a mother, and she exhibited a lot of resentment about the divorce. She did not understand why her and her sister's feelings were not considered by her father. She could not understand how her father could meet another woman and begin a second marriage so quickly.

Mary's psychological movement tended to indicate that she believes life is unfair and, therefore, she doesn't have to cooperate in the new family. This belief was discussed, including the implications for improving the relationship with her father and his wife.

At the second meeting, the Children's Life Style Guide was used (Dinkmeyer, Pew, & Dinkmeyer, 1979). This inventory, as discussed earlier in the chapter, explored with Mary her family's atmosphere, the family constellation, her early recollections and her priorities in life. The information was then summarized into the following life-style assessment:

Mary is the older daughter in a family of two girls.

Her major problem or challenge is accepting the divorce of her parents and the loss of her mother. She does not accept her stepmother.

Mary sees herself as intelligent, hard-working, responsible, with high standards, critical of herself, and stubborn.

Basic Perceptions

1. I expect the worst.
2. I am not sure you can trust men.
3. Life is unfair.
4. When I am restricted, I must rebel to be independent.

Basic Priorities

1. Control.
2. Superiority.
3. Comfort.
4. Pleasing.

Assets

1. Intelligent and develops insight readily.
2. Sense of humor. Can see her part in creating trouble.
3. Her stubbornness can become an asset when she is determined.

The following is an excerpt from Session 5:

> *Mary:* Dad is happier now that Lisa (stepmother) is around.
>
> *Therapist:* But how are things going between you and him?
>
> *Mary:* Well, after he talked with you he said he understood me a lot better, but I think he needs to come more times to understand how I feel.
>
> *Therapist:* You're not feeling understood by your dad.
>
> *Mary:* Well, he said I shouldn't feel that way.
>
> *Therapist:* Oh, he said you shouldn't feel . . .
>
> *Mary:* Yeah, the resentment toward Lisa.
>
> *Therapist:* You're very hurt and he doesn't recognize it.
>
> *Mary:* Sometimes I'm afraid to discuss it, because he gets uptight.
>
> *Therapist:* How do you feel now toward Lisa?
>
> *Mary:* I'm not as nervous around her, but I don't feel it is right. It seems unfair.
>
> *Therapist:* You had been concerned and anxious, wishing she wouldn't come. Why are you anxious?
>
> *Mary:* I feel I have to meet her standards. I feel I have to pretend I am happy she is here, and I am uncomfortable.
>
> *Therapist:* It feels like she doesn't understand your feelings.
>
> *Mary:* Yeah, I don't want to change.

Therapist: You feel like everyone is forgetting your mother and you feel abandoned.

Mary: Yes, and no one seems to care, especially Dad.

Therapist: Yes, it is like your belief that you can't trust men. I can understand your unhappiness about losing your mom and at the same time you're very unhappy about Lisa.

Mary: Yes, she's different. She comes into a bad situation and can adjust.

Therapist: Maybe she doesn't think of it as bad.

Mary: It's not bad, just hard.

Therapist: Tell me more why it is hard.

Mary: Well, trying to win me over.

Therapist: Oh yes, I wouldn't want that challenge. It would be almost impossible if you decided not to cooperate. Seems like you are determined not to have her win you over.

Mary: [Recognition reflex smile.] Well, sort of . . . that's a good question!

Therapist: Yes, and what we need to consider is why you resist her.

Mary: I have to learn to like her more.

Therapist: What really causes the problem? Who do you think it could be?

[Long pause.]

Mary: Me; but why am I doing this?

Therapist: I guess you might think it is unfair. You lost Mom and now it feels you're losing Dad, too. Maybe this is a way to get even with Dad.

Mary: It's possible; but I don't think I plotted the whole thing.

Therapist: It's not that you do it intentionally.

Mary: I wonder if my Dad and Lisa think I'm doing it intentionally, though.

Therapist: You feel they may think you're doing this to get even?

Mary: Well, I'm not. I just don't want to . . . [pause].

Therapist: Don't want to give in?

Mary: Yes, I feel they aren't doing it the way I would.

Following this interview, a meeting was scheduled with Mary's father, Lisa, and Mary. The purpose of the sessions that followed was to examine the relationships in the family and seek to resolve the conflict.

The case illustrates several counseling techniques:

1. Meeting with the parents to identify the major issues and goals.
2. Meeting with the child to establish a cooperative, goal-aligned relationship.
3. Being empathic to develop the counselor-client relationship while identifying feelings, beliefs, and goals.
4. Diagnosing the life-style.
5. Processing life-style information back to the child and showing how the faulty beliefs may interfere in relationships.
6. Working with the total family unit to improve the relationships and explore the real issues.

ANNOTATED BIBLIOGRAPHY

Dewey, E. (1983). *Basic applications of Adlerian psychology.* Coral Springs, FL: CMTI Press.

A unique work by a former student of Dreikurs, Mosak, and other Adlerian mentors. Dewey has compiled readable "notes" from classes on topics such as life-style, early recollections, and dreams. This book is widely used by students in introductory courses.

Dinkmeyer, D., & Dreikurs R. (1963). *Encouraging children to learn: The encouragement process.* Englewood Cliffs, NJ: Prentice-Hall.

A basic work outlining the significance of encouragement as applied especially to children and adolescents. The book contains chapters essential for understanding discouragement and the encouragement process.

Dinkmeyer, D., Dinkmeyer, D., Jr., & Sperry, L. (1987). *Adlerian counseling and psychotherapy* (2nd ed.). Columbus, OH: Merrill.

A comprehensive overview of Adlerian counseling and psychotherapy. This deals with the theory, phases of the counseling process, techniques, and special applications. Chapters on DSM-III-R classification and gerontology have been added to this second edition.

Dinkmeyer, D., & Losoncy, L. (1980). *The encouragement book: Becoming a positive person.* Englewood Cliffs, NJ: Spectrum.

The theory of encouragement is set forth. Detailed attention is given to the specific skills of encouragement. Communication, focusing on strengths, and developing perceptual alternatives are among the skills set forth.

Dreikurs, R. (1953). *Fundamentals of Adlerian psychology.* Chicago, IL: Alfred Adler Institute.

The basic theoretical work by Dreikurs. A study of Adler, exploring theoretical concepts intrinsic to the understanding of Adlerian psychology. The book clarifies the theory which undergirds technique.

Kern, R., Matheny, K., & Patterson, D. (1978). *A case for Adlerian counseling: Theory, techniques, and research evidence.* Chicago, IL: Alfred Adler Institute.

The book sets forth in a unique way the basic Adlerian precepts and provides a summary of empirical research results in educational and clinical settings. Helpful guidance is provided for new directions in designing counseling research.

Shulman, B. H. (1973). *Contributions to individual psychology.* Chicago, IL: Alfred Adler Institute.

Shulman, one of the foremost Adlerian psychiatrists and a teacher at the Alfred Adler Institute in Chicago, provides a collection of his articles on theory, psychopathology, and therapy.

REFERENCES

Corsini, R. J. (1977). Individual education. *Journal of Individual Psychology, 33*(2a), 292-418.

Corsini, R., & Painter, G. (1975). *The practical parent.* New York: Harper and Row.

Dinkmeyer, D., Jr. (1981). *Parent responses to Systematic Training for Effective Parenting* (STEP). Unpublished doctoral dissertation, University of Florida.

Dinkmeyer, D., & Dinkmeyer, D., Jr. (1977a). Concise counseling assessment: The Children's Life-Style Guide. *Elementary School Guidance and Counseling, 12,* 117-126.

Dinkmeyer, D., & Dinkmeyer, D., Jr. (1977b). Adlerian family therapy. *American Journal of Family Therapy, 9,* 45-52.

Dinkmeyer, D., & Dinkmeyer, D., Jr. (1982). *Developing understanding of self and others (DUSO) 1 and 2, revised.* Circle Pines, MN: American Guidance Service.

Dinkmeyer, D., Dinkmeyer D., Jr., & Sperry, L. (1987). *Adlerian counseling and psychotherapy* (2nd ed.). Columbus, OH: Merrill.

Dinkmeyer, D., & Dreikurs, R. (1963). *Encouraging children to learn: The encouragement process.* Englewood Cliffs, NJ: Prentice-Hall.

Dinkmeyer, D., & Losoncy, L. (1980). *The encouragement book: Becoming a positive person.* Englewood Cliffs, NJ: Spectrum.

Dinkmeyer, D., & McKay, G. D. (1982). *Raising a responsible child* (2nd ed.). New York: Simon and Schuster.

Dinkmeyer, D., & McKay, G. D. (1976). *Systematic Training for Effective Parenting* (STEP). Circle Pines, MN: American Guidance Service.

Dinkmeyer, D., & McKay, G. D. (1983). *Systematic Training for Effective Parenting of Teens* (STEP/Teen). Circle Pines, MN: American Guidance Service.

Dinkmeyer, D., & McKay, G. D. (1989). *STEP: A new look.* Circle Pines, MN: American Guidance Service.

Dinkmeyer, D., McKay, G. D., & Dinkmeyer, D., Jr. (1980). *Systematic Training for Effective Teaching* (STET). Circle Pines, MN: American Guidance Service.

Dinkmeyer, D., & Muro, J. (1979). *Group counseling: Theory and practice* (2nd ed.). Itasca, IL: F. E. Peacock.

Dinkmeyer, D., Pew, W. L., & Dinkmeyer, D., Jr. (1979). *Adlerian counseling and psychotherapy.* Monterey, CA: Brooks/Cole.

Dreikurs, R. (1953). *Fundamentals of Adlerian psychology.* Chicago, IL: Alfred Adler Institute.

Dreikurs, R. (1953). A psychological interview in medicine. *Journal of Individual Psychology, 10,* 99-122.

Dreikurs, R., Grunwald, B., & Pepper, F. (1971). *Maintaining sanity in the classroom.* New York: Harper and Row.

Dreikurs, R., Grunwald, B., & Pepper, F. (1980). *Maintaining sanity in the classroom* (2nd ed.). New York: Harper and Row.

Dreikurs, R., & Soltz, V. (1964). *Children: The challenge.* New York: Meredith Press.

Kagan, J., & Moss, H. (1962). *Birth to maturity.* New York: John Wiley and Sons.

Kern, R., Matheny, L., & Patterson, D. (1978). *A case for Adlerian counseling: Theory, techniques, and research evidence.* Chicago, IL: Alfred Adler Institute.

McKay, G. D. (1976). *The basics of encouragement.* Coral Springs, FL: CMTI Press.

Shulman, B. H. (1973). *Contributions to individual psychology.* Chicago, IL: Alfred Adler Institute.

Chapter 5

Person-Centered Approaches

Helen B. Moore, Ed.D.

INTRODUCTION

Person-centered therapy is the term given by Carl Rogers and his associates in 1974 to the primary theme which expressed Rogers' professional life. Rogers considered a "person-centered approach" to be the most descriptive of his value framework, given the variety and increasing number of fields of application (Rogers, 1980). At the same time, he believed the term "client-centered" was still accurate when applied specifically to counseling and psychotherapy (Bohart & Todd, 1988). This chapter will use "person-centered" for consistency and as a means of incorporating modifications and extensions of Rogers' work.

Person-centered therapy assumes that, given a particular therapeutic climate, individuals can be trusted to choose for themselves a growth-producing and psychologically healthy direction for their lives. Historically, person-centered therapy grew out of the Rogerian revolution (Ivey & Simek-Downing, 1980) in the 1940s and 1950s. As the United States' first distinctly indigenous school of therapy (Belkin, 1980), it was originally called *nondirective* in revolt against the diagnostic, interpretive, past-oriented methods and mystique of the psychoanalytic school and the directive vocational counseling methods. Rogers' book *Client-Centered Therapy* (1951) ushered in both a new term and a wave of humanistically oriented therapists. The effects have been felt not only in counseling and therapy, but also in education, social work, business, pastoral training, group process, human relations skills programs, race relations, conflict resolution, and politics. This chapter is concerned with the current status, extensions, innovations, and applications of the person-centered approach to therapy with children and adolescents.

History and Status

In the preface to a book which he published at the age of 75, Carl Rogers spoke of a recent time when the sentence, "I walk softly through life," flashed into his mind (Rogers, 1977). As he speculated later on this experience, he saw how it described his professional life. His associations took him back to his childhood reading of Indians and frontiersmen who would "glide noiselessly through the forest without stepping on a dead twig or disturbing the foliage. No one knew their whereabouts until they had reached their destination or accomplished their mission" (p. xi). Viewed with suspicion by the therapeutic establishment, despite prestigious academic appointments, Rogers persistently broke new ground during his long career and often did not realize his impact on the field. A tribute to his pioneering accomplishments and to the open and growing person he continued to be was in seeing his colleagues, his students, and their students over several decades take off from his theoretical and process orientation, expanding his work to new areas and developing their own models and theories. "One of the facts that has always given me great satisfaction is that client-centered therapy, by its nature, has always provided a congenial home for the development of creative hunches" (Rogers, 1970a, p. viii).

The years between 1928 and 1939 were times of experimentation for Rogers. After completing his education at Columbia Teacher's College in New York City, he moved to Rochester, N.Y., to work for the Child Study Department of the Society for Prevention of Cruelty to Children. At Rochester he was influenced by the social workers of the Rankian school, especially Dr. Jesse Taft, to value the therapeutic relationship and to emphasize the present, rather than the past. Rogers was also growing away from the therapist behaviors of coercion, advice giving, judging, and questioning, seeing these as unfruitful.

Gradually, he relied more and more on the client providing the direction in therapy, trusting the client's wisdom and experience. His first major book, *The Clinical Treatment of the Problem Child* (1939), was written before he left Rochester.

In 1940, Rogers accepted a full professorship at Ohio State University. His book *Counseling and Psychotherapy* (1942) was written shortly thereafter. It was heavy on technique, characterizing the nondirective phase in his thinking. Although it was not a popular book, attacking as it did the time-honored ways of most therapists of the time, students began to flock to Ohio State to study with him.

One of his greatest contributions to the training and supervision of counselors and therapists was his use, for the first time, of electronically recorded interviews which could become actual case transcripts. This greatly demystified the process of psychotherapy. Rogers exposed his own counseling sessions to the scrutiny of colleagues and students, gave his own critical feedback, and welcomed the same from others.

During the 1940s and 1950s, while at the University of Chicago, he and his students, many of whom later established their own reputations, turned out more research on psychotherapy than had ever before existed (Kirschenbaum, 1979). In 1951, his third major book, *Client-Centered Therapy,* was published. The establishment virtually ignored it; it was challenging and controversial, yet students and practitioners applauded it.

Rogers went to the University of Wisconsin between 1957 and 1963 with a joint appointment in psychology and psychiatry and a dream of working together with professionals of both disciplines on cooperative training and research projects. He made a valuable contribution through his work with chronic patients and collaborated on the book *The Therapeutic Relationship and Its Impact: A Study of Psychotherapy with Schizophrenics* with several authors who became famous in their own right in subsequent years (Rogers, Gendlin, Kiesler, & Truax, 1967). His most successful publication during this time was the book *On Becoming a Person: A Therapist's View of Psychotherapy* (1961a), a collection of essays which synthesized his work and applied his principles to many different kinds of relationships.

Rogers moved to California in 1964 at a time when Humanistic Psychology was having an impact on education, counseling, pastoral studies, group process, and other areas. The popularity of group work at that time gave him an opportunity to be with "normal" people and test out his hypothesis that, given the same therapeutic conditions, all people could be helped. He made tapes and films of his work and wrote a popular book called *Carl Rogers on Encounter Groups* (1970). Again, he demystified what happens in counseling, this time in groups, by describing his own behavior as a facilitator, letting it be viewed on film and heard on tape.

In 1978, Rogers and some of his associates formed the Center for Studies of the Person, where members carried out their own projects, from drug education to interracial encounters, to helping unskilled people into the working world. Rogers himself became actively involved in applying his insights to the field of education, working with school systems and publishing the books *Freedom to Learn: A View of What Education Might Become* (1969) and *Freedom to Learn for the 1980s* (1983).

Rogers remained active during the 1970s, with his books on marriage and its alternatives (1972), personal power (1977), and his personal reflections, experiences, and future perspectives (1980) reflecting his range of interests. On his 80th birthday, Rogers announced his intention to devote the remainder of his life to working toward world peace. At the time of his death on February 4, 1987, at the age of 85, he had been focusing his energies on conflict resolution and on applying his methods to politics and international relations. To this end he traveled widely, working with Catholics and Protestants in Ireland, with blacks and whites in South Africa, with Soviet, and with Central American leaders. The Carl Rogers Institute for Peace was founded in 1983 at La Jolla with the purpose of providing occasions for political and lay leaders to meet person-to-person in informal, intensive, and spontaneous dialogues, using profound listening and nonjudgmental valuing as a means of resolving differences and reaching understandings.

During his long professional life, Rogers was a leader in many prestigious professional groups and received numerous awards including the American Psychological Association's first

Distinguished Professional Contribution Award in 1972. Rogers has had a tremendous impact on the field of counseling and therapy.

OVERVIEW OF THEORY

Basic Theory and Assumptions

From his therapeutic work with a variety of persons, Rogers developed a view of people at variance with the more pessimistic, deterministic theory of the Psychoanalytic School and the tabula rasa orientation of the Behaviorists. He believed it was in the nature of people to strive toward self-fulfillment or self-actualization. The self-actualization tendency is the "inherent tendency of the organism to develop all its capacities in ways which serve to maintain or enhance the organism" (Rogers, 1959, p. 196). This is the viewpoint of the school of Humanistic Psychology, the diverse "Third Force" group which Carl Rogers, Abraham Maslow, and others are credited with pioneering and popularizing during the 1950s. Humanistic psychologists view people as being rational and basically trustworthy and as having dignity and worth, striving to grow and enhance their potentialities and to become socialized in harmony with others in their environment.

Person-centered counselors and therapists are usually referred to as *self-theorists* or *phenomenologists*. Self-theory holds that individuals exist at the center of a changing world of experience, termed the *phenomenological field*. The best vantage point for understanding the behavior of others is from their internal frame of reference, as only they can know how their private world is perceived. Much is unconscious, yet more is available to consciousness. People react as organized wholes to their unique perceptions and experiences. Pain, struggle, and emotion accompany growth as individuals try to satisfy their needs and move toward greater socialization, independence, and integration. The basic motivational force is the drive toward self-actualization, which means that people try to meet not only their physiological needs but also their needs to relate to others, to feel self-esteem, and to become productive and self-regulated.

As children develop, a part of their perceptual field becomes differentiated as the self—the "I," the "me." This sense of self becomes the self-concept and is made up of children's internal experiences and environmental perceptions, especially how others respond to and interact with them. The needs of children for the positive regard of others, their needs to be prized, to be accepted, to be loved, are so addictive that they become the most potent of all needs (Prochaska, 1979). Children who receive positive regard develop a sense of self-worth. When parents and others give the impression that their love is dependent on whether children please them, children begin to doubt their own internal feelings and thoughts and then begin to act to satisfy those significant adults. The behavior of children comes to be guided, not by whether their experience feels good and right to them, but by whether it is likely to result in their receiving love. For example, if anger is frowned upon in the home, children will deny their angry feelings despite their inner sensations and bodily reactions to the contrary. When children incorporate the values of others just to please the others and to receive regard, they have developed conditions of worth and feel good about themselves only when they live up to the expectations of others.

Theoretically, children could develop positive self-concepts if there was congruence between what they valued and prized in themselves and what was valued and prized by parents and others. "If an individual should experience only unconditional positive regard, then no conditions of worth would develop, self-regard would be unconditional, the needs for positive regard and self-regard would never be at variance with organismic evolution, and the individual would continue to be psychologically adjusted and would be fully functioning" (Rogers, 1959, p. 227).

VIEW OF PSYCHOPATHOLOGY

Pathology develops from the reactions of children to conditional love. The core of maladjustment is the incongruence between self, on the one hand, and, on the other hand, experiences which occur as children try to please their parents and significant people to receive more self-regard. "Psychopathology reflects a divided personality, with tensions, defenses, and inadequate functioning that accompany such lack of wholeness" (Prochaska, 1979, p. 114). The individual develops defenses to deal with incongruities, to cope with threats to self-esteem, and to lessen anxiety. Defenses, however, distort and deny the reality of experiences and result in inaccurate perceptions. Sometimes all that happens is a cognitive rigidity; at other times personality disorganization occurs and anxiety becomes overwhelming. "Whether a person goes into therapy because of a breakdown, or because defensive symptoms are hurting too much, or because of a desire for greater actualization, the goal is the same—to increase the congruence between self and experience through a process of reintegration" (Prochaska, 1979, p. 116).

General Therapeutic Goals and Techniques

Person-centered therapy can be understood as an evolution in the thinking of a group of humanistically oriented therapists influenced by the leadership of Carl Rogers. Emphasizing the striking change in this therapy over several decades, Hart and Tomlinson (1970) state: "The professional therapist who knows only early versions of client-centered therapy has seen the seeds but not the pumpkins" (p. 3). As Rogers grew and developed new insights in his work with clients, groups, and institutions, so did his emphasis change in regard to the process of counseling. Ivey and Simek-Downing (1980) chart identifiable stages which represent the development of person-centered therapy:

> *Stage 1: NON-DIRECTIVE (1940-50).* This stage emphasized the acceptance of the client, the establishment of a positive and non-judgmental climate, trust in the client's wisdom, permissiveness, and used clarification of the client's world as the main technique. His [Rogers'] writings give a central emphasis to skills in the counseling process.
>
> *Stage 2: CLIENT-CENTERED (1950-61).* This stage centers on reflecting the feelings of the client, incorporates resolving incongruities between the ideal self and the real self, avoids personally threatening situations for the client, and uses reflection as the main technique. Skills are not emphasized; rather a major emphasis focusing on the counselor as a person is evolving.

> *Stage 3: INCREASED PERSONAL INVOLVEMENT (1961-present).* While maintaining consistency with all past work, Rogers moved increasingly to emphasizing present-tense experience, a more active and self-disclosing role for the counselor, group as well as individual counseling, and consideration of broader issues in society, such as cultural differences and the use of power. The emphasis on skills remained low as Rogers emphasized the counselor's attitudes rather than interview skills. Coupled with this is an extensive emphasis on experiencing oneself as a person in relation to others. (p. 262)

During the 1940s, Rogers was developing his hypothesis about help seekers as responsible clients rather than dependent patients and his hypothesis about therapy as assisting them to achieve their own insights through a permissive, accepting, and nonauthoritarian atmosphere. The caricature of a Rogerian therapist during this nondirective period was one of a passive, innocuous person addicted to "uh-huh's." As Hart and Tomlinson (1970) stated: "Such a stereotype has never been accurate, but it does convey, in a distorted way, one of the main features of the early approach" (p. 3). Perhaps in their attempts to keep from adopting traditional therapist behaviors such as analyzing, diagnosing, giving advice, judging, and asking questions, early practitioners erred in the direction of too much passivity and shallowness.

During the client-centered phase, Rogers began to focus on the therapeutic relationship as the most important variable in the counseling process. This emphasis on the *quality* of the therapeutic encounter has been widely accepted in generic therapeutic practice. In their refinement of client-centered counseling, Boy and Pine (1982) list the following characteristics of the relationship:

A face-to-face relationship

A person-to-person relationship

A human relationship

A relationship of reciprocity and commitment

A relationship in which the client is voluntarily involved

A relationship possessing mutual respect

A relationship possessing effective communication

A relationship possessing genuine acceptance of the client by the counselor

A relationship in which the counselor empathically focuses on the needs and feelings of the client

A relationship that is liberating

An open-ended relationship in which outcomes essentially emerge from the client, not from the counselor

A relationship in which the client's desire for confidentiality is respected

A professional service that calls for acquired attitudes and skills on the part of the counselor

A professional service based upon a substantive rationale reflecting philosophical and psychological principles emanating from theoretical and empirical considerations of the person, human behavior, and society

A relationship in which the counselor possesses a concept of the person

A relationship in which being precedes becoming. (p. 127)

In an important essay, Rogers (1957) hypothesized from his clinical experience and from the research he and his students had conducted the "necessary and sufficient" conditions which appeared to initiate client growth and personality change. He believed that these conditions worked for all types of clients in all settings and that they needed to exist and continue over a period of time. In the article, he suggested operational ways of defining and measuring them and advanced his belief that empirical studies would provide future refinements. The conditions are:

1. Two persons are in psychological contact.
2. The client is in a state of incongruence, being vulnerable or anxious.

3. The therapist is congruent and integrated in the relationship.
4. The therapist experiences unconditional positive regard for the client.
5. The therapist experiences an empathic understanding of the client's internal frame of reference and endeavors to communicate this experience to the client.
6. The communication to the client of the therapist's regard is to a minimal degree achieved.

Person-centered counselors and therapists extracted from the essay the term *core conditions,* which they have assigned to attitudes of empathic understanding, respect (unconditional positive regard), and genuineness (congruence). Following the lead of Rogers, they believe that all people have within themselves the potential to understand themselves, change their attitudes, thoughts and behaviors, enhance their self-concepts, and become more self-directing in a therapeutic climate where the core conditions are provided.

Empathic understanding means that the counselor is able to sense accurately the client's private world and internal frame of reference and communicate that understanding so that it is felt by the client. This type of communication is a process by which the counselor not only understands the clearly presented and explicit client meanings, but also accurately senses and conveys those of which the client may be only dimly aware.

Respect implies that there are no conditions of acceptance for clients; rather, the counselor feels warm, positive, and nonjudgmental toward whatever or wherever clients are at the moment and is able to grant permission for them to have their own feelings, both negative and positive. It is not possible for therapists to feel such caring at all times, but the attitude needs to be conveyed frequently for constructive change to take place. In addition, basic to the concept of respect is the viewpoint that people live in separate realities, and thus, one person is in no position to judge another's reality as incorrect, distorted, or inadequate (Rogers, 1980). At the same time, acceptance does not imply one's approval of or agreement with the actions of another.

Genuineness depends upon the awareness of counselors of their own experiencing-in-relationships and the degree to which their behaviors, nonverbal and verbal, and their inner feelings match. This does not mean that counselors are perfectly integrated in all of their life aspects, nor does it mean that all their feelings need to be expressed in counseling; but it does require that they be aware of any discrepant feelings and behaviors. Being genuine in a facilitative sense implies a basic honesty but stresses the responsibility of the counselor to continue providing a supportive, nonthreatening atmosphere in large measure.

A means of conveying the "core conditions" became the basic verbal tool of the counselor during this client-centered phase. "The most striking change in the actual practice of psychotherapy was the therapist's emphasis on responding sensitively to the affective rather than the semantic meaning of the client's expressions" (Hart & Tomlinson, 1970, p. 8). This skill became known as *reflection of feeling* and became important in conveying the *active listening* or *empathic listening* behavior taught in training programs and endorsed by modern counselors and therapists of many persuasions.

The third, and present, period of person-centered therapy has also been termed *experiential* (Hart & Tomlinson, 1970). Therapists are process-oriented and interested in the ongoing experience of their clients. The goal of therapy is to help clients become able to experience feelings and to listen to their experience (Bohart & Todd, 1988, p. 132). Person-centered counselors and therapists today are more expressive and outgoing with their clients and share moment-to-moment experiencing, personal meanings, and feelings. When therapists respond to clients by openly conveying their own immediate experiencing, they respond to clients as persons. Clients are free to accept or reject the therapist's communications but may eventually be touched and changed by them (Hart & Tomlinson, 1970).

This concept of genuineness has taken on new significance. In Rogers' (1977) words:

> The more the therapist is herself in the relationship, putting up no professional front or personal facade, the greater is the likelihood that the client will change and

> grow in a constructive manner. It means the therapist is openly being the feelings and attitudes that are flowing within the moment. The term transparent catches the flavor of this element—the therapist makes herself transparent to the client. The client can see right through what the therapist is in the relationship; the client experiences no holding back on the part of the therapist. As for the therapist, what she is experiencing is available to consciousness, can be lived in the relationship, and can be communicated if appropriate. (p. 9)

Gendlin (1974) represents the thinking of many modern-day person-centered counselors and therapists with his endorsement of the use of any skills and techniques which seem helpful, his emphasis on the experiential aspects and honesty of the therapeutic encounter, and, especially, his focus on continuous empathic listening:

> Listening, therefore, is never a one-shot response, but involves at least a few steps; a listening response, then again hearing, then again responding. When that first thing is really heard, wait. Let the person see what now arises. Respond to that. Several such steps, not just one turn, are listening in this sense of the word. (p. 221)

Responding should take off from and return to client-centered reflection of feeling as a necessary baseline for all other responses: "Only in this way can the therapist stay constantly in touch with what is occurring in the person, and thus know and help make good use of whatever beneficial results other therapeutic procedures may have" (Gendlin, 1974, p. 216).

Today, person-centered counselors work in diverse ways and use a variety of skills to enhance the counseling process. Their commonality is a trust in the therapeutic process and the belief that the growth potential of individuals of all ages and conditions tends to be released in a relationship in which the counselor feels and communicates genuineness, respect, a nonjudgmental attitude, and a deep empathic understanding toward the client. Counselors seek to understand fully their clients' phenomenological world and how it is affecting their present thinking and feeling. As authentic beings counselors express their own thoughts, feelings, and experiences with their clients when appropriate. The therapeutic climate is one of openness, safety, and freedom for clients to be as they are at the time and to become what they would like to be. Problem solving and making value judgments are primarily the job of the client, who can be trusted to act responsibly, given such a climate.

Therapist skills and techniques are valuable only to the extent that they enhance the therapeutic process and enrich the relationship. How something is said or what is said is less important than what is going on between the counselor and client and the feelings shared. The process of effective counseling, however, is undergirded by a foundation of skills possessed by the counselor that help to communicate empathy, respect, genuineness, and faith in the client's drive toward self-actualization.

Systematic Skills Training

The influence of person-centered theory has been felt in many training programs for counselors and therapists. Regardless of the theoretical stance of trainers or trainees, person-centered attitudes and concepts remain the foundation for relationship building, developing trust and a facilitative working alliance. Most process work in therapy and counseling, at the least, begins from a person-centered framework.

Students today are taught in an experiential manner and through some method of systematic skills training. In experiential training, cognitive learning is not ignored, but there is an emphasis on helping trainees get in touch with their own experience and feelings, while working either in simulated or actual counseling situations. Experiential training is thought to foster congruence, genuineness, and self-understanding in future counselors, which in turn will better enable them to build relationships of trust, openness, and mutuality with clients.

Systematic skills models have roots in the research attempts of Rogers and his associates to quantify and demonstrate the effectiveness of the "core conditions" of empathy, respect, and genuineness. A great part of the effectiveness of any one orientation to counseling can be accounted for by the central core of facilitative conditions that each of these orientations holds in common (Carkhuff, 1969; Truax & Carkhuff, 1967). Carkhuff and Berenson (1967) demonstrated that those who possess academic knowledge and credentials may not be the best helpers and that, indeed, helping can be for better or worse. Egan (1975) suggests that overly cognitive, nonsystematic training programs, run by individuals who themselves lack basic helping skills, can be a devastating combination.

The *Carkhuff Model* (1969) divides the counseling process into two parts: the initial or facilitating stage based largely on Rogers' "core conditions," and the action stage which extends Rogerian theory. According to Carkhuff, counselors who offer high levels of empathy, genuineness, respect, and concreteness (the direct expression of specific feelings and experiences), as judged on a five-point scale, help clients move toward self-exploration and eventual behavioral change. Counselors who demonstrate low levels of the above conditions may increase client defensiveness and actually block client growth. Low levels are associated with counselor behaviors such as judging, moralizing, giving advice, asking questions, changing the focus of the client, and attending only to content.

Egan's first edition of *The Skilled Helper* (1975) became a popular three-stage model in person-centered concepts, particularly in Stage 1 and Stage 2. In Stage 1, the helper responds with empathy, respect, genuineness, and concreteness to the world of the client in order to aid that person's self-exploration. In Stage 2, the helper uses advanced skills of accurate empathy, self-disclosure, confrontation, and immediacy to help the client achieve more objectivity and realize a need to change. Helpers aid in the choosing and implementing of constructive action programs and support behavioral change in Stage 3.

In general, the systematic skills training programs, of which only two have been cited, can be characterized as person-centered in that they stress the importance of the relationship in counseling, the attitudes of the counselor, including the Rogerian "core conditions," and the self-determination of the client. They discourage counselor behaviors which are nonfacilitative, and they stress empathic listening and responding, entering the phenomenological world of the client and exploring it in a nonthreatening manner.

INDIVIDUAL PSYCHOTHERAPY/ COUNSELING WITH CHILDREN

Person-centered counselors work with children with developmental, remedial, and crisis concerns by providing a safe climate which encourages free and open expression of feelings and thoughts. The counselor believes in the child's potential to move in a forward direction toward greater responsibility and socialization. The relationship established between adult and child is one of acceptance, regardless of how "bad" the child's behavior is considered to be by the child, parents, teachers, or other children. The counselor conveys empathy, respect, genuineness, and honesty and does not have a hidden agenda for the child; nor does the counselor hold to a blanket acceptance of another adult's agenda or expectations. This precludes, for the most part, the use of indirect methods by a counselor who "knows" what the "problem" is but doesn't bring it out into the open.

This is a big order for a counselor; it implies faith in the capacity of the child to become self-directing, and it respects the right of the child to choose to change or not to change attitudes and behaviors which bother other people or appear to be self-defeating for the child. It takes considerable time to create a truly person-centered atmosphere and develop such a relationship.

The Counseling Process in Elementary Schools

Writing from a person-centered orientation, Reisman (1973) defined psychotherapy as the communication of person-related understanding, respect, and a wish to be of help:

> "Person-related understanding" refers to all communications that attempt to comprehend the client's or other person's thoughts, feelings, or behavior. . . . "Respect" denotes a positive regard for the individual's dignity, rights, uniqueness, and capacities for constructive change. "A wish to be of help" is simply that, and it implies that the professional is motivated by some desire to contribute to the welfare of the public. (p. 10)

A definition of the school counseling process would be similar to Reisman's definition of psychotherapy with children. Reisman believes psychotherapy is appropriate for comparatively mild to moderate childhood problems. Counselors in school settings work with children to enhance their development, foster their autonomy, and help them through developmental concerns. They will usually spend less time with children who require extensive or long-term help and will make referrals to clinics or private practitioners when such therapy is indicated.

In schools, counselors will find their work with children easier if they have fully explained their role and functions to administrators, teachers, and parents and have established collaborative relationships with those important adults. In addition, school counselors need to explain to all children, usually through classroom visitations, what they offer and what can be expected in counseling. All children experience developmental concerns, and self-referrals should be encouraged. Reisman (1973) underscores the child's perception of what is wrong as the most important perception because the child is the client. A person-centered counselor helps the child understand the counseling process, its purposes and goals, and accepts the child's experience and attitudes in regard to the reason for referral.

In school settings, time constraints, the pressing concerns of teachers and other adults, accountability, and other pressures may make person-centered counselors more action oriented. In the context of a warm, caring, and nonjudgmental atmosphere, the counselor feels free to give the child honest feedback in regard to what is going on in the relationship between the two of them and what seems to be taking place in the child's life. Because of the dynamic, changing nature of person-centered theory, counselors in schools can be comfortable with extensions of their basic theoretical stance in areas of information giving and mutual goal setting and decision making with children. Counselor behaviors which continue to be undesirable and should be avoided are those which tend to cause a child to become more defensive or feel less self-worth: moralizing, judging, lecturing, and asking "why" questions. Testing and a diagnosis of schoolchildren can be helpful, and school counselors work as team members with other professionals, but the process of counseling remains the same. In the actual counseling situation, the counselor's first job is relationship building, establishing an atmosphere where the child feels there are no conditions for acceptance. Person-centered counselors seek ways to understand the child's world and the child's perception of problem areas. Inviting children to decide how to use their time with the counselor is one way to proceed. Although Rogers and other person-centered therapists have more recently deemphasized techniques in favor of emphasizing the attitudes of the counselor and the counseling relationship, there are skills which research and practice have identified as helpful in getting children to express their feelings about themselves, their world, and others, and to understand these feelings and their experiences in relationship to their behaviors. In general, the techniques and skills are those used in systematic skills training programs for helpers: These skills enrich the relationship and set the stage for change.

Nelson (1972) states that counseling transcripts with children have identified at least five characteristic client-centered skills: simple acceptance, reflection, clarification, summarization, and confrontation. To these can be added immediacy, self-disclosure, open-ended questions, silence, and reflection of deeper feelings. The skills are defined as follows:

1. *Simple acceptance.* The counselor gives a minimal, encouraging, verbal or nonverbal response such as a head nod.
2. *Reflection.* The counselor expresses in different words the feelings and attitudes expressed by the child. When children hear back what they have said, they feel understood and their feelings accepted.
3. *Clarification.* The counselor checks out what the child has said and what is meant. Clarification can "make clear" and concrete what a child may have difficulty expressing in words.
4. *Summarization.* The counselor summarizes in a few words the essence of what a child has said. Children often jump around in their expression of ideas, feelings, and experiences and are helped to tie things together

with a summary from the counselor. Summarization can also help maintain a counseling focus, expecially when the child likes to engage in "story telling."

5. *Confrontation.* The counselor tentatively and gently confronts discrepancies, distortions, or game playing which the child reveals. Confrontation, when caring and gentle, invites children to examine their behavior and decide if they want to change.
6. *Immediacy.* The counselor responds with feedback about the relationship between the child and the counselor. The counselor shares honest feelings and thoughts in an attitude of helpfulness and genuineness.
7. *Self-disclosure.* The counselor shares similar feelings, experiences, and thoughts in an effort to help the child gain more understanding. Self-disclosure is not an attempt to change the focus to the counselor's own problems but a means of deepening the relationship.
8. *Open-ended questions.* The counselor asks questions designed to get at the feelings of children and keep them exploring events, experiences, and thoughts. These questions are the opposite of fact finding or a "20-questions" approach which usually results in brief and less thoughtful responses from children.
9. *Silence.* Silence is used to allow both counselor and child to think about what has been said. Using silence can also convey to children that they can really say what they want.
10. *Reflection of deeper feelings.* The counselor responds with a feeling which seems under the surface or implicit in what the child is saying. The response is used to help promote more understanding on the part of the child.

In capsulated form, the following transcript illustrates how these skills might be used:

Child: My daddy took me to see a movie about spaceships.

Counselor: [Nods head.] I see . . . [Minimal encouraging lead.]

Child: Yes, he bought me a new softball, and Barbara got books about cats, and he didn't bring Mommy a single present and she didn't go the movie, either.

Counselor: Maybe you wonder why everyone but Mommy got a present . . . [Clarification.]

Child: Daddy doesn't live with us anymore. Mommy and Barbara cry a lot.

Counselor: How does it make you feel to have your daddy gone? [Open-ended question.]

Child: Sad. He could come back.

Counselor: You feel sad when he's not home and you'd like him to live with you. [Reflection of feeling.] [Silence.]

Child: When he comes back home, he's gonna take me to lots of movies and the circus. I saw a circus once and there were elephants and horses and clowns and they all got into a little car and kept coming out. I counted them.

Counselor: You think your dad would do things with you if he lived with you again. [Summarizing to keep the counseling focus.]

Child: [Silence.]

Counselor: Johnny, from what you've told me, your daddy loves you and likes to do things with you. You really want him to live with you and Barbara and your mom. But maybe that's not possible right now. . . . What do you think? [Gentle confrontation.]

Child: He could if he wanted to. I'd be real good all the time.

Counselor: When my father and mother got divorced, I used to think it was my fault and that if I'd been really good it wouldn't have happened. I wonder if that's a little bit how you feel? [Self-disclosure.]

Child: Once I saw a circus on TV, and a lady got shot out of a cannon.

Counselor: When you talk about the circus on TV, I get confused and wonder if you were listening to me or if you just want to stop talking about Daddy now. Could you tell me how you're feeling? [Immediacy.]

Child: I want to tell you about the circus.

Counselor: It's hard to talk about things that hurt.

[Reflection of deeper feeling.]

[Silence.]

With young children or those having trouble expressing themselves, person-centered counselors offer activities which build rapport and help them see into the child's world. The child may draw, respond to stimulus pictures, or listen to a story picked by the counselor as offering an opportunity to elicit feelings, thoughts, and experiences. As children begin to feel secure with the counselor, accepted, and understood, many open up, expressing frustrations, hurts, and ambivalent feelings. Children who see their problems as caused by others are confronted to further their tendencies toward responsibility and self-direction. This is done with respect for the child's right to deny or disagree with the counselor's assessment. As counseling progresses, person-centered counselors in the schools help children design and implement plans for working on their (the children's) expressed concerns. At this point, counselors are pragmatic in using what works and fits with the needs and wishes of children.

If there was one problem common to the many clients he had helped over the years, Rogers considered that problem to be that they did not accept themselves (Kirschenbaum, 1979). They believed they were not "OK"—not capable or good enough. Counselors working with children have found this problem central to other symptoms and behaviors, and have incorporated into counseling sessions experiences designed to identify and enhance the child's positive feelings and strengths. The child is encouraged in finding ways to feel good, accepted, and worthwhile. In this way, person-centered school counselors resist the role of "fixer" and offer something more fundamental to the growth and development of children. They know that as counselors they can only create the conditions for children to learn or relearn the attitudes and behavior that result in positive identity (Muro & Dinkmeyer, 1977).

Counselors are occasionally not as honest and genuine in their dealings with children as they are with adults. It is a truism that children can "spot a phony," yet often they are treated as fragile creatures who must be shielded from reality, at least until a so-called "good relationship" is established. Children usually sense manipulation and a holding back of the "bad news." Person-centered counselors try to be as open as possible with children and encourage parents and teachers to be the same. The following brief transcript illustrates genuineness as a two-way communication process.

> Lynn and her supervisor were discussing Lynn's concern about a child she was seeing in counseling whom she described as being phony with her. The child had been referred by her teacher for classroom behaviors he found bothersome.
>
> *Lynn:* Janie is so sweet and nice with me, and I thought we had a good relationship; but when I asked her how things were going in class, she lied and denied any problems. Then I found out from her teacher how bad her behavior really was.
>
> *Supervisor:* You are concerned about Janie's phoniness with you, but I wonder if you've been completely honest with her? It sounds to me like she doesn't really know why her teacher referred her to you; so perhaps it's not surprising that she wants to put up a good front. Maybe she thinks you won't like her if she tells you about her misbehavior.
>
> *Lynn:* I hadn't thought of it that way. I was afraid I wouldn't be able to establish a warm relationship with her if I told her right out what her teacher had said or why she was referred. Maybe I wasn't genuine with her.

Elementary counselors are often asked by administrators, teachers, or parents to work with a child on a particular issue which disturbs or worries the adult. The person-centered counselor feels uncomfortable using indirect methods of getting at the problem issues because such hedging would violate the important attitude of counselor genuineness in a relationship. One solution is for the adult who feels a concern for a child to meet with the counselor and child and openly express the concern, perhaps with prior support and collaboration between the counselor and the adult. The following is an example of such an effort; here the teacher, the child, and the counselor come together.

> *Teacher:* Jimmy, I am bothered by seeing you pick on some of the smaller children on the playground. I noticed today that you pulled Mary's hair and made her cry, and later I saw you hit Billy pretty hard. I'd like you to talk with Mr. Jones about this.
>
> *Mr. Jones:* [To Jimmy.] Let's go to the counseling room so we can talk by ourselves for a while. I'd like to know how you feel about what happened today on the playground.
>
> *Mr. Jones:* [To Jimmy, in counseling room.] We can be comfortable in here and you can tell me what you want to. What we talk about here is between the two of us. Your teacher would like us to discuss what happened on the playground today. I'd like to hear you tell me about it.

The Counseling Process in Clinic Settings

The person-centered counselor in a clinic setting may work with children who display disturbed behavior or deep-seated anxieties, requiring more time for the solution of the problem. The disturbance is often a matter of degree and depends to a large extent on how adults in the life of the child are being affected. Supervisors of counseling and therapy interns often hear their students express their belief that the parent, not the child, has the problem. As practitioners know, this may indeed be the case, and the parents may need to be consulted and involved in the treatment program.

In clinics, as in schools, the child's assessment of what is wrong is most important because the child is the client. Yet responses of adults shape behaviors, influence the self-concepts of children, color their expectations for how others will treat them, and are important in determining the nature of their disturbance (Reisman, 1973). In the decision-making procedure of whether to begin the lengthy and demanding process of psychotherapy, the professional's assessment, the parents' assessment, and the child's assessment of the problem are all needed. This does not contradict the belief of the person-centered therapist that, regardless of diagnosis, the process of treatment is the same; rather, it respects the child and the situation or context in which the questionable behavior is occurring and in which the child is living. With adequate assessment, therapy may not be indicated; rather, changes in the child's environment or in the attitude or responses of adults in the child's life may be all that is required.

Reisman (1973) has set forth seven principles of psychotherapy with children, as follows:

1. The therapist assesses the client as a precondition to psychotherapy and as an integral part of the process of psychotherapy.

2. The therapist listens to the client and allows ample opportunity for the latter to express feelings and beliefs.

3. The therapist communicates his [or her] understanding of the client, his respect, and his wish to be of help.

4. The therapist negotiates with the client a purpose or goal for their meetings.

5. The therapist makes clear what is unusual or inconsistent in the client's behavior, feelings, and beliefs.

6. When dealing with behaviors that are supported within a given system, the therapist may modify the behaviors by negotiation within the system.

7. The therapist negotiates termination with the client when he [or she] believes that the advantages of ending the meetings outweigh what may be gained by their continuance.

As can be seen, person-centered beliefs are incorporated into these principles. It is assumed that the child is capable of reasonable behavior, so limits in therapy are mentioned only as the need arises. Therapists let children know the reason for referral and that they understand and want to help. In deciding on goals, the child and therapist seek a mutual agreement, which may not necessarily adhere to the goals of the referral source. The therapist respects the child's attempts at self-direction and points out ways in which there are inconstencies in beliefs, actions, and feelings. When the behavior of the child is inappropriate and ineffective, the child receives honest feedback, but not in the context of a judgment or threat to the child's self-esteem. Whenever possible, the client selects the termination date. In terminations, the courage, faith, and confidence of both the client and the therapist are put to the test (Reisman, 1973).

Play as a Therapeutic Medium with Children

Play techniques have been used with children in clinics and in private therapy for many years; its use in schools has been more recent and more limited. One of the author's earliest experiences with this approach occurred some years ago in an elementary school with Joey, a 7-year-old boy, referred by his teacher for lack of motivation and disturbing behavior in the classroom.

Joey arrived promptly at nine-thirty in the morning, twice a week, said little or nothing, often rocked in an old rocking chair for a time, and then accepted the ongoing invitation to play with any of the materials available. He usually chose clay as his medium. He made clay people, including his teacher and classmates, and he dropped clay bombs on them or pushed them aside with his hand. The counselor responded initially only to what seemed to be taking place: "That took care of them." Gradually, Joey decreased his aggressive play, and his clay teacher and students began doing things together. The time spent in counseling over several months was largely in silence, spotted by simple reflective statements and open questions. To this writer's amazement, the teacher continually gave feedback such as: "I don't know what you're doing with Joey, but I wish you saw him every day; he's so good when he comes back to class." In retrospect, it can be seen that the relationship made no demands on Joey; he was accepted and allowed to choose the direction of the sessions, and the counselor tried to communicate an understanding of his actions and feelings during the session.

Person-centered therapy assumes children can solve their own problems as they re-create their world and their relationship to it in play. It can be particularly useful for young children with short attention spans, or who have difficulty expressing themselves verbally, or with those who are emotionally or developmentally immature. Using play with such children provides them with freedom and reduced pressure. It facilitates communication and helps the counselor or therapist enter the world of the child.

Early client-centered counselors who wrote on the use of play therapy with children include: Axline (1947), Dorfman (1951), and Moustakas (1953). Axline advocated play as a more natural medium for self-expression with children than verbalization and saw it as an opportunity for them to "play out" feelings and problems just as adults "talk out" their difficulties. She suggested eight principles to guide play sessions with individuals, groups, and classrooms:

1. The therapist must develop a warm, friendly relationship with the child, in which good rapport is established as soon as possible.

2. The therapist should establish a feeling of permissiveness in the relationship so that the child feels free to express his or her feelings completely.

3. The therapist should accept the child exactly as he or she is.

4. The therapist should be alert to recognize the "feelings" the child is expressing and reflect those feelings back to him (or her) in such a manner that he will gain insight into his behavior.

5. The therapist should maintain a deep respect for the child's ability to solve his (or her) own problems if given an opportunity to do so. The responsibility to make choices and to institute change is the child's.
6. The therapist does not attempt to direct the child's actions or conversation in any manner. The child leads the way; the therapist follows.
7. The therapist does not attempt to hurry the therapy along. It is a gradual process and is recognized as such by the therapist.
8. The therapist should establish only those limitations that are necessary to anchor the therapy to the world of reality and to make the child aware of his (or her) responsibility in the relationship.

Nelson (1972) urges counselors "to treat play behavior as if it were verbalized—reflecting, summarizing, confronting, and so on—yet remaining true to 'the givens' of the situation rather than extending into the interpretive realm" (p. 215). In an initial play situation where a child is pounding a girl doll with a mother doll, the counselor's response: "I wonder how the girl doll feels when the mother doll hits her like that?" is much less threatening than: "How do you feel when your mother hits you?"

In the permissive atmosphere of the play room, only realistic, necessary limits are set (such as no physical behavior toward the counselor or therapist, no destroying of toys, etc.), and the child begins to feel valued in the presence of an empathic adult. Whereas early nondirective therapists advocated complete freedom for children to choose toys with which to play, counselors and therapists with elementary school children may maximize time by putting into view toys which have the potential to elicit feelings and thoughts concerning problem areas already identified. For example, a doll family and a few props may be all that is needed for productive sessions, as with Mary:

> Mary, age 6, had been deserted by her mother and began acting out in her highly structured first-grade classroom. The counselor observed Mary and asked to work with

her. When Mary first saw the counselor, she looked at her with obvious suspicion and asked: "Whose mama are you?" The counselor worked with Mary ½ hour weekly. The first 3 weeks were spent virtually in silence while Mary played. After 3 weeks she began to talk, using the doll family. She buried the mother doll three times that day, and it remained buried for 2 weeks after which Mary laid it in a "coffin." The counselor reflected what she observed Mary doing and created the permissive atmosphere for Mary's feelings to come to the surface.

In the above example, it required time for the child to work through her feelings and cope with her school and home situation. Ideally, in such situations, the school and remaining family members cooperate in providing the needed support and security.

Some young children in school and clinic settings can best express their feelings through play activities, using puppets, art media, games, and other materials. Person-centered counselors may choose unstructured or structured means of facilitating the counseling process as long as a climate of trust, acceptance, and empathy is consistently applied. Using play has been effective with both normal and troubled children. The process may be slow, but a modification in the child's attitude and behavior often results as the child begins to feel more OK and competent.

INDIVIDUAL PSYCHOTHERAPY/ COUNSELING WITH ADOLESCENTS

Counseling with Adolescents in School Settings

The high school counselor with a reputation for keeping confidences and for being accepting, nonjudgmental, and empathic is likely to be a busy person, whether an adolescent needs help with a personal concern or has a need for career exploration and information. Person-centered counselors in school settings must operate within institutional guidelines and policies and support the academic and vocational goals of education. Fortunately, most educators today agree that physical, personal, social, emotional, academic, and vocational aspects are intertwined; and they focus on educating the student as a "whole" person. Guidance has become an integral part of the educational system in the United States with counseling as one of its primary components.

In a competitive, constantly changing society with confusing values and messages, adolescents struggle to grow and develop into responsible, cooperative, productive adults. Problems abound for them: emotional swings, peer pressures, eating disorders, changing sexual mores, family disorganization, drugs, college and job decisions. Though idealistic, many lack confidence, not only in themselves but in the world outside of school.

Counselors with a person-centered philosophy convey to these students their faith that they, the students, can become self-directing and capable of finding viable solutions and coping strategies. This communication of faith in the student is not a passive process of merely listening and waiting for the adolescent to take the initiative. The person-centered counselor provides a relationship with attitudes of empathy, respect, and genuineness (the "core conditions") and incorporates the skills which are used with children, except in more sophisticated form as consistent with the increased cognitive and abstract thinking processes of youth. Listening in an accepting, empathic manner is still fundamental to the process of counseling with adolescents and cannot be rushed. Students are the best judges of their current experience and must be allowed sufficient opportunity to explore who they are and what they want. "The client must feel free enough to reveal his innermost feelings without fear of contradiction or reprisal from the counselor. . . . In a truly permissive atmosphere he can explore his innermost feelings, sift them, accept them, or reject them" (Boy & Pine, 1963, p. 48). Adolescence is a time of contradictory thoughts, feelings, values, and behaviors; and the person-centered counselor may help students obtain more objectivity through gently encountering and confronting them.

Despite time constrictions during the school day, the person-centered counselor will still refrain from falling into a pattern of advice giving (as opposed to information giving, which is often desirable and necessary). For example, the open-ended question, "What do you see as your options in this situation?" is more respectful than, "Here are your options. . . ." Skilled counselors ask few questions, especially avoiding those which seem to be based on curiosity and fact finding or which ask why. Teenagers often receive "why" questions with defensiveness or hostility.

Dimensions are added in counseling adolescents in accordance with the expressed needs and concerns of the adolescent. The implication here is that counselors may use vocational interest tests and information systems as tools for self-exploration and that counselors are knowledgeable and helpful in career as well as personal, social, and emotional areas. In educational and vocational counseling, the person-centered counselor expects students to make the choices and contacts which will result in their feeling confident and responsible. In essence, the person-centered counseling relationship is primarily one of talking together and experiencing together; however, the school counselor uses skills, activities, materials, and interventions to enhance self-concept development, to aid in self-understanding, and to foster independence and decision making for young people.

School counselors may not have the option to prolong exploration during school time of students' deeper problems; yet frequently, the relationship provided and the attitudes given in a few sessions may help students define for themselves a direction. Sensitive and competent school counselors need to be knowledgeable concerning referral sources for students who have problems that are more appropriately handled in longer term therapy.

Counseling with Adolescents in Agency Settings

Agencies provide a regular, specified time for adolescents to receive help in a setting apart from their family, school, peers, and neighborhood. Agency counselors can often be more objective and able to see a broader picture of the adolescent's functioning than is possible in the structure of a school setting. Many adolescents prefer to disclose themselves to an individual not connected with their everyday lives. On the other hand, the agency counselor often needs parental and school collaboration in meeting specific adolescent needs in therapy.

When an adolescent voluntarily seeks counseling or agrees to a referral suggested by a concerned adult, the person-centered counselor provides the facilitative conditions, uses skills which enhance the exploration of feelings, attitudes, and behaviors, and conveys trust in the potential wisdom of the youth to choose the direction of therapy and the areas to be examined. Adolescents frequently find a nonjudgmental adult who really listens to them without interrupting, giving advice, or judging their behavior to be a welcome relief from their encounters with adults they feel do not understand them.

Adolescents seen in counseling often find their thoughts, feelings, and behaviors confusing even to themselves. Depression and suicidal thoughts are not uncommon, and the astute counselor searches out these possibilities. Teenagers worry about their mood swings and unpredictability. Inferiority feelings plague them, and small failures in relationships loom as major obstacles in their lives. Parents and other authority figures become symbols of their lingering dependence and sometimes rebellion. A person-centered counselor tries to see into this experience of teenagers to help them sort out beliefs, feelings, values, and behaviors. The basic skill remains that of reflection; the counselor reflects in an accurate, succinct, and organized manner first the explicit and later, as the relationship develops, the implicit expressions and personal meanings of youthful clients. Short summaries also help systematize the adolescent client's thinking. As adolescent clients feel understood and better focused on the core of their concerns, they often begin to explore in more depth. The counselor risks gently confronting any mixed messages, ambiguities, and discrepancies perceived in the relationships in order to help young people see their behavior more clearly, both with the counselor and with others in their lives. After sufficient exploration has taken place and understanding begins to occur, the modern-day, person-centered counselor is ready to help the adolescent assess alternatives, make decisions, and formulate action plans.

Counselors often find that therapy with teenagers occurs in ups and downs as the young people "test them out," throw out roadblocks and other resistances: they are late, they "forget" appointments, they talk about inconsequential things. Person-centered counselors remain mindful of their own experiencing when adolescents are inconsistent and avoidant; they behave in spontaneous fashion, perhaps showing humor, perhaps displaying frustration. The attitude of genuineness is the most important posture they offer at such times. Use of the skill of immediacy (disclosing the therapist's immediate feelings about the relationship) lets the client know that the counselor can be relied upon not to manipulate but to be honest and open and to give accurate feedback. Immediacy creates a "you and me in this together" feeling which many teenagers long for.

If all adolescents were ready and willing clients, the agency counselor's job would be well rewarded. Perhaps the more usual case is the "reluctant," or involuntary, youth who is referred by the parents, school, or court system. Beier (1975) suggests that client-centered counselors generally deal with involuntary clients in one of three ways: (1) counselors indicate their faith and confidence in the ability of potential clients to make their own decisions but refuse to accept them as clients until they are ready to seek help on their own; (2) counselors accept them and actively engage in reflecting their resistances ("It must make you resentful to be here; you feel forced to do something you don't want to do"); (3) counselors accept them and discuss in an aboveboard fashion the fact that they are considered to be clients and the ways they can go about helping themselves.

Counselors choosing the first alternative may find adolescent clients not ready to make a decision for help. These adolescents may interpret refusal to accept them for treatment as indifference rather than respect. The second choice finds the counselor being permissive and nonjudgmental in reflecting what is not expressed by the silent client but seems to be "in the air." Some counselors have successfully used silences spotted by short reflective statements such that the involuntary client gradually comes to the belief that there is no threat and that no demands will be made by the therapist. Beier refers to the third method as "anxiety-arousing" and an expansion of traditional client-centered views. In effect, it puts responsibility on involuntary clients to accept the reality that they, not their parents, their teachers, their probation officers, or society, are the clients and that help is available and is freely offered. In choosing any of the three types of initial approach with referred adolescents, person-centered counselors cannot be certain as to outcome, but in all cases can offer in nonverbal and verbal ways the attitudes of empathy, respect, and genuineness.

GROUP PROCEDURES WITH CHILDREN AND ADOLESCENTS

Rogers once stated that he believed the intensive group was "the most rapidly spreading social invention of the century, and probably the most potent" (Rogers, 1970b, p. 1). As he had done for the process of therapy with the introduction of recordings and transcripts of sessions, he opened up group process to public scrutiny with the use of tapes and films. He believed that groups were unique opportunities for "normal" people to have honest and open interactions, intimacy, and the freedom to drop their facades. He thought that the group climate of safety, openness, risk taking, and genuineness fostered a trust which helped members recognize and change their self-defeating behaviors, test out more innovative and constructive behaviors, and begin to relate in a more adequate and effective fashion in everyday life situations.

The group setting provided an opportunity for Rogers to continue his own personal growth as he entered his sixties. He had never been a very spontaneous person, despite his lifelong beliefs in openness to expression of feeling and genuineness of relationships. Now he developed the quality of spontaneity as he participated in and facilitated groups during the 1960s and 1970s. The Rogerian group was unstructured; participants were encouraged to express their immediate experience and feelings and to share whatever they wished.

The process evolved in stages: At first there was confusion, awkwardness, an emphasis on past experience, and a resistance to personal exploration and sharing of feelings. Gradually, negative feelings began to be expressed in the group and personally meaningful material began to be explored. Then facades cracked, and confrontation and feedback occurred. Finally, deeper feelings and personal meanings began to be expressed and stirrings of self-acceptance and commitment to change would begin.

Rogers came to believe through his group work that people had tremendous capacities to be therapeutic and healing with one another. Group workers with children and adolescents have seen these potentialities come to life as the participants show accepting and empathic attitudes toward one another and offer their personal help. Rogers, whose work with groups extended to people in many professions and of all ages, ranked the group relationship as more easily developed with children because of their greater spontaneity and openness. He made the following ranking of difficulty, from greatest to least, in initiating group process and expressing feelings: administrators, college faculty, high school faculty, elementary teachers, college students, high school students, elementary school students (Rogers, 1969).

Group work with children is perhaps more likely to take place in a school setting than in an agency setting because of the greater possibilities school counselors have for getting children of an age group together with regularity. Counseling groups may consist of referred children or may be composed of children who voluntarily respond to invitations to be members of a small group. In any setting, potential group members should be screened by the counselor for suitability; for example, a seriously disturbed child may be inappropriate for a particular group. Person-centered counselors trust the group process, are optimistic about the forward-growth strivings of children, convey this belief, and provide the "core conditions" to children in group settings. They use the same verbal skills and techniques in groups as they use with individuals.

The unstructured group is seldom used with younger children in schools; rather, counselors plan activities which support their beliefs that children's self-esteem is enhanced as they identify, clarify, and understand their feelings; talk freely about their ideas and concerns; and experience more rewarding relationships with peers. Even when misbehavior or lack of motivation is the presenting concern of teachers or parents, person-centered counselors believe that children's behavior changes for the better as they feel better about themselves (develop more positive self-concepts) and receive positive feedback from others.

Group counseling provides an opportunity to talk about common concerns such as developing friendships, getting along with siblings, and clarifying a value system. "Feeling" groups are especially popular with person-centered counselors working with young children. In these groups, a feeling vocabulary is developed, feelings are discussed, with examples from the students' lives, and often situations involving feeling states are role-played. Self-concept groups are also popular, and the counselor may decide to open each session with an activity similar to those presented in the book *100 Ways to Enhance Self-Concept in the Classroom* (Canfield & Wells, 1976). If peer relations is the area for exploration, the counselor may provide initial structure by encouraging children to tell one thing they like in a friend or something about themselves that makes them a good friend. Listening is encouraged, and sometimes the counselor may have one child repeat what another has said to reinforce their attentiveness.

Counselors with young children need to control the process and be sure that all children are included and experience no threat. In school settings it is not advisable to probe into deeper problem areas or encourage self-disclosure which might harm children if confidences are not kept. Confidentiality can be a problem with child groups, and it is probably best for counselors to assume that children will talk about what they did in the group. On the other hand, group members should be encouraged not to reveal what others say. In starting a group, the counselor might begin with an introduction such as:

> This is our group and our special time together to talk about how we feel, what we think about, and what we do. We'll feel freer to talk if we make a plan not to talk outside this group about what anyone else says in the group; then we'll know we can trust one another. Do you think we could do that? [Discussion would follow.] First, let's get acquainted by telling one another about one thing we can do well.

Person-centered counselors must experiment with size, duration, and composition of groups and with various ways of facilitating the process with children. There are few strict guidelines other than adherence to the philosophy that growth occurs in a therapeutic climate of empathy, respect, and openness.

A more unstructured group can often be used with older children in upper elementary and middle school. In this type of "growth" group, children may choose topics for discussion and may even take turns being facilitators. Person-centered counselors may use the small group setting to help children learn the same facilitative conditions and skills in communication taught to adults; and, in fact, children can become "peer counselors" and assist others in and out of the group. Establishing and maintaining confidentiality is also easier with older children, but it needs to be continually reinforced.

Nelson (1972) has listed a set of behavioral expectancies for children participating in small groups:

1. *Deep listening.* Members of the group are encouraged to listen to the comments being made to see if all the meaning and feeling seems to be expressed.

2. *Helping each other talk.* Members of the group are encouraged to help the person talking to continue to express him- or herself in order to be sure that the meanings and feelings behind his or her comments are clear.

3. *Discussing problems and concerns.* Group members are encouraged to focus on matters of concern to them with which they believe the group can help.

4. *Discussing feelings.* Group members are encouraged to think through and to discuss their feelings about the concerns for which they believe the group can provide insight, understanding, or assistance.

5. *Confronting.* Members of the group are encouraged to point out when they feel the individual is not being entirely truthful or accepting responsibility, or when they feel that an obvious solution is being overlooked.

6. *Planning and reporting.* Group members are encouraged to test out in the group their ideas for solving their concerns, to formulate these into plans for action, and to report on the success or failure of their undertakings. (pp. 228-229)

These expectancies are consistent with the person-centered counselor's group work and can be applied with older children and adolescents in school or agency settings.

It is unfortunate that there is not more group work provided for adolescents in school settings, as their strong peer ties, social inclinations, and need to explore their values could be invaluable. Adolescents and youth may be initially more uncomfortable, embarrassed, and resistant in a group setting than children in a group setting, and, therefore, person-centered counselors need patience, understanding, and, above all, faith in the group process. Whether or not structure is provided in the form of exercises or activities is an individual matter; counselors working from a person-centered orientation have been successful with both unstructured and structured groups for teenagers.

When agency counselors can get together a small group of children or adolescents, they have fewer limitations on time and duration of sessions, the depth of explorations, and the issue of confidentiality. Children or teenagers who meet only once a week together in a clinic setting without seeing one another daily in school and knowing each other as friends or neighbors will usually feel freer to discuss the deeper problems they have at home or in school or their worries in regard to their feelings and behaviors. The person-centered counselor works to provide the safety, permissiveness, and intimacy that make children and youth comfortable in exposing themselves and their problems. The counselor facilitates the process, modeling deep respect, empathy, and genuineness. As the process develops, children and teenagers become effective helpers for one another.

Groups in schools and agencies today are often organized around common needs of children and adolescents, such as coping with divorce or establishing appropriate independence. In both settings, parents of children need to be informed that such a group is offered and can be helpful. Their permission is needed for the child's inclusion. Person-centered counselors accept the mixed feelings of children and adolescents who are experiencing common problems such as alcoholism or family disorganization, helping them to explore and understand how they really feel and what is happening in their lives. Often knowing that others in the group have similar thoughts, feelings, and experiences is enough to stimulate coping strategies.

In summary, group procedures in schools and agencies offer the potential for children and adolescents to help one another and to grow together toward a better self-understanding, better relationships with others, and a better adjustment to their environment.

CLASSROOM AND EDUCATIONAL APPLICATIONS

Rogers had been influenced, since his days at Columbia Teachers College (1924-1928), by the idea that people learn best through experience. He believed that his own personal experiences had provided for him the most meaningful and significant learnings in his life. In his own teaching he applied insights, becoming a facilitator rather than an expert or authority. Students were not accustomed to his unstructured classes and methods, and they often experienced frustration, even trying to change him. He continued to believe that they were the best selectors and judges of their learning, and that if a nonthreatening atmosphere of freedom were provided, they could be trusted to learn and evaluate themselves. He defined the elements involved in significant or experiential learning as follows (Rogers, 1969):

> *It has a quality of personal involvement*—the whole person in both his feeling and cognitive aspects being *in* the learning event. *It is self-initiated.* Even when the impetus or stimulus comes from the outside, the sense of discovery, or reaching out, of grasping and comprehending, comes from within. *It is pervasive.* It makes a difference in the behavior, the attitudes, perhaps even the personality of the learner. *It is evaluated by the learner.* He knows whether it is meeting his need, whether it leads toward what he *wants* to know, whether it illuminates the dark area of ignorance he is experiencing. The locus of evaluation, we might say, resides definitely in the learner. *Its essence is meaning.* When such learn-

ing takes place, the element of meaning to the learner is built into the whole experience. (p. 5)

Rogers believed that teachers preferred to facilitate this type of learning but were locked into traditional, conventional approaches. "When we put together in one scheme such elements as a *prescribed curriculum, similar assignments for all students, lecturing* as almost the only mode of instruction, *standard tests* by which all students are externally evaluated, and *instructor-chosen grades* as the measure of learning, then we can almost guarantee that meaningful learning will be at an absolute minimum" (Rogers, 1969, p. 5).

In his book *Freedom to Learn* (1969), Rogers emphasized the belief he had held for some years, which was that he was interested only in *facilitating* the process of learning for individuals, not in teaching or instructing them. Thus, students would set their own goals and decide how they wanted to reach them. For teachers who wished to grant this freedom, he advocated: (1) providing many resources; (2) using learning contracts; (3) helping students conduct their own inquiries and make their own discoveries; (4) using simulation activities for experiential learning; (5) using programmed instruction when students wished to learn more efficiently; and (6) having students evaluate themselves. The first chapter in *Freedom to Learn* is of special interest to educators of children; it describes the attempts of a sixth-grade teacher to apply many of Rogers' beliefs on education to her classroom.

During the 1960s and 1970s views similar to Rogers', if not as radical, were advanced by humanistic, person-centered educators who were seeking more democratic learning climates for students consistent with their beliefs in the drive toward growth, health, and self-actualization in individuals. These educators believed that the curriculum should include an affective component and that students should be helped toward self-awareness, self-understanding, and self-responsibility. Fostering creativity, divergent thinking, inquiry learning, and problem solving became goals of these teachers and educators. A respect for the uniqueness of student perceptions, values, feelings, and beliefs was promoted.

At the same time, education was being greatly influenced by the behavioral school of psychology which emphasized programmed learning, specific behavioral objectives, contingency management, management by objectives, and accountability. Perhaps both schools of thought went to extremes. Today there appears to be a trend toward a "return to basics" in education; however, the humanistic, person-centered influence is too compelling in a democratic society to be discarded, and much of the earlier influence continues to be felt.

Person-centered educators work together today in many school systems, not only in the cognitive domain, but in helping children and adolescents develop positive self-concepts through encouraging their accomplishments and personal strengths, helping them clarify their beliefs and values, and conveying a trust in the ability of students to make their own choices and assume responsibility for their actions. These educators also try to improve communication within school systems, both horizontally and vertically. Gazda's *Human Relations Development: A Manual for Educators* (1973, 1977) is an example of one model for communication in education which draws heavily on person-centered theory and technique. Another person-centered model focusing on the teacher-student relationship is Gordon's *Teacher Effectiveness Training* (1974).

Person-centered counselors, especially in the elementary and middle schools, have influenced the curriculum in at least four ways: (1) by helping teachers conduct classroom meetings such as advocated by Glasser (1969) where children can communicate openly and honestly and develop personal responsibility; (2) by encouraging teachers to incorporate within the school day opportunities for students to explore their feelings, beliefs, values, and attitudes through planned activities or by taking advantage of spontaneous opportunities during regular content instruction; (3) by compiling and demonstrating affective programs and materials for use in the classroom to complement the cognitive learning; and (4) by actually conducting classroom guidance activities on a regular basis. High school counselors have been directly involved in the curriculum through offering minicourses on topics such as clarifying values, understanding relationships, and resolving conflicts, in addition to their regular counseling and guidance functions.

Person-centered counselors firmly believe that early and continued classroom guidance activities can serve a preventive as well as a growth-enhancing function and help in the future adjustment of adolescents and youth. Many materials are consistent and suitable for the counselor's work in classroom guidance. Among the books which contain helpful activities are *100 Ways to Enhance Self-Concept in the Classroom* (Canfield & Wells, 1976), *Guidance Activities for Counselors and Teachers* (Thompson & Poppen, 1979), *Real Learning: A Sourcebook for Teachers* (Silberman, Allender, & Yanoff, 1976), and *Values Clarification* (Simon, Howe, & Kirschenbaum, 1972). Another valuable resource is the book *Counseling Children* (Thompson & Rudolph, 1988), which lists many interventions for use with problem behaviors of children. The activities presented in these books cover a broad range; taken together, there are activities to help build self-esteem, develop effective peer relationships, resolve conflicts, clarify values, and encourage listening skills and the skills of communicating feelings and wants.

Counselors with a person-centered orientation also use materials in elementary classroom guidance such as the Magic Circle Program (Bessell, 1970; 1969-1974) which focuses on: (1) awareness—knowing what your thoughts, feelings, and actions really are; (2) mastery—knowing what your abilities are and how to use them; and (3) social interaction—knowing other people. Structured programs used by person-centered counselors include Developing Understanding of Self and Others (DUSO) (Dinkmeyer & Dinkmeyer, 1982) and Toward Affective Development (TAD) (Dupont, Gardner, & Brody, 1974). These kits offer daily activities for a school year and are especially helpful in stimulating classroom discussion.

A number of film-strip series such as *First Things: Values* (1972) and *First Things: Social Reasoning* (1974) have been useful for classroom guidance. Counselors have also made use of stories such as *I Am Loveable and Capable* (IALAC) (Simon, 1973), to work with a classroom on self-concept. Most important, person-centered counselors use their own creativity in designing activities and materials for specific classroom needs.

In summary, person-centered approaches have had an impact on education by calling attention to learning climates for children and adolescents where they can explore their feelings, values, and beliefs, see themselves as capable and trustworthy, and experience their own power to make choices and take responsibility. Educators have been influenced to look at their own patterns of communication and methods of teaching to see if they are enhancing all aspects of student development. Counselors have helped to bring into the curriculum of elementary, middle, and high schools guidance experiences that encourage continued personal, emotional, and social growth of students.

PARENTING SKILLS

Person-centered counselors help parents individually, but the group approach has demonstrated the power of parents to help one another as they share together their struggles and successes in developing more effective ways of raising responsible children. As in other forms of person-centered helping, counselors create a climate of psychological safety for parents based on attitudes of empathic understanding, respect, and genuineness. Trust in the resources of parents to develop and implement their own goals is conveyed by the group leader.

Group approaches range from the unstructured Rogerian type to structured training models. In the less structured group, the counselor serves as a facilitator, letting the group go through the expected initial feeling of lack of direction and frustration, and trusting the group process. The belief is, and experience confirms this, that as trust develops parents will drop their defenses and choose what is most significant for them to work on in the group. Person-centered counselors use self-disclosure and confrontation and give feedback when appropriate, always in the attitude of caring, respect, and challenge of the parents' resources. Counselors believe that as members feel safe and understood, they will develop insights which will motivate them to change ineffective attitudes and behaviors toward their children and adolescents.

The most influential, structured person-centered program for parents was developed by Thomas Gordon, a graduate student of Rogers. Gordon began to offer courses for parents in the 1960s, beginning in his own community in California. The success of his course is attested to by the increased number of individuals who have received special training as instructors and the thousands of parents across the country who completed his Parent Effectiveness Training (P.E.T.) programs. The book *Parent Effectiveness Training* (1970) presented his insights to the public at large, consistent with a person-centered educational philosophy that individuals can and will learn what has meaning for them.

Since developing the Parent Effectiveness Training model, Gordon has expanded his work into education with courses for teachers, into organizational development with courses on Leadership Effectiveness Training, and into youth work with a program called Youth Effectiveness Training. His purpose has been to make available to individuals, parents, teachers, executives, administrators, and young people the principles of humanistic, democratic relationships so that effective and positive benefits could result.

Specific to parents, Gordon believed that they were more often blamed than trained, that parenthood was a difficult, demanding job, and that the skills of more effective parenting could be taught. He demonstrated faith in the ability and willingness of parents to learn attitudes, methods, and skills used by professional counselors and therapists in establishing relationships and working with children.

Gordon (1970) stressed the importance of parents being congruent and sending clear and honest messages that match their true feelings:

> Real parents will inevitably feel both accepting and unaccepting toward their children; their attitudes toward the same behavior cannot be consistent; it must vary from time to time. They should not (and cannot) hide their true feelings; they should accept the fact that one parent may feel accepting and the other unaccepting of the same behavior; and they should realize that each will inevitably feel different degrees of acceptance toward each

> of their children. . . . While children undoubtedly *prefer* to be accepted, they can constructively handle their parents' unaccepting feelings when parents send clear and honest messages. (pp. 27-28)

A valuable and often-quoted contribution of Gordon's has been his list of twelve typical ways parents respond to the feelings and problems of their children. These are the verbal behaviors which person-centered counselors and therapists try to avoid. Sometimes dubbed "the dirty dozen," the categories are:

1. *Ordering, directing, commanding.* Telling the child to do something, giving him or her an order or a command.
2. *Warning, admonishing, threatening.* Telling the child what consequences will occur if he or she does something.
3. *Exhorting, moralizing, preaching.* Telling the child what he or she *should* or *ought* to do.
4. *Advising, giving solutions, or suggestions.* Telling the child how to solve a problem, giving him or her advice or suggestions, providing answers or solutions for the child.
5. *Lecturing, teaching, giving logical arguments.* Trying to influence the child with facts, counter-arguments, logic information, or your own opinions.
6. *Judging, criticizing, disagreeing, blaming.* Making a negative judgment or evaluation of the child.
7. *Praising, agreeing.* Offering a positive evaluation or judgment, agreeing.
8. *Name-calling, ridiculing, shaming.* Making the child feel foolish, putting the child into a category, shaming him or her.
9. *Interpretation, analyzing, diagnosing.* Telling the child what his or her motives are or analyzing why he or she is doing or saying something; communicating that you have the child figured out or diagnosed.
10. *Reassuring, sympathizing, consoling, supporting.* Trying to make the child feel better, talking the child out of his

or her feelings, trying to make those feelings go away, denying the strength of those feelings.

11. *Probing, questioning, interrogating.* Trying to find reasons, motives, causes; searching for more information to help you solve the problem.
12. *Withdrawing, distracting, humoring, diverting.* Trying to get the child away from the problem; withdrawing from the problem yourself; distracting the child, kidding him or her out of it, pushing the problem aside.

In place of these twelve communication styles, Gordon advocates responding to children in ways that increase the chance that they will feel free to keep talking, feel less guilt and inadequacy, reduce defensiveness and resentment, and help the parent-child relationship. He popularized the term *active listening,* which is now used widely to describe Rogerian listening, or the empathic listening which involves entering the world of another and reflecting feelings and meanings. This manner of listening is especially useful when children have problems they recognize, when they "own" their problems and need to feel understood.

Gordon differentiates between the *you message* ("you're always late," "you're lazy," etc.) sent by parents to their children which may make them feel resistant and unworthy, and the *I message,* which confronts children with their parents' feelings and places responsibility on the children to modify their behavior. *I messages* are essentially those employed by person-centered counselors using immediacy with their clients, expressing their own feelings and thoughts about the here-and-now counseling relationship. Parents are taught by Gordon to use this type of verbal message when they are feeling annoyed or frustrated by something that is occurring and, thus, "own" the problem. An example of *you* and *I messages* for the same situation is given by Gordon (1970):

Situation: A child has just kicked his parent in the shin.

Parental "you" message: That's being a very bad boy. Don't you ever kick anybody like that!

> *Parental "I" message:* Ouch! That really hurt me—I don't like to be kicked. (p. 118)

Gordon has been concerned about the negative effects of parental power tactics on children and believes that parents continue to use power out of a lack of knowledge and experience with any other method of resolving conflicts. His own method for parents is called the *no lose* method and assumes a relatively equal power between those involved in a conflictual situation. As Gordon (1970) describes it:

> Parent and child encounter a conflict-of-needs situation. The parent asks the child to participate with him in a joint search for some solution acceptable to both. One or both may offer possible solutions. They critically evaluate them and eventually make a decision on a final solution acceptable to both. No selling of the other is required after the solution has been selected, because both have already accepted it. No power is required to force compliance, because neither is resisting the decision. (p. 196)

The *no lose* method of conflict resolution is considered successful by Gordon because: (1) the child is motivated to carry out the solution; (2) there is more chance of finding a high-quality solution; (3) it develops thinking skills in children; (4) it reduces hostility and generates warm feelings; (5) it requires less effort; (6) it eliminates the need for power; (7) it gets to the *real* problem; (8) it treats children as individuals to be trusted to make responsible, mature choices. The trust and goodwill offered by parents toward their children in the *no lose* method is similar to the person-centered attitudes offered by counselors and therapists. Therapeutic changes often take place in children whose parents use the P.E.T. principles and philosophy.

Another popular program for parents emphasizing democratic and positive parenting is the Systematic Training for Effective Parenting, or STEP program (Dinkmeyer & McKay, 1976). Although this program is based on the Adlerian family counseling model, it incorporates many person-centered attitudes, such as listening for feelings, offering acceptance and encouragement, and showing confidence and trust in children to make responsible choices. The program also advocates person-centered counseling skills such as reflective listening, open responses, and the use of *I* statements to express authentic parental feelings. STEP calls attention to ineffective styles of communication similar to Gordon's "dirty dozen." It emphasizes parental attitudes which relate closely to those which person-centered counselors and therapists convey in their relationships with clients. In place of the *no lose* method of solving conflicts, STEP teaches the use of natural and logical consequences in helping children take responsibility for their behavior. This program does not require the training that is part of becoming a P.E.T. instructor.

Helping parents has become a necessary part of the work of counselors and therapists in both school and agency settings. The desire and need of parents to become more effective in their communication with and discipline of their children have been satisfied by these professionals through systematic training programs as well as through individual and group counseling.

FAMILY INTERVENTIONS

Person-centered counselors help families in the following ways: (1) counseling with children and adolescents; (2) establishing parent groups and parenting programs; (3) doing consultation with parents; (4) counseling with parents; (5) training parents as therapists for their own children; and (6) doing family therapy. Counseling with children and adolescents and parenting programs have been discussed in prior sections of this chapter. This section will address parent consultation, parent counseling, training parents as therapists, and family therapy.

Consultation with Parents

Reisman (1973) defines consultation as "an interaction process between two individuals, one of whom has a specialized area of knowledge that is sought or valued by the other, who has a problem in this area" (p. 212). Counselors and therapists are often asked by parents for help in understanding their children's problems and behavior and in considering ways to cope more effectively as parents. In consultation, information and ideas are exchanged, and the counselor collaborates in meeting the specific goal as articulated by the parent. When parents desire consultation, the counselor does not assume therapy is needed or should be provided. As consultants, person-centered counselors believe that parents can achieve insights and solve their problems with their children in an atmosphere of empathy and respect and an open, genuine exchange of ideas and information.

In Reisman's definition of psychotherapy as a form of communication of person-related understanding, respect, and wish to be of help, the distinction between consultation with parents about their children and psychotherapy with parents may become blurred. "Psychotherapy can be employed in consultation, and consultation can be employed in psychotherapy" (Reisman, 1973, pp. 220-221). The difference lies in the parents' goal which, in consultation, is to receive help related to their role as parents. The therapist-consultant accepts and understands what it is the parents want. It may become appropriate for the therapist to invite parents to join a parenting group for additional support and assistance. Should it become apparent that one or both parents desire more than consultation, and, in fact, want personal counseling, the therapist would need to either refer them or renegotiate for counseling services.

Counseling with Parents

When a counselor is seeing a child or adolescent individually, it may be advisable to see the parent or parents for personal therapy also. This is especially problematic when it is an older child or adolescent being seen by the counselor. These clients need to feel that their counselor is their own, is objective and impartial, and can be trusted to maintain confidentiality. When parents feel the need for more help than is given in the consultation process and desire to explore their marital relationship or their personality functioning, a referral can be made.

In the process of individual therapy, the families of clients often reap benefits. In his essay "The Implications of Client-Centered Therapy for Family Life" (Rogers, 1961a), Rogers discussed his observations for some of the ways clients changed in their family living as a consequence of counseling. Clients became more expressive of their true feelings with family members and became better at accepting their own real feelings without defensive pretenses. Communication improved and mutual understanding developed as clients began to listen empathically and to respond to their families with respect. Another dividend was a willingness on the part of clients to let other family members be separate persons with their own feelings, values, and beliefs, and to trust in the potential of these family members to become responsible and self-directing.

Training Parents as Therapists

An innovative person-centered approach for helping emotionally disturbed children up to age 10 is *filial therapy* (Guerney, 1964), which trains small groups of parents as play therapists for their children. The advocates of filial therapy regard "the essence of the filial technique to be that of systematically tapping a relatively neglected but potentially powerful resource: the energy of parents in working for the betterment of their children" (Guerney, Guerney, & Andronico, 1966, p. 886). In filial therapy, parents are trusted and helped to effect change in their children in their homes, rather than in clinic settings. The training process for parents is extensive, combining didactic instruction with supervised experience in the methods of person-centered play therapy and a person-centered group experience. In group counseling, parents observe the modeling of communication skills and are helped to cope with feelings and difficulties as these emerge during the course of filial therapy (Andronico, Fidler, Guerney, & Guerney, 1967).

In learning the process, parents in the small groups watch demonstrations, role-play, observe one another conducting play sessions with their own children, and give and receive feedback. Parents are taught to encourage, accept, and reflect all feelings expressed by their children and to convey person-centered attitudes of empathy, acceptance, and understanding. After training they continue the sessions in their own homes, using a particular room, time, and group of toys. The direction of play is left to the child; the only limits are that children cannot extend the time of the sessions, break expensive toys, or physically hurt the parents.

A more recent program focusing on adolescent-parent relationships is PARD, Parent-Adolescent Relationship Development (Guerney, 1977). PARD grew out of the filial therapy program and was begun to help dysfunctional parent-adolescent relationships. PARD uses both didactic and experiential instruction, but it differs from filial therapy in that the adolescents as well as their parents are trained in self-expressive and empathic skills. PARD therapists work with both individual dyads and groups of youths and parents. Carkhuff (1971) first proposed the concept of "training as treatment," and, following this lead, person-centered therapists and counselors explain the therapeutic process and help clients develop those skills that enhance any relationship. PARD is an example of this trend. Although relatively new, it has also been employed as a preventive and developmental program for use with normal families (Lavant, 1978a).

FAMILY THERAPY

Person-centered family therapists find the family systems paradigm consistent with their beliefs in the inherent resources for growth and self-understanding of individuals. The family-as-client is offered respect, empathy, and a genuine therapist who is concerned with the family's movement toward wholeness. In fact, the spontaneity and humor of the experiential school of family therapy is made-to-order for person-centered therapists who value responding to the moment-to-moment experience of a family in therapy.

Person-centered family therapists do not begin with preconceived notions of family pathology, nor do they see themselves as skilled diagnosticians calling the shots (Raskin & Van deer Veen, 1970). The therapist interacts freely and genuinely with family members, responding empathically but leaving with the family members the locus of responsibility for interpretation and action.

Whereas the person-centered family counselor is actively involved, expressive, and interested in facilitating a genuine, honest encounter among family members, the essential philosophy remains the same: family members are trusted to assume responsibility for their own change and growth. Although not reluctant to state a preference based on experience with families, the therapist respects their ability to make decisions which are best for each about all aspects of the therapy, such as: Who will participate and to what extent, what the significant areas for discussion will be, what meaning will be derived from the experience, and what action(s) will be taken, if any (Lavant, 1978b). The counselor trusts the group process, enters the phenomenological world of the family, communicates an empathic understanding of family experiences, and acts as a facilitator and model of therapeutic attitudes and behaviors.

Person-centered family therapy is an underdeveloped area in terms of theoretical and clinical writings and empirical research (Lavant, 1978a), but it is being used by individual practitioners who believe in the relationship conditions of empathy, respect, and genuineness. These therapists emphasize the experiencing of family members and trust the self-determination and drive of the family members toward healthy individual and family growth.

EFFICACY

Rogers' emphasis on the therapeutic relationship has become almost universally adopted (Bohart & Todd, 1988). Person-centered attitudes and skills have become givens for therapists and counselors of many orientations. This is demonstrated by the wide acceptance and adoption of systematic skills training, which includes training in warmth, empathy, respect, and genuineness, in most current counselor training programs. Person-centered ideas thus become the process whereby therapists of differing theoretical bases can establish the type of relationship and attitudes which will help them proceed in fostering client change and development. Keat (1974) sees the client-centered relationship as a necessary condition to therapeutic change in children and, therefore, it precedes the use of specific behavioral interventions. He estimates that the relationship alone has been not only necessary but sufficient in about one-fourth of child-counseling cases, especially when the child is emotionally deprived.

Person-centered counselors hold beliefs that children, adolescents, and adults can become responsible and self-directing and thus actively help them set their own goals and find ways to achieve these goals. These counselors are involved and spontaneous as they seek to understand the feelings and attitudes of clients of all ages, using many skills and interventions in their desire to help and encourage client growth. Thus, a "pure" type of person-centered counseling that can be subjected to rigorous research is hard to come by today. Studies which purport to compare or contrast client-centered counseling with children and adolescents to other therapeutic orientations still conceive of the client-centered counselor as leaving out the "action" part of helping. Much of the efficacy of the person-centered approach lies in the counseling relationship, in the use of core attitudes on the part of the counselor which research has demonstrated to facilitate client growth, and in the flexibility and openness of the person-centered counselor to discover with clients what will best help them meet their goals.

A major contribution of Rogers to the field of psychotherapy was his willingness to state his formulations in testable hypotheses and submit them to research efforts (Corey, 1982). He conducted and stimulated many research studies; at least 140 separate therapy studies are known, most of them published; and if the research on groups, play therapy, education, and leadership were included, there might be as many as 200 (Kirschenbaum, 1979). Patterson (1973) has observed that "the client-centered approach has led to, and is supported by, a greater amount of research than any other approach to counseling or psychotherapy" (p. 12).

Rogers consistently modeled an unusual combination of a phenomenological understanding of clients and an empirical evaluation of therapy. He and his colleagues demonstrated that a humanistic approach to doing therapy and a scientific approach to evaluating it need not be incompatible (Prochaska, 1979). When he began his research attempts, there were few precedents, and his first significant contribution was in taping, transcribing, and publishing therapy sessions verbatim. Initial research efforts consisted of classifying responses from transcripts to see what happened in therapy. The next phase involved the use of recognized clinical tests in attempts to validate therapy results. Finally, researchers put their minds to the major goal of testing hypotheses that the *process* of therapy results in change and that the therapeutic conditions of empathy, unconditional positive regard, and congruence foster the process.

Rogers received large-scale grants while at Chicago and worked with 15 to 20 researchers over several years, about 10 of whom stayed involved the entire time. Designs were created to address earlier research problems of small population samples, lack of controls, and lack of instrumentation to measure changes in client attitudes.

Some of the research results were presented in *Psychotherapy and Personality Change* (Rogers & Dymond, 1954). Rogers and a colleague developed a seven-point Process Scale to demonstrate where individuals were at the beginning of therapy, at points during the process, at termination, and at follow-up (Rogers & Rablen, 1958). The scale described behavior in the areas of feeling and personal meanings; manner of experiencing; degree of incongruence; communication of self; manner in which experience is construed; relationship to problems; and manner of relating (Corsini, 1979). The scale was used subsequently in many studies, including those with schizophrenics (Rogers et al., 1967). Reporting on validation studies, Rogers (1961b) wrote: "Studies with the Process Scale have reliably correlated process movement in therapy with outcome, as well as correlating positive process movement with the presence of the three therapist conditions: genuineness, caring, and understanding" (p. 33).

Research in person-centered therapy has demonstrated that certain skills used by counselors directly influence the degree to which clients will explore their concerns (Carkhuff, 1969; Rogers et al., 1967; Truax & Carkhuff, 1967). Carkhuff called these skills "responding skills" and "the core of facilitating dimensions." His five-point scales (1969, Vol. II) have stimulated much research and are widely used in training and supervision. Truax and Carkhuff (1967) believe that from 20% to 50% of the variability of a variety of outcome indices may be accounted for by these primary core dimensions, essentially those which person-centered counselors convey in providing the "core conditions."

Recently, Rogers and Sanford (1984) summarized research done in foreign countries on psychotherapy, the student-teacher relationship, and the use of encounter groups. They reported the studies as demonstrating the efficacy of the person-centered approach. In general, research has supported the effectiveness of client-centered therapy (Smith, Glass, & Miller, 1980). As he neared the end of his long and productive life, Rogers was concerned about the lack of humanistically oriented research. In a significant article (Rogers, 1985), he reemphasized his call over the years for new models of science which would allow for research methodology more appropriate for person-centered, phenomenological and humanistically oriented concepts and beliefs. He believed that new models were beginning to appear and that there was "clearly no one best method for all investigations . . . one must choose the means or model best adapted to the particular questions being asked" (Rogers, 1985, p. 7). Rogers' continued modeling of the artist/scientist by his own life is a legacy for all person-centered and relationship-oriented practitioners.

CONCLUSIONS

Person-centered counselors seek to provide a therapeutic climate with attitudes of empathy, respect, and genuineness where clients of all ages and with a variety of concerns can be themselves and feel cared about and safe. Given this atmosphere, counselors trust that the process will release the vast resources for growth and behavioral change which people possess.

Counselors with a person-centered orientation believe that children and adolescents are capable of self-direction and self-responsibility. In facilitating the development of children and youth, person-centered therapists listen with care and patience, use skills which convey the core attitudes of empathy, respect and genuineness, and are prepared to use a variety of interventions and materials to enhance the counseling process and relationship.

CASE STUDIES

Child Case Study

The following case demonstrates how person-centered counselors work with children today, making use of a variety of skills and interventions, using consultation, observation, verbal approaches, and various media and activities. The case demonstrates how one counselor, a school psychologist, sought to discover what would work best with a particular child to aid that child's process of self-discovery and development. The person-centered philosophy of trust in the child's capacity to change, given the conditions of empathy, respect, and genuineness, is illustrated.

Client: Charlie, age 11

Reason for Referral: Charlie was referred to the school psychologist for counseling by the teacher of his class for behaviorally handicapped students. The counselor's primary intent was for Charlie to develop a positive relationship with an adult who could provide support if or when Charlie "lost it" in school. A secondary goal was to explore the emotions contributing to Charlie's identified misbehaviors.

Background Information: When he was a third grader, Charlie had received learning disabilities tutoring. His tutor considered him to have severe attitudinal problems as manifested by his: (1) refusal to acknowledge errors in his work; (2) refusal to accept help with his work; (3) sullen, angry facial expressions; and (4) unreasonably high expectations. Based on the tutor's and teacher's recommendations, Charlie was placed the following year in a classroom unit for students with severe behavioral handicaps.

Initial Session: The counselor wanted to build rapport in the first sessions, so he chose a setting in which the client was very comfortable—the out-of-doors. During the session, the client was extremely talkative. A main focus was the disappointment he had experienced in his family, such as his parents forgetting his last birthday and his father refusing to let him go to the funeral of his grandmother with whom he had lived for two years. The counselor listened and reflected his feelings.

Second and Third Sessions: Because the client had been very verbal during the initial session, the counselor decided to use a sentence completion exercise to evoke more feeling responses. Charlie did not respond well to this exercise (his answers were brief and nonpersonal), so the next session began completely unstructured. This bored Charlie and he became very fidgety. Observation in his classroom showed that one of his favorite activities was drawing. Consequently, during the third session, structure was again provided by the counselor; Charlie was asked to fill in the sections of a personal Coat of Arms. This activity is one included among suggestions for enhancing self-concept (Canfield & Wells, 1976) and allows for artistic rather than verbal expression. Charlie's interest was high as he commented: "This is great! I love to draw." However, he refused to draw without the aid of a ruler. The counselor hypothesized that this refusal indicated a need for structure and/or control. On the section of the shield which was to depict what Charlie wanted to be in the future, he became very angry and impatient with not being able to draw a fireman's hat the way he wanted it. He finally threw his marker across the room and refused to continue drawing, at which time the following dialogue occurred:

Counselor: It looks like you get angry when you can't make things the way you want them to be.

Charlie: I'm mad!

Counselor: You're really angry now.

Charlie: When I'm mad, I hate people.

Counselor: Can you tell me more about that?

Charlie: I hate people who think I can't do things right. I can do it.

Counselor: It really bugs you when other people think you can't do things right when you know you can. [Silence.] Do you want to finish the shield now, Charlie?

Charlie: It's stupid. It doesn't look right. I'm not doing it.

Counselor: You're not satisfied with it. Maybe sometimes you get angry with yourself, too, when you think you goof up.

[At this point, Charlie's wishes to discontinue were respected and the session was terminated.]

Subsequent Sessions: The above session paved the way for weekly sessions, twenty in all. The counselor provided an atmosphere of acceptance and permissiveness. Charlie was allowed to direct the sessions in the sense that drawing was always the activity and he chose what to draw. The content usually was guns, foreign legion hats, or rescue vehicles. Often Charlie's verbalizations indicated his involvement in some type of conflict to which there was no expressed resolution. As sessions progressed, his comments changed from description of the content ("this is a gun") to participation in the content ("Pow! Pow! I gotta get the bad guy before he gets me"). The client's need for structure decreased, as exhibited by his declining dependence on the ruler. Another change was seen in his attitude. Instead of continuing to be sullen and defensive, he became enthusiastic and usually cooperative, smiling instead of frowning. Eventually, more specific content was suggested by the counselor for the purpose of eliciting feelings in the area of family dynamics. Although verbalization was not elaborate, much of the anger formerly expressed began to dissipate.

Final Session: The end of the school year marked the termination of counseling. During the final session, Charlie was particularly exuberant. He wanted to draw a picture for the counselor. He began by drawing the often-depicted foreign legion hat. He then drew a series of snow skis, each of which represented a skier who fell, was injured, and then was taken away in an ambulance. Finally, Charlie drew another pair of skis. The following monologue ensued:

Charlie: This is me. Close your eyes. [The counselor complied.] Open your eyes! [Pause.] Surprise! You thought

I was going to get hurt, too, but I didn't! I had a parachute! I'm OK!
It was the opinion of the counselor that Charlie was, in fact, much more OK than he was when he first began counseling. He had begun to see that he could think ahead, control his behavior, and become more responsible.

Epilogue: At a placement-team meeting at the end of the year, it was the consensus of the team members that Charlie's substantial progress made it appropriate for him to return to the regular classroom the next year. Provisions were made for the teacher and the psychologist to be available to provide support as needed.[1]

Adolescent Case Study

The following case is presented to demonstrate person-centered counselor attitudes in working with adolescents, especially the attitude of genuineness. The case offers the additional vantage point of demonstrating supervisory experiences of a person-centered nature which help counselors to stay in touch with their own experiencing in counseling relationships and to work toward understanding the experience of their clients.

Donny,[2] age 16, was referred to the clinic for psychoeducational evaluation by the Juvenile Court at the request of his father and stepmother who termed his behavior "incorrigible." One of the recommendations for the diagnostic evaluation was for counseling, and Donny was assigned to a counselor-trainee. Donny appeared resistant and reluctant during early sessions, and the counselor felt frustrated. In the counselor's own words:

Donny was my first adolescent case. I knew my philosophical stance toward counseling was essentially a humanistic, Rogerian blend, but I had not yet developed a sense of my own "style" as a counselor. Words such as genuine, accepting, empathic, etc. sounded good and

---

[1]This case was contributed by Joyce Clinton Moore, school psychologist for the Mariemont, Ohio, school system.

[2]This case, contributed by Duncan Adams, occurred while he was a counselor-trainee at the Child Development Clinic at James Madison University.

> made a lot of sense to me, but I had not had a real chance to see them work for me. This, coupled with the fear that Donny would perceive me as yet another judgmental authority figure in his life, had the effect of causing me to rely very heavily on technique. I felt like I was playing the role of counselor, I wasn't very effective, I wasn't very genuine, and most of all, I wasn't very comfortable.

Donny had not shown up for his second appointment. At the beginning of the next one, the counselor said, "I missed you last week." Donny replied, "Well, I had to talk with Mr. Jones, and I kinda forgot about it." While reviewing videotapes of the sessions, a supervisor helped the counselor develop insight into Donny's feelings by role-playing what Donny might like to be saying if he were honest and also what he might be revealing through his body language. The counselor was encouraged to role-play what he had experienced during the sessions, and, most important, what he wished he had said. An example is as follows:

> *Counselor:* Donny, I was angry last week when you didn't show up or call me. I spent about half an hour just sitting and waiting for you to come.
>
> *Supervisor:* [as Donny] I wish you had admitted you were mad instead of just saying you missed me, because I knew you were anyway. I need you to be honest and real with me. . . . I don't need someone to talk with who hides his feelings like I do.

Another supervisory session went a step further. The clinic setting was fairly sterile and probably intimidating to Donny. It was decided that the two would begin meeting in a more natural setting—walking outdoors, going for a drive, etc. The counselor reported that the binding "counselor-client" role was loosened, and he and Donny became closer. Donny was more at ease, talked more, and made substantially more eye contact.

During the last session, the counselor and client drove to the country to talk. The day before had been Donny's birthday. The following dialogue took place:

Counselor: So, how was your birthday?

Donny: All right, I guess.

Counselor: What happened?

Donny: Not much.

Counselor: Well, I mean, did you have a birthday cake, or did anyone say, "Happy Birthday"?

Donny: Nope.

Counselor: How did that feel?

Donny: All right, I reckon . . . don't bother me none.

Counselor: Good grief, Donny! It would make me mad as hell . . . hurt my feelings, all kinds of stuff!

Donny: Well, yeah, I did kinda expect my Dad to do something. [Pained expression.] I didn't figure my stepmother would. The hell with 'em.

Counselor: Well, *I'd* like to wish you a happy birthday.

The two talked more about Donny's anger, particularly toward his father, a taboo area before this time. Donny allowed himself the experiencing of his emotions and went on to reveal some of his dreams and hopes for the future, about leaving the past behind, coping with the present, and planning a better life ahead. In the counselor's words: "I felt like we were closer at this point than at any other time in our relationship, and although we had more sessions scheduled, we both seemed to sense that this was the right time to terminate counseling and let Donny get on with his life."

ANNOTATED BIBLIOGRAPHY

Hart, J. T., & Tomlinson, T. M. (Eds.). (1970). *New directions in client-centered therapy.* Boston: Houghton Mifflin.

Resulting from the collaboration of a number of distinguished authors, this book demonstrates the theoretical sophistication and complexity that have come from Rogers' original system. Areas of theory, practice, and research are explored. All of the writers have practiced from a client-centered background and have done research related to therapy. The book includes sections on parenting, family therapy, filial therapy, and groups.

Rogers, C. R. (1951). *Client-centered therapy.* Boston: Houghton Mifflin.

Written in a personal rather than an academic style, Rogers describes changes in his thinking and practice and, for the first time, attempts to organize and systematize his insights to other fields such as education and counselor training. Colleagues contributed chapters on play therapy, group-centered psychotherapy, and group-centered leadership and administration.

Rogers, C. R. (1961). *On becoming a person: A therapist's view of psychotherapy.* Boston: Houghton Mifflin.

A collection of twenty-one of Rogers' essays, this book was, of all of his own books, his favorite. Not just a book on psychotherapy, it synthesizes the work of his career and applies his therapeutic principles to a variety of human relationships. The essay titled "The Characteristics of a Helping Relationship" has been reprinted in journals of many professions, and the questions Rogers asked at that time are still being asked by those who choose a person-centered approach toward helping.

Rogers, C. R. (1980). *A way of being.* Boston: Houghton Mifflin.

A compilation of personal experiences, thoughts, feelings, and beliefs, this book is a testament to Rogers' ever active mind, keen intellect, honesty, integrity, and faith in people and community. The book also provides final thoughts on person-centered theory and its extensions.

REFERENCES

Andronico, M. P., Fidler, J., Guerney, B. J., Jr., & Guerney, L. F. (1967). The combination of didactic and dynamic elements in filial therapy. *International Journal of Group Psychotherapy, 17,* 10-17.

Axline, V. (1947). *Play therapy.* Boston: Houghton Mifflin.

Beier, E. G. (1975). Client-centered therapy and the involuntary client. In W. Walsh (Ed.), *Counseling with children and adolescents: An anthology of contemporary techniques.* Berkeley, CA: McCutchan.

Belkin, D. S. (1980). *Contemporary psychotherapies.* Chicago: Rand McNally.

Bessell, H. (1970). *Methods in human development: Theory manual.* El Cajou, CA: Human Development Training Institute.

Bessell, H. (1969-1974). *Human development program: Activities guides—Level BI, II, III, IV, V, VI.* El Cajou, CA: Human Development Training Institute.

Bohart, A. C., & Todd, J. (1988). *Foundations of clinical and counseling psychology.* New York: Harper and Row.

Boy, A., & Pine, G. J. (1963). *Client-centered counseling in the secondary school.* Boston: Houghton Mifflin.

Boy, A. V., & Pine, G. J. (1982). *Client-centered counseling: A renewal.* Boston: Allyn & Bacon.

Canfield, J., & Wells, H. C. (1976). *100 ways to enhance self-concept in the classroom: A handbook for teachers and parents.* Englewood Cliffs, NJ: Prentice-Hall.

Carkhuff, R. R. (1969). *Helping and human relations: A primer for lay and professional helpers* (Vols. I & II). New York: Holt, Rinehart & Winston.

Carkhuff, R. R. (1971). Training as a preferred mode of treatment. *Journal of Counseling Psychology, 18,* 123-131.

Carkhuff, R. R., & Berenson, B. G. (1967). *Beyond counseling and therapy* (1st ed.). New York: Holt, Rinehart & Winston.

Corey, G. (1982). *Theory and practice of counseling and psychotherapy* (2nd ed.). Monterey, CA: Brooks/Cole.

Corsini, R. J. (1979). *Current psychotherapies* (2nd ed.). Itasca, IL: Peacock.

Dinkmeyer, D., Sr., & Dinkmeyer, D., Jr., (1982). *Developing understanding of self and others (DUSO) 1 and 2, revised.* Circle Pines, MN: American Guidance Service.

Dinkmeyer, D. D., & McKay, G. (1976). *Systematic training for effective parenting.* Circle Pines, MN: American Guidance Service.

Dorfman, E. (1951). Play therapy. In C. Rogers, *Client-centered therapy.* Boston: Houghton Mifflin.

Dupont, H., Gardner, O. S., & Brody, D. S. (1974). *Toward affective development.* Circle Pines, MN: American Guidance Service.

Egan, G. (1975). *The skilled helper: A model for systematic helping and interpersonal relating.* Monterey, CA: Brooks/Cole.

First things: Social reasoning. (1974). Pleasantville, NY: Guidance Associates.

First things: Values. (1972). Pleasantville, NY: Guidance Associates.

Gazda, G. M. (1973). *Human relations development: A manual for educators.* Boston: Allyn & Bacon.

Gazda, G. M. (1977). *Human relations development: A manual for educators* (2nd ed.). Boston: Allyn & Bacon.

Gendlin, E. T. (1974). Client-centered and experiential psychotherapy. In D. Wexler & L. Rice (Eds.). *Innovations in client-centered therapy.* New York: John Wiley.

Glasser, W. (1969). *Schools without failure.* New York: Harper and Row.

Gordon, T. (1970). *Parent effectiveness training.* New York: Peter H. Wyden.

Gordon, T. (1974). *Teacher effectiveness training.* New York: David McKay.

Guerney, B. G., Jr. (1964). Filial therapy: Discussion and rationale. *Journal of Counsulting Psychology, 28,* 304-310.

Guerney, B. G., Jr., (1977). *Relationship enhancement.* San Francisco: Jossey-Bass.

Guerney, B. G., Jr., Guerney, L. F., & Andronico, M. P. (1966, March). Filial therapy. *Yale Scientific Magazine.*

Hart, J. T., & Tomlinson, T. M. (Eds.). (1970). *New directions in client-centered therapy.* Boston: Houghton Mifflin.

Ivey, A., & Simek-Downing, L. (1980). *Counseling and psychotherapy: Skills, theories, and practice.* Englewood Cliffs, NJ: Prentice-Hall.

Keat, D. B. (1974). *Fundamentals of child counseling.* Boston: Houghton Mifflin.
Kirschenbaum, H. (1979). *On becoming Carl Rogers.* New York: Dell.
Lavant, R. F. (1978a). Client-centered approaches to working with the family: An overview of new developments in therapeutic educational, and preventive methods. *International Journal of Family Counseling, 6,* 31-44.
Lavant, R. F. (1978b). Family therapy: A client-centered perspective. *Journal of Marriage and Family Counseling, 40,* 35-42.
Moustakas, C. (1953). *Children in play therapy.* New York: McGraw-Hill.
Muro, J., & Dinkmeyer, D. (1977). *Counseling in the elementary and middle school: A pragmatic approach.* Dubuque, IA: William C. Brown.
Nelson, R. (1972). *Guidance and counseling in the elementary school.* New York: Holt, Rinehart & Winston.
Patterson, C. H. (1973). *Theories of counseling and psychotherapy.* New York: Harper and Row.
Prochaska, J. O. (1979). *Systems of psychotherapy: A transtheoretical analysis.* Homewood, IL: Dorsey Press.
Raskin, N. J., & Van deer Veen, F. (1970). Client-centered family therapy: Some clinical and research perspectives. In J. T. Hart & T. M. Tomlinson (Eds.), *New directions in client-centered therapy.* Boston: Houghton Mifflin.
Reisman, J. M. (1973). *Principles of psychotherapy with children.* New York: John Wiley.
Rogers, C. R. (1939). *The clinical treatment of the problem child.* Boston: Houghton Mifflin.
Rogers, C. R. (1942). *Counseling and psychotherapy.* Boston: Houghton Mifflin.
Rogers, C. R. (1951). *Client-centered therapy.* Boston: Houghton Mifflin.
Rogers, C. R. (1957). The necessary and sufficient conditions of therapeutic personality change. *Journal of Consulting Psychology, 21,* 95-103.
Rogers, C. R. (1959). A theory of therapy, personality, and interpersonal relationships as developed in the client-centered framework. In S. Koch (Ed.), *Psychology: A study of a science (Vol. III): Formulations of the person and the social context.* New York: McGraw-Hill.
Rogers, C. R. (1961a). *On becoming a person: A therapist's view of psychotherapy.* Boston: Houghton Mifflin.
Rogers, C. R. (1961b). The process equation of psychotherapy. *American Journal of Psychotherapy, 15,* 27-45.
Rogers, C. R. (1969). *The freedom to learn: A view of what education might become.* Columbus, OH: Charles Merrill.
Rogers, C. R. (1970a). Forward. In J. T. Hart & T. M. Tomlinson, *New directions in client-centered therapy.* Boston: Houghton Mifflin.
Rogers, C. R. (1970b). *Carl Rogers on encounter groups.* New York: Harper and Row.
Rogers, C. R. (1972). *Becoming partners: Marriage and its alternatives.* New York: Delacorte Press.
Rogers, C. R. (1977). *Carl Rogers on personal power.* New York: Delacorte Press.
Rogers, C. R. (1980). *A way of being.* Boston: Houghton Mifflin.

Rogers, C. R. (1983). *Freedom to learn for the 1980s.* Columbus, OH: Merrill.
Rogers, C. R. (1985). Toward a more human science of the person. *Journal of Humanistic Psychology, 25,* 7-24.
Rogers, C. R., & Dymond, R. (1954). *Psychotherapy and personality change.* Chicago: University of Chicago Press.
Rogers, C. R., Gendlin, E. T., Kiesler, D. J., & Truax, C. B. (Eds.). (1967). *The therapeutic relationship and its impact: A study of psychotherapy with schizophrenics.* Madison, WI: University of Wisconsin Press.
Rogers, C. R., & Rablen, R. (1958). *A scale of process on psychotherapy.* Unpublished manuscript, University of Wisconsin.
Rogers, C. R., & Sanford, R. C. (1984). Client-centered psychotherapy. In H. I. Kaplan & B. J. Sadock (Eds.). *Comprehensive textbook of psychiatry* (Vol. 4). Boston: Williams & Wilkins.
Silberman, M. L., Allender, J. S., & Yanoff, J. M. (1976). *Real learning: A sourcebook for teachers.* Boston: Little, Brown.
Simon, S. (1973). *I am loveable and capable: A modern allegory on the classical put-down.* Niles, IL: Argus.
Simon, S., Howe, L., & Kirschenbaum, H. (1972). *Values clarification: A handbook of practical strategies for teachers and students.* New York: Hart.
Smith, M. L., Glass, G. V., & Miller, T. I. (1980). *The benefits of psychotherapy.* Baltimore: Johns Hopkins University Press.
Thompson, C. L., & Poppen, W. A. (1979). *Guidance activities for counselors and teachers.* Monterey, CA: Brooks/Cole.
Thompson, C. L., & Rudolph, L. B. (1988). *Counseling children* (2nd ed.). Pacific Grove, CA: Brooks/Cole.
Truax, C. B., & Carkhuff, R. R. (1967). *Toward effective counseling and psychotherapy.* Chicago: Aldine Press.
Wexler, D., & Rice, L. (Eds.). (1974). *Innovations in client-centered therapy.* New York: John Wiley.

Chapter 6

Behavioral Approaches

Douglas T. Brown, Ph.D.
H. Thompson Prout, Ph.D.

INTRODUCTION

The behavioral approach to therapeutic change is rooted in learning theory concepts, originally formulated in experimental psychology laboratories. The terms *behavior modification, behavior therapy,* and *cognitive behavior therapy* refer to the types of intervention utilized by behaviorally oriented practitioners. Although the terms are used interchangeably, behavior modification often refers to operantly oriented procedures whereas behavior therapy is more often associated with classical conditioning-based procedures. The entire field of behavior therapy represents a wide variety of learning theory-based techniques. Much of the terminology and many of the basic concepts used by behavior therapists in conducting interventions are borrowed from learning principles first demonstrated by psychologists doing research with animals and humans in well-controlled experimental settings. In fact, the methodology and procedures of behavior therapy were well known before they were widely applied to clinical problems.

The behavioral view of human functioning is based on the assumption that most behavior, abnormal or undesirable and normal or desirable, is the result of learning. Environmental influences and factors, which include how people respond to our behaviors, are seen as the key etiological factor in most psychological disorders. Relying heavily on the scientific approach to problem solving, the behavioral therapist will use a systematic, objective, and data-based approach to developing interventions. Behavioral treatment involves the application of learning principles to help the client eliminate maladaptive behaviors or to learn more adaptive modes of functioning.

History and Status

John Watson (Watson & Raynor, 1920) is generally viewed as the father of behaviorism as a result of the now-classic experiment with a child known as "little Albert." Albert was a child who had previously not demonstrated any fear when presented with white, furry, animal-like objects. In the experiment, Albert was exposed to a white rat and, at the same time, a loud noise. After several trials of pairing the rat with the noise, Albert showed a strong fear response when presented with the rat alone. The fear response also generalized to other white, furry objects (e.g., cotton, rabbits). This experiment was significant because it clearly demonstrated that human emotional responses could be developed through a learning paradigm. This circumstance was in contrast to the dominant psychoanalytic views of the time that focused on intrapsychic and unconscious drives which allegedly accounted for most significant human emotions.

Shortly after the "little Albert" experiment, Mary Cover Jones (1924) reported a case study of a rabbit-phobic child. Jones, through a gradual, graded exposure of the child to a rabbit and the association of the exposure with food for the child, was able to eliminate the fear response to the point that the child was able to pet the rabbit at the end of the treatment. This case is recognized as one of the first applications of learning principles to a clinical problem and is viewed as a precursor of systematic desensitization and other fear- and anxiety-reducing procedures.

While experimental research continued, it was not until the 1950s that behaviorists began to look more closely at human problems. During this decade, three important works were published that essentially provided the theoretical base for most of the behavior therapy and behavior modification techniques utilized today. In 1950, Dollard and Miller published *Personality and Psychotherapy,* which attempted to integrate psychoanalytic theory and learning theory. They reformulated and translated the then popular psychoanalytic theory and concepts into learning theory, stimulus-response language. Although this work did not refute or dismiss psychoanalytic theory, it offered an alternative behavioral view of interpreting personality and the psychotherapeutic process. B. F. Skinner's book *Science and Human Behavior* (1953) extended the use of operant principles to solving human problems. Skinner's work provided the base of operant methodology, criticized the psychoanalytic view of human functioning, and strongly advocated a scientific approach to clinical work, emphasizing observable behavior as the focus of therapeutic change. Skinner did not deny the existence or importance of private, internal events but felt that these events were too subjective to deal with effectively in a scientific approach to changing human behavior. In 1958, Joseph Wolpe published *Psychotherapy by Reciprocal Inhibition,* which dealt with learning theory approaches for treating adult neurotic disorders. Utilizing a classical conditioning base and viewing anxiety as a key determinant in neurotic disorders, Wolpe developed the basic procedures for systematic desensitization.

Bandura (1969) is credited with the recognition of the importance of observational learning in both the acquisition and change of behavior. Bandura (1977) has also developed a social learning theory that involves elements of operant, classical, and observational learning to explain behavior. This approach emphasizes multiple influences on behavior and the importance of the environment and social context and offers a comprehensive framework for explaining behavior in general (Kazdin, 1980). The social learning view probably best represents what would be the orientation of an eclectic behavior therapist. Lazarus' (1976) multimodal behavior therapy, which emphasizes a comprehensive behavioral view of problem definition and intervention, is quite compatible with the social learning view.

Meichenbaum (1977) is generally credited with developing the area of cognitive behavior modification. His procedures involve the use of behavioral techniques for modifying thought patterns generally associated with dysfunctional or abnormal behavior. Meichenbaum believes that thought patterns and environmental influences are interactive in producing behaviors.

Thus, behavioral interventions should concentrate on both areas in order to be effective.

From the late 1960s to the present, an enormous number of behavioral techniques were developed, applied, and researched. Techniques have included systematic desensitization, relaxation training, anxiety management training, emotional flooding, self-control procedures, aversive procedures, token economies, behavioral contingency contracting, modeling, and cognitive behavior modification, to name a few. Behavioral approaches have been applied to problems of anxiety, depression, aggression, lack of assertiveness, psychosis, social skill difficulties, addiction, sexual dysfunction, eating disorders, psychosomatic disorders, academic skill difficulties, marital and family dysfunctions, delinquency, withdrawal, enuresis, encopresis, etc. Thus, with the wide variety of techniques and applications, it is rather difficult to point to one set of procedures and say that they are representative of behavior therapy.

The "explosion" of behavior therapy in the last 20 years has yielded a number of journals that present almost exclusively articles on behavioral approaches to human problems. Among these journals are *Behavior Research and Therapy, Behavior Therapy, Journal of Applied Behavior Analysis, Cognitive Therapy and Research, Behavioral Assessment, Behavioral Counseling Quarterly,* and *Behavior Modification.* Many of the major professional groups have divisions or interest groups on behavioral approaches. The *Association for the Advancement of Behavior Therapy* (AABT), located in New York City, is the largest and most established organization dedicated to behavior therapy. It is a multidisciplinary organization that holds an annual convention, publishes journals and other publications, and sponsors training for those interested in behavior therapy.

OVERVIEW OF THEORY

Basic Theory and Assumptions

The behavioral approach to counseling and psychotherapy rests on a number of basic assumptions (Rimm & Masters, 1979):

1. *The behavioral approach tends to focus on specific behaviors rather than on presumed internal, underlying causes.* Where-

as other approaches view behaviors as symptoms of underlying psychopathology, the behaviorist sees these behaviors as the primary focus of intervention. Internal and unobservable events such as cognitions, self-verbalizations, and physiological reactions (e.g., anxiety) are considered in treatment but by virtue of how they mediate observable behaviors. The behavioral approach considers external stimuli or events as being the most influential of the behavioral determinants, rejecting the medical model or traditional psychodynamic view of internal stimuli or states as being primary factors. Further, behavior therapists do not accept the concept of psychological traits as primary behavioral determinants. More emphasis is placed on the situational aspects of behavior. The behavior therapist will not focus on changing these internal states as a goal of treatment. These internal states, as compared with overt behaviors, are seen as less accessible and reliable and more subjective; and apparent changes in these internal psychological states do not necessarily result in behavior change and improved functioning.

2. *Maladaptive behaviors are acquired through the same principles of learning as are "normal" behaviors.* The way an individual learns behaviors is a product of the environment and the individual's unique learning history. However, the basic learning mechanisms are the same for "normal" and for "abnormal" behavior. Other theories view pathology as a result of a different psychological process. For example, behavioral research has shown that aggressive behaviors can be learned through observation of an adult model (Bandura, Ross, & Ross, 1963). Similarly, we know that more appropriate social behaviors (e.g., social skills) are also learned through modeling. Thus, two behaviors, one undesirable and the other desirable, are learned through the same mechanism of learning–modeling.

3. *The behaviorist uses psychological and learning principles as the basis for developing interventions to modify maladaptive*

behavior. Because the behavioral approach assumes that most behaviors are acquired via learning, the behaviorist further assumes that maladaptive behaviors can be modified by employing the learning principles that apparently resulted in the maladaptive behavior and will use established principles in developing treatment categories.

4. *The behavioral approach involves setting specific, defined goals for intervention.* Goals of treatment are often stated in a form that allows for objective, preferably measurable, assessment of treatment progress. The alleviation of specific problems, the reduction of certain problem behaviors, or the acquisition of new, desirable behaviors would be appropriate goals. The behavior therapist would attempt, for example, to identify specific situations and problem areas related to a client's reported generalized "unhappiness."
5. *The behavior therapist selects his or her intervention techniques to deal specifically with the client's unique problems.* Some forms of traditional counseling and psychotherapy utilize essentially the same approach, regardless of the client's presenting problems. For example, a nondirective play therapist might treat both an anxious child and an aggressive child in a similar fashion. The behavior therapist, on the other hand, might provide desensitization for the anxious child and develop a reinforcement program for the aggressive child. These two sets of techniques are vastly different, yet both have a learning theory base.
6. *Behavior therapy focuses on present behavior and social contexts.* The notion of psychological insight as being curative is generally rejected by behaviorists. Individual historical data are seen as important only as they relate directly to the current problem behaviors from a learning theory standpoint. The behavior therapist will focus on present behaviors and current social context factors which seem to be maintaining problematic behaviors.

Learning or Conceptual Bases

As has been mentioned several times above, the behavioral approach utilizes learning principles to assess problem behaviors and develop interventions. The four major types of learning or conceptual bases are classical conditioning, operant conditioning, observational learning, and cognitive learning.

CLASSICAL CONDITIONING. Classical conditioning focuses on involuntary or reflex behaviors. Various stimuli in the environment automatically evoke or elicit reflex responses. Startle responses to loud noises and salivating with food in the mouth are respondents or unconditional responses. These are learned, automatic, or involuntary responses. However, responses can also be learned through classical conditioning in which a previously neutral stimulus begins to yield a reflex response, usually through repeated associations of the stimulus with some unconditional stimulus. Phobias are often respondent behaviors. The famous "little Albert" case noted above is an example of a classically conditioned fear response. In classical conditioning, the stimuli or events which *precede* the behavior are viewed as the controlling influence in behavior. Wolpe's (1958) systematic desensitization is a behavior therapy procedure based on classical conditioning principles (Kazdin, 1980).

OPERANT CONDITIONING. Operant behaviors are viewed as voluntary behaviors which are spontaneously and freely emitted by the individual. These behaviors are developed and controlled by the consequences which follow them. Whether a behavior is strengthened (increased) or weakened (decreased) is a function of the consequences or events that follow the behavior. In general, behaviors that increase following a desirable consequence are strengthened by positive reinforcement. Behaviors that decrease following an undesirable consequence are weakened through punishment. Behaviors that decrease because reinforcement has ceased to occur are weakened by extinction. For example, children who receive teacher praise for homework completion and who increase their completion rate might be said to have had their academic behaviors strengthened by positive reinforcement. If, on the other hand, the teacher gives no praise for the desirable behavior (i.e., does not strengthen the behavior by positive reinforcement), the behavior would decrease. A comprehensive set of operant procedures and technology is available to the practitioner. (See Kazdin, 1980, and Sulzer-Azaroff & Mayer, 1986.) Most everyday behaviors are operants, and operantly based intervention programs are most often used in applied settings like schools, institutions, and correctional facilities (Kazdin, 1980).

OBSERVATIONAL LEARNING. Observational learning is concerned with learning that occurs when an individual observes another person (i.e., a model) engaging in a certain behavior and then acquires and displays the same or similar behavior. The behavior is learned through the individual's watching the model, and the behavior is said to be imitated. The individual who acquires the new behavior does not have to receive any direct consequences of the behavior for learning to have taken place. For example, a small boy observes his father working with tools. Later, the boy is seen hammering on a piece of wood. The boy has imitated his father's (i.e., the model's) behavior. A variant of observational learning is vicarious reinforcement in which an individual observes a model receiving reinforcement for certain behaviors. The effects of the reinforcement "spread" to others in the environment. For example, a child sees an older sibling receive parental praise for doing household chores. An increase in the younger child's completion of chores would be attributed to vicarious reinforcement (Kazdin, 1980).

In reality, most behaviors are not attributable to any one single type of learning. Most situations have elements of classical, operant, and observational learning, and most problem behaviors are probably acquired through a variety of learning mechanisms. For example, school phobia has been explained from all three learning viewpoints, as follows: a classical view—a child acquires a fear response through associational learning; an operant viewpoint—a child is not reinforced or is punished (e.g., peer taunting) for school attendance; and an observational view—a child observes other children's fear responses. Social learning theory (Bandura, 1977) utilizes elements of the three types of learning to explain behavior and emphasizes multiple influences on behavior that occur in most social contexts. This allows learning theory to account for a broader range of behaviors than the more simplistic explanations provided by any one type of learning alone.

COGNITIVE LEARNING. The cognitive approach in behavior therapy represents one of the more recent developments in the field. The cognitive approach (e.g., Mahoney, 1974; Meichenbaum, 1977), is concerned with cognitions or thoughts, the thinking process, and how cognitions influence emotions and behavior. In part, the cognitive-behavioral view is behavior therapy's response to the criticism that behaviorists are concerned only with observable and measurable behaviors and that important internal events are ignored in treatment and planning. Behavior is viewed as being mediated by cognitions, and, thus, behavior can be modified by a change in thoughts. For example, an impulsive child hurries through his or her schoolwork and the resulting work is sloppy and full of errors. The child is then taught to self-verbalize or silently say to him- or herself cues like "slow down" or "take your time," with the result being neater, more correct work. In this situation, the thought or self-verbalization yielded an observable behavior change. Other cognitive-behavioral approaches focus more on the thought process and how it contributes to maladaptive behaviors and emotions. These approaches are quite similar to rational-emotive therapy and to Beck et al.'s (1979) cognitive therapy.

The behavioral approach in general has not focused much attention on developmental variables. Ross (1980) notes the importance of genetic-constitutional factors and temperamental characteristics in the development of behavior. Social learning theory offers a comprehensive framework for looking at how environmental and learning factors contribute to development. The behavioral approach, however, does not have a developmental age- and stage-bound theory similar to that offered by psychoanalytic theorists. Most behaviorists do consider developmental variables in treatment planning but use them largely in determining the expected ranges of behavior for different age groups and in setting goals. For example, social skills training must be planned with consideration of cognitive and language development variables. We should not expect a 6-year-old to have the vocabulary to conduct a complex social interaction, although the strategies for teaching those skills are available. The behaviorist, lacking a specific developmental theory, must interface interventions with data from child and adolescent development.

VIEW OF PSYCHOPATHOLOGY

Abnormal behavior or psychopathology is not considered as distinct from normal behavior in terms of how it develops and how it is maintained (Kazdin, 1980). It is not a disease process that overwhelms the normal personality. The behavior therapist will shy away from diagnostic labeling and a search for underlying causes for abnormal behavior. The same learning principles that explain normal behavior can also account for abnormal behavior. The determination of what is abnormal is often subjective and influenced by the social context of where the behavior occurs. Crying hysterically at a funeral might be considered normal behavior, but doing the same thing throughout a party might be looked upon as abnormal behavior.

Erwin (1980) noted that the medical model concept of "mental illness" is rejected by behavior therapists, who prefer to substitute terms such as "abnormal behavior," "deviant behavior," "maladaptive behavior," and "problems in living." Although Erwin notes problems with these terms, they do convey meanings different from "mental illness." Abnormalcy and deviance connote both a statistical difference as well as deviance from some social criterion or norm of acceptable behavior. Maladaptive implies that the behavior is preventing optimal functioning or interferes with the acquisition of certain desired goals. Problems in living refer to a similar concept, focusing more on behavior that impedes routine functioning. Erwin further notes that the term "maladaptive characteristics" probably comes closest to covering the concerns focused on by behavior therapists because it includes not only unwanted behaviors, but also images, feelings, and thoughts.

Ross (1980) notes that there is no absolute definition of a psychological disorder. Children's behavior is considered normal when it conforms to the prevailing consensual norm, a norm set by both peers and adults in the environment. Ross has proposed a definition of psychological disorders in children:

> A psychological disorder is said to be present when a child emits behavior that deviates from an arbitrary and relative social norm in that it occurs with a frequency or intensity that authoritative adults in the child's environment judge, under the circumstances, to be either too high or too low. (p. 9)

Implicit in this definition is the concept of viewing behaviors as either deficient or excessive. Rather than utilizing diagnostic labels or global descriptions, the behavior therapist may assess or classify behaviors into one of these categories. A deficit behavior occurs not at all or at too low a rate, with too little intensity, or too slowly. Conversely, an excess behavior occurs at too high a rate, with too much intensity, or for too long. A withdrawn child who fails to approach other children might be termed deficient in pro-social behavior. A hyperactive child might be considered as displaying excessive motor activity.

General Therapeutic Goals and Techniques

Behavior therapy follows a systematic and data-based model of intervention. The assessment and diagnostic phases are not seen as separate components, but as part of a total process. Gottman and Leiblum (1974) and Brown and Brown (1977) have conceptualized counseling and psychotherapy in a systematic step-by-step process. In fact, both approaches use flowchart models to assist the practitioner in systematically planning, developing, and making decisions about interventions. This allows looping back either to reassess a problem or to modify strategies. Although their approaches are not totally intended for the behavior therapist, they are consistent with and based on behavioral intervention principles.

The first step in the intervention process involves deciding who is to be involved in the assessment and intervention phases. This decision is made by determining the setting where the problem is occurring and who are the significant individuals in those settings. For example, if a child is displaying problem behavior both at home and at school, it will be best to see both parents and teachers at some point. It is also important to determine who initiated the referral, how the decision was reached to come for treatment, and what the differing opinions are of those involved on the need for treatment and whether a problem exists.

The second step involves definition and operationalization of the problem. This step may include formulation of target behavior definitions into measurable and/or observable terms. At this point, some general assessment will be made regarding whether the problem represents an excess or deficit behavior. However, the assertion that a problem exists as the result of a performance discrepancy may mean that the child's performance or behavior does not match the expectation of another individual. Although the behavior can be objectively measured and quantified, expectations are more subjective and value based. The discrepancy can exist when, for example, a child's behavior is genuinely excessive or deficient, or when the expectation of the adult is too rigid. A child who receives a *B* on a report card with all the rest of the grades *A* would not generally be considered academically deficient. Yet, a parent with an expectation of all *A*s might label this a problem. This would appear to be a problem of very high expectations, rather than a child behavior difficulty. Thus, the assessment at this phase focuses not only on the behaviors, but also on the norms of the referral sources.

The third step involves collecting base-line data on the problem or target behaviors. In behavioral therapies, this may include direct observation with collection of frequency data to more subjective ratings of the intensity of a problem. This step has a goal of obtaining a representative sample of the current level of the problem behavior, with this level assessed in a quantifiable fashion. An overactive child's problem may be described by the number of times the child is out of his or her seat in school. An anxious high school student may report ratings from 0 to 10 to describe anxiety experienced at various times during the day. Related to this data collection phase may be an assessment of the environments the child is in to determine what environmental factors may be contributing to the problem and to determine what learning mechanisms may be operating.

A fourth step involves negotiating a contract with the clients and setting treatment objectives or goals. The goals will ordinarily be stated in quantifiable form so that both client and therapist can agree that the goal has been met.

The fifth step is the beginning of the actual intervention. Depending on the results of the previous assessments, the therapist will choose from the variety of behavioral techniques available. The intervention will be designed to meet the unique problems presented. The overactive child may respond to a reinforcement program, whereas desensitization may help the anxious adolescent.

The sixth step involves the monitoring of the intervention. Data is collected periodically and systematically during the intervention phase. The process permits modification of the behavioral strategy if change does not occur, as well as determining when the goals have been met.

Finally, the behavior therapist plans strategies to insure that desirable changes are maintained and that these changes are transferred to settings other than those where the treatment may have been focused. At this point, the therapist is concerned with insuring that a reduction in overactive behavior in the classroom is generalized to the home and other environments. The therapist teaches coping skills to the adolescent who has become anxious about current problems so that he or she will be better able to handle anxious situations in the future.

The behavioral approach to therapy presents some distinct practices:

1. It is systematic, objective, and orderly.

2. Assessment and intervention are interrelated and interdependent functions.

3. It focuses on monitoring of change and modifying of strategies if necessary, i.e., the flowchart conceptualization.

4. It is data-based, emphasizing operationalization of problems.

5. It emphasizes interventions which are based on learning principles but which are uniquely designed to deal with the specific problems presented.

APPLICATIONS WITH CHILDREN

Children present a unique challenge to the applied behavior therapist. Although most of the behavior of young children appears to be governed by operant conditions which are externally controlled, the rapid development of cognition changes the nature of therapeutic interventions across various mental age levels. However, for the most part, behavior analysis with children is highly performance-based (Sulzer-Azaroff & Reese, 1982). Thus, all of the terminology used to define pathology is operationalized so that its rate and duration may be accurately measured. Intervention techniques are designed to provide experimental paradigms which result in the identification of the antecedents and consequences surrounding a given behavior. Thus, although a behavior therapist may look at the precipitating factors leading to a child's pathological behavior, the focus is on identifying specific procedures which will yield more acceptable behavior patterns. With younger children the procedure utilized is usually highly "noncognitive." That is, little attempt is made to use intrinsic reinforcement systems and to modify behavior by modifying cognitive structures. A high degree of precision in controlling external environmental stimuli is thus required.

Operant Techniques

In very young children, operant techniques have been utilized for modifying vocalization behavior such as crying and tantrums (Etzel & Gewirtz, 1967). It has been demonstrated that the level of vocalization in infants is dependent on specific patterns of adult reinforcement (Weisberg, 1963). It has also been established that social learning principles control a wide array of deviant behaviors in very young children, including uncontrolled crying, anxiety, regressed motor development, and delayed language.

Behavior therapy has been particularly successful in dealing with incontinence and toilet training in young children. Foxx and Azrin (1973a) have described a technique for the rapid toilet training of young children. Their technique requires that the child be able to respond to verbal instructions and to exhibit a minimal amount of social imitation skill. Generally, the technique requires that the following procedures be implemented:

1. Disturbing stimuli be minimized during the operant conditioning phase.
2. A high number of urination trials be produced by increased fluid intake in order to increase the number of positive reinforcements provided per unit time.
3. Precise delivery of operant reinforcement for correct toileting behavior. This includes exact timing of reinforcement so that it is delivered at the termination of the appropriate behavior.
4. Reinforcement of all component skills such as raising of pants, flushing of toilet, etc.
5. Use of high-quality reinforcers such as food and physical contact.
6. Use of a variety of reinforcers with a high level of frequency (continuous reinforcement).
7. Use of a high degree of verbal instruction.
8. Negative reinforcement for "accidents," such as continuous reprimands, etc.
9. Gradual fading of all prompts and reinforcers.

Utilizing this training technique, Foxx and Azrin have been able to demonstrate that children can be effectively toilet trained in 1 to 2 days and that this behavior can be stabilized within 1 month. Physiological maturation and developmental age level are important factors, with children in the 26- to 36-month range being most susceptible to this technique.

Generally, operant techniques have been very successful with overt behavior in very young children. At this age, however, most behaviors have readily identifiable antecedents. It is difficult to label a given behavior as "pathological" because few behaviors meet the criterion of being enduring personality characteristics.

In addition, language per se is not necessary to implement a behavior therapy approach with young children. These techniques are also utilized primarily by adults in the child's ecological milieu rather than by professional therapists working in more restrictive environments. The relative susceptibility of young children to operant techniques significantly improves the likelihood of success using behavior therapy.

Fears and Phobias

Fears and phobias have been studied more widely in adults than in children. It is only with the relatively recent realization that children suffer from various anxiety disorders that childhood phobias have been investigated more intensely. In behavior therapy, Watson first described phobic reactions in the case of "little Albert" (Waston & Raynor, 1920) discussed above. Watson was able to demonstrate that nonfearful stimuli can be made fearful through association and that such phobic reactions tend to generalize to a number of similar stimuli. Thus, in the case of little Albert almost all furry objects produced phobic responses.

Longitudinal studies indicate that fears and phobias of children persist into adulthood and possibly worsen (Ollendick, 1983; Ollendick & Cerny, 1981). Persistent maladaptive fears are present in an estimated 3% to 8% of children. In many cases, fears and phobias drastically interfere with the child's academic and social development or play a role in the development of behavior problems that adversely affect the family and school systems. A number of studies (Fox & Houston, 1983; Houston, Fox, & Forbes, 1984) have shown that state anxiety, trait anxiety, and high stress in children are related to decrements in performance in a variety of settings. In addition, those children with high cognitive state anxiety tend to exhibit somatic disorders either in childhood or in later life. Reynolds and Paget (1983) have suggested that self-esteem is also adversely affected by high states of stress and anxiety and that, in turn, stress and anxiety are affected by low levels of self-esteem.

Between the ages of 48 and 72 months, children develop fears of imaginary objects. Fears of this type are complex and tend to vary across a number of dimensions including health, race, socioeconomic status, and parental upbringing (Kennedy, 1971).

Some of the more common phobias include fear of school, of bodily injury, of the dark, of animals, of other children, of adults, and of strange places. Phobias tend to be acquired along several dimensions. First, children tend to acquire many of their parents' fears. Second, learned fear of a given object tends to generalize easily to other similar objects. And finally, it appears that phobias can be conditioned and unconditioned with relative ease by using operant techniques.

A number of general approaches have been used with fears and phobic reactions in children. These approaches include systematic desensitization, emotive imagery, muscular relaxation, reciprocal inhibition, and reinforced practice. In addition, self-monitoring and self-control have been stressed by recent studies (Ollendick, 1983; Ollendick & Cerny, 1981; O'Mara & Graziano, 1974). In this technique children are taught to monitor and record their fear reactions and to utilize pleasant scenes to inhibit the fear.

Systematic desensitization involves teaching the child relaxation skills and then exposing the child to a hierarchy of fears beginning with the least emotionally arousing stimulus. This exposure can be "in vivo" or through the use of films or imagery. As the therapist progresses through the hierarchy of fears, the child is taught how to relax in the presence of fear-evoking stimuli. Some children have difficulty achieving deep muscle relaxation either through lack of attention, cooperation, or motor ability. They may also be unable to achieve vivid enough images to allow for deconditioning with relaxation. Other more concrete counter-conditioning agents may be necessary such as food, music, or play therapy.

SCHOOL PHOBIA. Children who are school phobic suffer extreme anxiety when faced with the prospect of going to school. They may be unable to eat, may complain of a variety of somatic ailments (e.g., stomachaches, headaches, fatigue) and may experience high rates of tardiness, absenteeism, and illness (Rhine & Spaner, 1983). Some children who are school phobic may also be depressed and withdrawn, frequently remaining at home, often without the parents' knowledge (Boyd, 1980; Trueman, 1984). Many school-phobic children exhibit anxieties regarding school performance. They constantly seek approval and worry excessively about their competence in a variety of areas. Children with school phobia are also often in an enmeshed relationship with one or both parents, most often the mother.

Kennedy (1965) has suggested that two classes of school phobia exist: Type I and Type II. Type I school phobia is described as an actual school-related phobic reaction. Type II school phobia is a more generalized phobic reaction related to school and numerous other environments. Children exhibiting Type I school phobia have a number of characteristic behaviors including acute onset of the phobic reaction, lower grades in school, questionable physical health of their mother, and expressed concern about death. In general, Type I phobics have parents who have questionable health but are otherwise well-adjusted. Type II phobics tend to be more chronic, are more likely to occur in the upper elementary grades, and come from families in which the communication patterns are poor and in which a more generalized disturbance is present.

Kennedy suggests that a number of conditions must be met in the behavioral treatment of school phobia in order to achieve success. These include:

1. The establishment of good professional interaction between the school system and the behavior therapist.

2. Enforced school attendance through the cooperation of the parents and behavior therapist.

3. The amelioration of the child's somatic complaints by refusal to deal with them on the part of both parents and the behavior therapist.

4. An intensively structured home-based program for the parents in order to give them the confidence necessary to deal with the child.

5. A brief interview/interaction with the child by the behavior therapist to explain the contingencies of the treatment.

6. Continuous follow-up with the parents by the behavior therapist and, if necessary, in-home intervention by the

behavior therapist to provide modeling and instruction regarding appropriate parental behaviors.

Children with Type I phobias are more successfully treated by the above techniques than those with Type II phobias. It is often necessary to use more intensive anxiety desensitization procedures with children suffering from Type II phobias in order to treat them effectively.

DIRECT DECONDITIONING OF CHILDHOOD PHOBIAS. Wish, Hasazi, and Jurgela (1975) have described a process for the direct deconditioning of a variety of childhood phobias. Whereas deconditioning techniques have been utilized extensively with adults, it is only recently that they have been used with childhood phobic reactions. In this procedure, feared or phobic stimuli are paired with pleasant events. In addition, systematic desensitization is used. The first step in the procedure is to establish a fear hierarchy. This is done by having the child rate the level of fear associated with a variety of similar stimuli. In the second step of the procedure, the child undergoes progressive relaxation utilizing a modified technique such as that described by Keat (1979). The third step of treatment involves the self-administration of the deconditioning procedure. Here the feared stimuli are paired in some meaningful way with pleasurable stimuli over successive trials. Wish et al. (1975) describe this procedure specifically for a child experiencing phobic reactions to loud sounds:

> The deconditioning procedure was accomplished in the following way. The record album, a pleasurable record album, which was forty minutes in length, was recorded on four tracks of an 8 track stereo tape. The remaining four tracks of the tape were used to superimpose the feared stimuli (sounds in the fear hierarchy) upon the ongoing music. Each sound was presented five times on the tape with an average of approximately 30 seconds between sounds. Order of sound presentation was based upon the subjective unit of disturbance ratings, with least feared sounds being presented earliest in the tape. Feared sounds were obtained from a series of profes-

> sional sound effects recordings. After the tape was completed, it was transferred to an 8 track stereo tape cartridge and given to the child. (p. 298)

Utilizing this technique it is possible to reduce most learned phobic reactions in a relatively short time. Basically, the success of systematic desensitization rests on the ability of the behavior therapist to recondition responses passively by associating them with other responses which are incompatible with anxiety (i.e., relaxation). As incompatible responses are paired with increasing levels of the phobic stimulus, they eventually displace the fear reaction. As we will see later, this general technique is used to reduce a number of anxiety-related behaviors.

Social Isolation and Withdrawal

Some children develop fears and phobias of being ignored, ridiculed, or attacked by other children. Such a child can be described as socially isolated (Ross, 1980). Like other phobias, this behavior tends to worsen over time and to result in considerable withdrawal behavior on the part of the child. It is critical that intervention be undertaken as soon as possible in order to break this cycle. A number of techniques have been developed for this purpose, including the teaching of social skills through modeling and other forms of therapy which maximize peer interaction. Strain, Shores, and Timm (1977) developed a social skills training procedure in which other children were used as confederates in increasing overt social behavior of isolated children. They asked their confederates to approach withdrawn children and solicit social contact. Gresham (1980) has described a variety of modeling techniques which can be used with withdrawn children. These include verbal, symbolic, and live modeling. He has described several procedures, including symbolic modeling through videotapes, abstract modeling, covert modeling through imagery, participant modeling, and self-modeling. Lowenstein (1982) reduced general anxiety in withdrawn children by developing assertiveness in the child's behavior and promoting an improved ability to communicate effectively. Family patterns were investigated to determine factors in the environment that maintained the children's shy and withdrawn behavior. Lowenstein employed implosive therapy in order to prompt and reinforce emotions other than shyness and withdrawal in the presence of discriminative stimuli.

Research with withdrawn children indicates that substantial progress is possible through the consistent use of behavior therapy. As the level of withdrawal increases, however, the number of potential training sessions necessary to effect change increases dramatically. The presence of adequate language is another critical variable in predicting the rate of success with these children.

Enuresis and Encopresis

Enuresis describes a condition in which urine is involuntarily discharged and in which there is no organic pathology present. Nocturnal enuresis occurs in approximately 20% of young children and constitutes a serious violation of social folkways in the perception of most parents. Therefore, the stress placed upon the child regarding this behavior is significant, resulting often in a secondary anxiety condition with other symptoms being exhibited. These symptoms may include somnambulism, eating disorders, and a wide variety of anxiety reactions.

Instrumental conditioning methods have been used with success in the treatment of enuresis (Mowrer & Mowrer, 1938). A number of commercially manufactured devices are available for this purpose. Generally the devices consist of a urine-sensitive pad which is connected to some sort of auditory or tactile stimulus. When the device senses wetness, it responds with either a bell, a mild shock, or a buzzer. It is then the child's responsibility to turn off the alarm.

The general procedure for instrumental conditioning of enuresis involves the gradual shaping of the desired behavior (bladder retention) followed by appropriate reinforcement. This process involves increasing the time frame in which bladder distention cues are present without urination occurring (Kimmel & Kimmel, 1973). The presence of an alarm provides feedback in this process. In the first day of training the child is asked to refrain from urination for approximately 5 to 10 minutes. The child is promised a reinforcement if the task is accomplished.

It is important that this first retention activity be a success and, therefore, be followed by a reward. The time demand is then gradually increased with appropriate reinforcements following successful trials. At night the alarm device provides feedback and, therefore, reinforcement for retention. This process can be supplemented by direct social reinforcement from the parents.

Houts, Liebert, and Padawer (1983) provide convincing experimental evidence on the effectiveness of the bell and pad method for training bladder retention control. Their study included 60 enuretic children ages 4 through 12 involved in 1-hour group training sessions and treatment at home. Some subjects in the study were also treated with imipramine (a drug commonly used to control enuresis). An interesting finding of the study is that the subjects who later relapsed were more likely to have been treated with imipramine than subjects who showed long-term bladder control.

Cognitive control theory has also been used in conjunction with more traditional operant techniques in the treatment of enuresis. Cotugno (1987) reports a study in which children's "self talk" was successfully modified in order to help them achieve better bladder control.

In summary, the procedure for control of enuresis includes: (1) teaching the children to hold urine for longer and longer periods of time before going to the bathroom; (2) introducing large amounts of fluids in order to increase the number of trials; (3) reinforcing the child after urination in an appropriate setting; (4) keeping a careful chart of progress and making the chart available to both the parent and the child; (5) having the child practice starting and stopping the urination stream; and (6) shaping toward independent practice trials on the part of the child.

Encopresis is a term which defines any disturbance of bowel evacuation or retention. This can include either soiling or constipation. In either of these cases, prior to the use of behavior therapy, the child should undergo a thorough physical examination. Although the behavioral etiology is not well understood, it is assumed to be a stress reaction which falls in the general class of anxiety disorders. In some instances it may be an attention-getting device on the part of younger children. Much of the early work of Mowrer and Mowrer (1938) relates directly to the treatment of encopresis. In encopretic children the feedback mechanisms which signal the need to defecate are often dulled or missing. The child becomes unaware that his or her rectum is full. The normal response is that of evacuation, but this response occurs in inappropriate settings. The task of behavior therapy is to develop a stimulus-response link which is socially appropriate. Neale (1973) has described a method of treatment in which instrumental conditioning is used to cause decay of the anxiety response. This is done through reciprocal inhibition where the child is taken to the bathroom at least four times daily and permitted to void while simultaneously receiving positive reinforcement or associating other positive circumstances (e.g., candy) with the experience. As soon as the child has become accustomed to using the bathroom four times a day, this procedure is gradually faded and the child is allowed to use the bathroom as needed. A careful record is kept of defecation, and this record is reviewed by both the behavior therapist and the child.

Other researchers have used cathartics or suppositories in conjunction with behavior therapy. O'Brien, Ross, and Christophersen (1986) investigated a combination of cathartic and behavioral treatment procedures for eliminating diurnal and nocturnal encopresis. They found that independent toiletings resulted after 8 to 39 weeks of treatment using a combination of suppositories, positive practice, time-out, and hourly toilet visits. Ultimately, in the case of all subjects, the suppositories were systematically faded. Brown and Doolan (1983) emphasized the need for detailed analysis of the etiology of individual cases of encopresis and the need for sustained treatment approaches sometimes over lengthy time periods.

The general procedure for the treatment of encopresis includes (1) complete physiological examination to determine any medical abnormalities; (2) correction of any physiological difficulties (i.e., constipation, impaction) by the use of appropriate suppositories or cathartics; (3) use of instrumental conditioning techniques for feedback and reinforcement during appropriate evacuation; (4) the systematic fading of treatment contingencies when bowel control is accomplished; and (5) the use of reciprocal inhibition techniques to associate positive circumstances with evacuation rather than punishment.

Autism and Childhood Psychosis

Autism and childhood schizophrenia are serious child behavioral disturbances which have not been susceptible to traditional modes of therapy. The etiology of these disorders is not agreed upon by various professionals. Thus, specific strategies for their treatment vary tremendously. Although autism is considered a relatively rare disorder, it does have a number of specific behavioral characteristics. Webster (1980) has described these characteristics, including affect isolation, unrelatedness to others, inconsistent developmental continuity, self-destructive behavior, temper tantrums, self-identity confusion, concrete thinking, perceptual inconsistencies, echolalia, physical uncoordination, and language deficits. Kanner (1945) described autism as the inability of the child to relate to people in a natural way that is evident from the beginning of maturation. In addition, the autistic child shows an obsessive-compulsive desire for sameness coupled with perserverative activity.

Childhood schizophrenia is considered by most theorists to differ from autism. Ross (1980) lists several defining characteristics: (1) distorted interpersonal relationships, (2) a distorted concept of self and the relationship of one's body to the environment, (3) preoccupation with specific objects without regard to their use, (4) demand for consistency in the environment, (5) use of speech to communicate bizarre and meaningless content, (6) poor motor coordination and locomotion, and (7) the appearance of retardation with occasional periods of "normality."

Interventions with autistic and other psychotic children are similar. Ferster (1961) has indicated that psychotic children experience a decrement in their developmental process which reduces the general efficiency of reinforcers. Thus, psychotic children do not produce behavior which solicits reinforcement from parents, and this reciprocally reduces the amount and variety of reinforcement which parents provide their children. In the case of autistic children, the absence of language eliminates totally the use of verbal interchange and reinforcement. With other psychotic children the use of bizarre language may severely limit the ability of the parent to provide verbal reinforcement. The primary focus of most behavioral interventions has been on the area of selective attention. Autistics and some childhood schizophrenics develop over-exclusive attention. Thus, these children attend in a perseverative manner to a limited array of stimuli within the environment. Other psychotic children exhibit overinclusive attention on a subset of environmental stimuli. Thus, a major goal for behavior therapy is to generalize the attention span or make it more susceptible to specific environmental stimuli. This goal is accomplished through traditional operant discrimination training techniques.

Foxx and Azrin (1973b) have described a technique called positive practice overcorrection. It has the objective of interrupting self-stimulatory behavior evident in many psychotic children. By injecting an annoying or punishing consequence we teach the child that self-stimulatory behavior is not rewarded. Positive reinforcement is provided for appropriate social interaction and behaviors which are directed to the outward environment of the child. Lovaas, Koegel, Simmons, and Long (1973) have delineated several of the most effective behavioral procedures for use with psychotic children. These include (1) use of food as a contingent primary reinforcer, (2) use of reinforcement withdrawal when necessary, (3) aversive stimulation for self-stimulatory and injurious behavior, (4) modeling of appropriate behaviors, (5) reinforcement of incompatible behaviors, and (6) use of socially reinforcing language experiences.

Brawley, Harris, Allen, Fleming, and Peterson (1973) have described procedures for intervention with autistic children. They first identify appropriate and inappropriate behaviors in a given child. The appropriate behaviors include verbalization of words and phrases, use of objects in their intended mode, and compliance with requests or commands. Inappropriate behaviors include self-stimulation such as hitting, slapping, random verbalizations, withdrawal, and temper tantrums. These behaviors are recorded for a sufficient period to develop an appropriate base line. In the first reinforcement phase, a number of reinforcers are used to determine those which will be most effective. Next, the therapist determines which behaviors the child is capable of imitating and reinforces all appropriate imitations performed by the child (i.e., mimicking of sounds and gestures). In order to encourage appropriate use of materials, the child is directed and reinforced in a number of activities, including hopping, skipping, ball throwing, balance beam walking and other similar tasks. Verbal commands are constantly paired with gestural stimuli. In order to determine if reinforcements have been effective, a reversal period is used to elicit an extinction response. This is followed by a second reinforcement period for a total of 20 to 30 sessions. Brawley and his colleagues have demonstrated an average of 80% success using this methodology.

Autistic and schizophrenic behavior requires utilization of fundamental operant techniques. However, unlike other disorders, the array of reinforcers available to the behavior therapist is limited. These reinforcers tend to saturate rapidly and may or may not have potency on a given day. A major goal of behavior therapy is to establish fundamental language control of the child's behavior. Research has tended to show that relatively lengthy behavioral programming is necessary to effect permanent change in psychotic children. In any case, fundamental goals include establishing social reinforcers and basic language.

APPLICATIONS WITH ADOLESCENTS

A wide variety of anxiety-related disorders occur in adolescence. For behavior therapists the term *anxiety* or *neurosis* refers to a dysfunctional behavior pattern which is under the control of a number of stimulus conditions, many of which are abstract. Some of these stimulus conditions may be totally unknown to the client. The task of the behavior therapist is to determine the environmental contingencies which are associated with the undesirable or dysfunctional behavior pattern. These stimuli may be both external (environmentally controlled) and internal (cognitively controlled). This fact has given rise to two varieties of behavior therapy: the traditional operant variety and cognitive behavior modification as proposed by Meichenbaum (1977).

Anxiety and Phobic Disorders

Ross (1980) has suggested that anxiety may be viewed as a construct. It functions to maintain avoidance behavior in the absence of specific aversive stimuli. Thus, anxiety takes the place of previously associated aversive stimuli. Anxiety in the absence of these aversive stimuli produces a variety of physiological and psychological phenomena, including heightened heart rate, blood pressure, and respiratory rate and a sense of distress. Mowrer (1947) has described anxiety as a classically conditioned autonomic arousal which is causally linked to instrumental avoidance behavior. Bandura (1977) has provided a social learning context for anxiety-related disorders in which children and adolescents acquire, through modeling, characteristics associated with anxiety reactions and irrational behavior.

Many dysfunctional behavior patterns in adolescents are anxiety based. One of the major treatment interventions for these disorders is a procedure called systematic desensitization, which was developed by Wolpe (1958). Wolpe's principle of reciprocal inhibition states that anxiety-related stimuli could be neutralized if they were elicited contiguously with other stimuli antagonistic to anxiety reactions. Thus, if anxiety-evoking stimuli could be associated with relaxation stimuli, then the probability of a generalized anxiety response to a given stimulus could be reduced. Wolpe's technique of progressive relaxation training is well known by many students of behavior therapy. This technique involves the training of the client to relax progressively various sets and subsets of muscles throughout the body and to experience simultaneously a feeling of psychological comfort and well-being. Since imaginary or cognitive stimuli are as effective in eliciting anxiety behavior as other environmental stimuli, Wolpe concluded that these cognitive stimuli could be replaced by other subjective feelings of well-being. A critical aspect of progressive relaxation is the creation of a hierarchy of responses. The client is asked to think of various anxiety-producing stimuli ranging from mildly anxiety producing to very anxiety producing. This is done while the client is deeply relaxed over repeated sessions ranging across the anxiety hierarchy. Each level of the hierarchy is presented until the client can visualize the anxiety-producing experience without responding negatively. Wolpe's desensitization technique has been one of the most effective techniques for anxiety and phobic reduction in adolescents and adults.

Weiner (1973) investigated the deconditioning of neurotic anxiety in adolescents. Obsessive-compulsive neuroses in this group are quite common. It is clear that in such disorders elimination of the conditioned autonomic drives is critical in order for the neurotic behavior to be eliminated. Because compulsive disorders are focused on habits which control the neurosis, it is the task of the behavior therapist to desensitize the person to these stimuli. Weiner described a 15-year-old boy with acute onset of obsessive-compulsive behaviors including washing, dressing, reading, and writing. The boy felt that if these behaviors were not executed something terrible would happen to him or his parents. The major treatment plan involved replacement of the obsessive, maladaptive rituals with a series of other, more delimited rituals that would interfere only moderately with normal activity. In this regard, the adolescent was asked to think of numerous positive reasons for carrying out the obsessive behaviors. In addition, a time limit was devised for each obsessive behavior. Thus, an attempt was made to develop positive environmental stimuli for the obsessive responses. An alternative technique would have been to desensitize the boy to the stimulus conditions themselves. With obsessive-compulsive disorders, it is important to modify conditions so that the link between stimulus and response is broken.

Behavior therapy has also been utilized to treat depressive reactions in adolescents. Depressive reactions are a common response to anxiety. Symptoms of depressive reaction include loss of self-esteem, somnambulism, lack of appetite, and unresponsive social interaction. Libert and Lewinsohn (1973) have demonstrated that clients with depressive reactions show considerably less social skill than their peers. Thus, depressive adolescents emit behaviors which are not positively socially reinforced. When these adolescents encounter traumatic experiences, they respond with depressive behavior. In addition, there is a tendency for prior depressive reactions to increase the future traumatic stimuli. Thus, depression tends to be a cyclical downward spiral in which the depressive behavior elicits nonsocial reinforcement on the part of adolescent peers. The primary behavioral treatment for depressive behavior involves the reinforcement of socially appropriate behaviors and the heightening of the potency of satiated reinforcers. Because the families of depressed adolescents tend inadvertently to reinforce passive and depressive behaviors, it is important to modify this pattern. Family and peer group members must be taught to elicit socially desirable behaviors and to reinforce them appropriately. In addition, the depressed adolescent must be taught to initiate social contact in a variety of situations and to receive reinforcement for this effort. Because many of the stimuli associated with depression are internal and self-generated, these cognitive mediators must also be modified. Cognitive theorists believe that distorted thinking is central to the development of depression in adolescents and children. Self-statement and self-management techniques are often used as means of cognitive restructuring in order to modify internal stimulus conditions which trigger depression and negative self-concept (Clarizio, 1985).

Many behavior therapy procedures described above can also be used with adolescents experiencing hysterical and psychophysiological reactions. In most instances, a social learning framework is the most appropriate vehicle for understanding these disorders. Modification of the external social environment and reinforcement system is critical, together with utilization of techniques such as desensitization, cognitive behavior modification (i.e., thought stopping, stimulus substitution), and, in some instances, aversion therapy.

Treatment of Delinquent Behavior: Aggression and Social Maladjustment

The treatment of antisocial and delinquent behavior has become a major focus in American society. Davidson and Seidman (1975) suggest that the treatment of juvenile delinquency through behavior modification is a relatively recent phenomenon. Behavioral interventions undertaken during the past two decades have shown promising results in modifying various delinquent behaviors. However, because most of the research undertaken with delinquent populations has occurred under poorly controlled conditions, it is difficult to ascertain precisely the impact of behavioral intervention techniques. Davidson and Seidman conclude that more careful delineation of specific delinquent behaviors is needed.

Wright and James (1974) have delineated some of the behavioral content which characterizes delinquent children.

These behaviors include (1) signs of early childhood behavior problems (e.g., excessive temper tantrums, enuresis, encopresis); (2) antisocial behaviors; (3) undisciplined or so-called delinquent behaviors such a school truancy, running away from home, and vandalizing property; and (4) eventual serious illegalities such as larceny, robbery, and assault. A number of environmental factors have been identified which promote delinquency. Delinquent homes typically have single-parent guardianship. In addition, family members are often themselves involved in quasi-legal activities (e.g., prostitution, excessive drinking). This circumstance is coupled with economic insecurity and poor parental supervision. The delinquent is likely to have experienced a number of negative interactions with schools and school personnel. Teachers in school settings are likely to have used negative or aversive stimulation as a means of physical control when dealing with delinquents. In addition, delinquents are likely to have few friends and relatively limited social contacts. Thus, the instances for receiving social reinforcement for appropriate behavior are severely limited.

Sutherland and Cressey (1970) have formulated several hypotheses with regard to the learning patterns of delinquents. They indicate that criminal behavior is learned through a variety of operant techniques including direct social reinforcement and through social modeling. Delinquent behavior is often learned through the adolescent's peer group because it is this group which provides the majority of social reinforcement. The specific group of delinquent behaviors which are learned is totally a function of the reinforcers available and the frequency of their occurrence. The atypical social norms acquired by most delinquents are a function of high rates of reinforcement for antisocial behavior in an environment of relative acceptance for these behaviors. Basically, the level of conditioning for a given delinquent behavior is directly contingent on the amount, frequency, and probability of reinforcement for that behvior. In this regard, Eysenck (1964) has suggested that certain personality traits lead to susceptibility in delinquents. These traits include (1) a high degree of suggestibility, (2) lack of emotional stability, and (3) lack of perseverance.

Basically, there are two behavioral etiologies suggested for the acquisition of delinquent behavior. The first states that delinquents have an inferior ability for socialization. In effect, they are not able to acquire rapidly the conditioned fear responses present in most persons. In the second, social learning theory is used to explain the rapid acquisition of psychopathic behavior present in many delinquents. Bandura and Walters (1963) feel that delinquents have few prosocial models operating in their environments and that they receive greater reinforcement for antisocial behavior both in peer groups and through social learning. Because the dominant subculture stresses aggressive and antisocial behavior, this mode is adopted by the delinquent adolescent.

Various behavioral treatment approaches have been utilized with delinquents. Several principles seem to relate especially well to delinquent populations. First, treatment should be directed toward reinforcement of achievement rather than toward obedience. The selection of positive reinforcers should be done very carefully in order to minimize any satiation effects. When punishment is utilized, it should be administered immediately and consistently when these rules are broken. After punishment, attention should be immediately refocused toward positive behavior with appropriate reinforcements. Generally, when dealing with delinquent populations, consistency is critical if unwanted behaviors are to be extinguished or counter-conditioned.

Bandura (1973) has suggested that much of the aggressive behavior acquired by adolescents is modeled by their peer group. He hypothesizes that new types of aggressive responses can be acquired through observational learning. Further, Bandura feels that the level of aggression may also be influenced by other factors such as frustration and the cultural relativity of the particular aggressive act. If we consider what is known about aggression, several conditions would reduce the probability of its acquisition in adolescents. First, environmental conditions which promote social learning of aggressive behavior should be reduced or eliminated. Second, training should be undertaken to inform parents that permissive treatment, on their part, of aggressive behavior actually acts to reinforce this behavior. Third, reinforcement contingencies should be set up to maximize nonaggressive, cooperative play in children. And finally, parents themselves should be taught not to model aggressive behavior to their children.

A number of other theorists have developed behavioral techniques for dealing with aggressive behavior in children and adolescents (Frankel & Simmons, 1985; Kettlewell & Kausch, 1983; Saylor, Benson, & Einhaus, 1985). Treatment strategies employed include extinction, differential reinforcement of other behaviors, time-out, physical punishment, environmental manipulations, and arousal reduction. Stress inoculation has also been used, including discussion of the components of anger, relaxation, modeling, and rehearsal of adaptive self-statements while in the presence of anger-provoking stimuli. Generally, the results of these studies indicated improved interpersonal problem-solving skills, decreases in fighting and aggressive behavior, and decreases in verbal aggression.

Behavioral contracting has been used extensively in working with delinquents. Contracting is simply a method for determining the exchange of positive reinforcement between two or more people. This is done by delineating the circumstances under which positive reinforcement will occur and, thereby, maximizing the probability that responses emitted by the delinquent will be socially acceptable. Phillips, Phillips, Wolf, and Fixsen (1975) describe a program which employs contracting in conjunction with a token system. The program, known as the *Achievement Place,* uses a three-pronged system in which (1) tasks are assigned, (2) performance is evaluated, and (3) consequences for performance are made explicit. Within the contracting framework, Phillips and his colleagues studied various methods for assigning tasks, including (1) individual versus group-assigned tasks, (2) consequences for individual performance versus consequences for group performance, and (3) a peer managership determined democratically by peers. Generally, their data show that as tasks and consequences are more individualized, they become more effective in producing the desired behavior. Group consequence conditions are not very effective when compared to individual consequence systems. No particular advantage was found to exist for democratically determined group leaders over those appointed on the basis of earned points. Generally, though, an elected managerial system was preferred by adolescents in this project.

Wright and James (1974) have reviewed the array of behavioral programs available to delinquents. These include (1) residential programs in which point economies are used together with response cost systems, (2) part-time residential, community-based programs in which point economies and contingency contracts are used in the programming effort, and (3) nonresidential community-based programs in which contingency contracts are used exclusively. Wright and James suggest that smaller, community-based programs provide the most efficacious solution for delinquent behavior, because behavioral programming can be more closely controlled and related to more realistic settings available in a community. They present cost-benefit data indicating that community-based programs are considerably less expensive than their institutional counterparts. In another community-based study, Stuart (1973) asserts that behavioral contracting may be the major intervention technique that can be acquired by parents and paraprofessionals. Techniques that are effective in home settings must require comparatively small amounts of time and be able to influence a broad array of behaviors. Behavioral contracting meets these criteria. Because the family plays a crucial role in the development and maintenance of delinquent behavior, teaching parents effective behavior management strategies could have significant long-term gains. Stuart has listed a number of assumptions that underlie behavioral contracting in families:

1. The receipt of positive reinforcements and interpersonal exchanges is considered a privilege rather than a right.
2. Effective interpersonal agreements are governed by the norm of reciprocity.
3. The value of an interpersonal exchange is a direct function of the range, rate, and magnitude of positive reinforcements mediated by that exchange.
4. Rules create freedom in interpersonal exchanges.

All behavior contracts are governed by these rules, and as a result many points of family debate are removed because they are covered contractually.

Eating Disorders

Obesity, bulimia, and anorexia nervosa are the major eating disorders associated with adolescent populations. Obesity appears to be familial in that multiple members of a given family are often overweight. A social learning model seems to be the best explanation for this behavior. Schacter (1971) suggests that obese people attend to external cues primarily for the triggering of eating behavior whereas persons of normal weight attend primarily to internal cues. This suggests that the treatment of obesity should focus on the management of external behavioral factors. Treatment of obesity involves a considerable amount of client contracting and, in some cases, family therapy. Successful weight control programs appear to include a combination of physical activity, contracting, maintenance strategies, and appropriate peer reinforcement for weight loss. The treatment of obesity involves a considerable amount of client involvement in the development of goals and in measuring weight change. The primary target behaviors are those which act as discriminative stimuli for eating. The behavior therapist assists the obese client in identifying the range of these cues available in the environment. This range is then narrowed significantly by eliminating the discriminative stimuli. In addition, the array of response behaviors involved in eating itself is modified in order to reduce the amount of food consumed. For example, slower eating behavior is heavily reinforced together with delay of gratification in eating. Some behavior therapists have used aversive stimuli in modifying eating behavior. The most common aversive stimulus applied is social disapproval. In a study by Lansky and Vance (1983), obese high school students were treated in a behavior therapy program. In this program it was found that behavior therapy resulted in significant weight reduction in the experimental group as compared with the control group. Parental participation in the treatment was positively associated with increased weight loss.

Bulimia refers to an eating disorder in which there are recurrent episodes of binge eating of large amounts of food in relatively short periods of time (under 2 hours). These episodes are usually terminated by social interruption, sleep, or self-induced vomiting. Bulimics undergo repeated attempts to lose weight by severely restrictive diets, self-induced vomiting, or the use of cathartics. They have an awareness that their eating pattern is abnormal and suffer chronic anxiety regarding their inability to control it. Depressed mood and reduced self-concept are common correlates of this disorder. Fairburn's (1984) cognitive behavior treatment has been shown to be effective in dealing with bulimia. This treatment involves the following: (1) control over eating patterns, including daily self-monitoring of all behaviors associated with bulimia, is exercised; (2) stimulus control techniques and behaviors incompatible with eating are used to counteract urges to binge; (3) cognitive behavior therapy is employed to identify dysfunctional thoughts and beliefs and obsessive behaviors associated with bulimia; (4) a maintenance program for self-monitoring of eating patterns is instituted.

Anorexia nervosa is a severe disorder characterized by restriction of food intake. Adolescents with this disorder have an intense fear of being obese. They also exhibit a distorted body image and refuse to maintain a weight near their ideal body weight. Social learning appears to be the determinant of this disorder (Crisp, 1984). Anorexics are often hospitalized because of severe malnutrition. Successful treatment of this disorder involves the use of reinforcement principles, social skills training, family therapy, and cognitive behavior therapy.

GROUP PROCEDURES WITH CHILDREN AND ADOLESCENTS

By virtue of the group members coming together, sharing experiences and problems, and interacting, behavioral group therapy offers many of the same "curative" factors as other types of group therapy. Group approaches also provide a variety of social models, allow the individual a format to try out new behaviors, and present a less isolated and more realistic situation than does individual therapy: The group itself may represent a microcosm of society, and working in a group may promote generalization more effectively than working on the same problems alone with a therapist. Various behavioral group therapies have been utilized with children and adolescents. Most techniques fall into one of four categories: (1) operant group therapy, (2) modeling and behavioral rehearsal, (3) social skills training, and (4) group procedures for reducing anxiety. In practice, it is likely that behavioral group therapy would employ more than one of these techniques.

Operant group therapy views the group as a micro-laboratory of a social environment in which the appropriate behavior of individuals can be increased or the inappropriate behavior decreased through the application of operant techniques and principles (Walker, Hedberg, Clement, & Wright, 1981). The therapist selects certain behaviors that also usually represent problem behaviors in the child's natural environment. The group serves as an environment over which there is more control and in which the behaviors can be modified and eventually generalized to other settings. The therapist may employ the operant techniques within the group such as positive reinforcement, punishment, tokens, time-out from reinforcement, response cost, shaping, or chaining to develop or increase adaptive behaviors or decrease maladaptive behaviors (Rose, 1972). For example, a withdrawn child may show little initiative in interacting with peers in the classroom. The larger classroom may also prevent the teacher from developing a systematic program to deal with the problem. In the small group situation, the therapist could use shaping techniques—first reinforcing any movement the child makes toward the group, then any attempt on the part of the child to interact with group members, gradually working toward normal peer interactions in the group. This would be paired and followed up with a classroom program to promote the transfer of these newly developed prosocial skills. Similarly, operant group procedures could be used to decrease aggressiveness in a group with the goal of reducing aggression in other settings.

Operant group techniques may also be used as an adjunct to other types of group procedures. Children, and adolescents to a lesser degree, may enter a group without the prerequisite skills necessary to benefit from group discussion. For example, a psychologist might wish to run an affectively oriented group for 10-year-old children with learning disabilities. Upon beginning the group, the psychologist finds that the children have difficulty staying in their seats, tend to interrupt each other, and generally engage in horseplay. Through the application of operant techniques, the psychologist can increase behaviors that promote group functioning and decrease those that hinder desirable group interaction. The operant techniques may allow more rapid movement toward effective group interaction, even though the focus of the group is nonbehavioral.

Modeling and behavioral rehearsal are based on social learning theory and the laboratory research on modeling and imitation. Because the group already contains individuals who serve as models and potential models, the systematic use of modeling is especially well suited to the group context. Observational learning assumes that individuals can learn simply by observing behavior and its consequences. The therapist serves as a model for group members and the members serve as models to one another. The therapist, cognizant of the different variables that help determine whether someone is an effective model (e.g., see Bandura, 1969), systematically sets up situations in which various models can engage in desirable behaviors. Similarly, the therapist may selectively reinforce by praise certain desirable behaviors that other group members might develop via vicarious reinforcement. For example, in a group for adolescents, one individual may be admired or respected by most group members. This adolescent may be an effective model for other group members. The group may, for a session, be focusing on interviewing skills. The therapist may select the admired group member to be the focus of a role play for a hypothetical job interview. During the role play, the therapist could systematically reinforce selected behaviors appropriate for the situation. The other group members would learn from observing their peer and also would be vicariously reinforced by the therapist's reinforcement of the model. The therapist may also model desired behaviors and may invite guest models to visit the group periodically.

Behavioral rehearsal is generally used in conjunction with modeling. Behavioral rehearsal requires group members to initiate (actually engage in) behaviors and receive feedback from the therapist and other group members. It is different from simple role playing in that someone else models the desired behaviors to show the client how the role should be played (Rose, 1972). It also allows the practicing of these behaviors, often relatively complex sequences, in a more protected and less anxiety-arousing situation. Behavioral rehearsal employs modeling and imitating, as well as direct reinforcement through feedback.

A typical modeling and behavioral rehearsal sequence might focus on asking a teacher for help and clarification on an assignment. Initially, the therapist or therapists (behavioral groups of this nature often utilize co-leaders) and the group members set up the situation by describing the scene. The initial role play might involve one therapist playing the teacher and the other therapist playing the student. The therapist playing the student displays the desirable behaviors for that situation. A discussion follows in which group members comment on the situation and the behavior, with the therapists highlighting certain desirable aspects (e.g., eye contact, requesting rather than demanding) of the sequence. Next, a group member volunteers or is selected to engage in a similar role play, also followed by feedback and discussion period. Depending on time, each group member might engage in the role play in front of the entire group, or the group might break into dyads for further practice. The group would conclude with a summary discussion of the important aspects of the situation and the appropriate behaviors.

Social skills training can occur either in a classroom teaching situation or in a group context. In the classroom, the teacher is more likely to utilize operant techniques to reinforce desirable social behaviors selectively, whereas group procedures will tend to use modeling and behavioral rehearsal techniques. In fact, the modeling and behavioral rehearsal sequence outlined above might be fairly typical of a social skills training group activity. The primary difference is that social skills programs often have a more structured, task-analyzed, sequential organization similar to a curriculum, whereas modeling and behavioral rehearsal groups might utilize group- or therapist-generated problem situations to a greater degree.

Goldstein, Sprafkin, Gershaw, and Klein (1980), in their book *Skillstreaming the Adolescent,* describe a structured group approach for teaching prosocial skills to adolescents. It provides the trainer (i.e., leader) with instructions for beginning and continuing group sessions, a checklist for determining areas for needed skill work, and a skill checklist summary to record progress. Skills are broken into categories ranging from beginning social skills (e.g., listening, asking a question) to planning skills (e.g., setting a goal, making a decision). Each skill is outlined in behavioral steps. For example, in the Beginning Social Skills area, the skill of "Starting a Conversation" is outlined as follows (p. 87):

Step	Trainer Notes
1. Greet the other person	Say "hi," shake hands; choose the right time and place.
2. Make small talk.	
3. Decide if the other person is listening.	Check if the other person is looking at you, nodding, saying "mm-hmm."
4. Bring up the main topic.	

SUGGESTED CONTENT FOR MODELING DISPLAY

A. School or neighborhood: Main actor starts conversation with secretary in school office.

B. Home: Main actor discusses allowance and/or privileges with parent.

C. Peer group: Main actor suggests weekend plans to a friend.

This type of format breaks down the specific skills into component parts and allows the teaching of the specific skill. A number of other similar programs are available for adolescents as well as younger children.

Procedures for reducing anxiety usually involve the teaching of relaxation techniques in the group setting. The leader first instructs the group in the relaxation techniques and then guides the group through the techniques. Most of the sets of instructions or relaxation scripts utilized in individual therapy can be adapted for group use. Two other anxiety-reducing procedures are appropriate for group work. First, group desensitization is useful for common anxiety situations. In group desensitization, the group is led through relaxation, followed by presentation of a standard hierarchy. This type of intervention has been particularly useful in dealing with test anxiety (Prout & Harvey, 1978). The second procedure involves anxiety management training. In this technique, children are taught how to relax and how to use relaxation procedures in real-life stressful situations.

A comprehensive review of the literature on cognitive behavior training for social skills in adolescents can be found in an article by Gresham and Lemanek (1983). Kazdin, Esveldt-Dawson, and Matson (1983) have also reviewed the effect of various instructional systems on the development of social skills.

CLASSROOM AND EDUCATIONAL APPLICATIONS

Behavioral principles have been extensively applied in the schools since the 1960s. Lindsley (1968) has suggested that the teacher can be considered a behavioral engineer in the classroom provided he or she has the proper tools. If one adopts the behavioral viewpoint that human activities are controlled by their environmental consequences, then many aspects of the classroom can be arranged and rearranged to produce specific desired behaviors. In this model the teacher becomes the major instrument for making use of the basic principles of behavior control in order to alter children's behavior. Fundamental reinforcement contingencies are examined and modified if necessary.

One of the more comprehensive methods for utilizing behavioral principles in the classroom has been developed by Ogden Lindsley (1972). His method is known as *precision teaching* and it utilizes operant techniques in the classroom. Basically, precision teaching provides exact means for measuring performance on a continuous basis. This is done by clearly delineating the desirable behaviors required of students and measuring these behaviors over time with the aid of behavioral charts. Precision teaching stresses accountability on the part of teachers as well as students. The rate of production or efficiency is a critical variable to be measured in precision teaching. In dealing with exceptional children, precision teaching seeks to define operationally wanted and unwanted behaviors. Children are given considerable involvement and responsibility in the learning process. All assessment of child disorders is done through adaptive behavior measures in order to make intervention possible.

Proficiency is a key concept in precision teaching. Proficiency is the frequency per unit of time at which competency is achieved for a particular skill. It is the expectation that proficiency increases over time and is, therefore, a measure of cost effectiveness. If in a given programming effort proficiency begins to decline, then modifications must be made in the program in order to make it efficacious. For behavior to be measurable it must contain movement cycles. Therefore, it must be observable and it must be repeatable and measurable in the scientific sense. For Lindsley, much of the current educational jargon (e.g., thinking, synthesizing, integrating, conceiving) does not lend itself to measurement. He suggests that output terminology (e.g., writing, saying, marking, doing, pointing) must be measurable in order for education to have accountability. Lindsley indicates that children go through four stages of learning. The first stage, *acquisition,* focuses on learning the information and skills necessary to perform a task. Performance at this level is characterized by a relatively high error rate and a relatively low rate of acquisition. In the second stage, *fluency building,* the child has acquired the basic skill but needs a variety of settings in which to practice that skill. At this stage the performance level increases as the child generalizes the skill to various situations. In the third stage, *maintenance,* intermittent reinforcement is provided in order to maintain the skill over a long period of time. In the final stage, *application,* the emphasis is on practical application of the skill to everyday life experiences.

Because precision teaching provides predictable contracted rewards for performance, it tends to increase motivation in formerly unmotivated children. The fact that it emphasizes intrastudent performance further helps to increase the efficiency of individual students while maintaining relatively low anxiety levels. The system provides an overall evaluation of the educational process within a given classroom that is data based and, therefore, aids in providing documentation regarding needs. The reciprocal reinforcement system inherent in precision teaching is a fundamental reason for its success. In this system both teachers and students provide reinforcement for one another based on mutually agreed-upon behavioral contracts.

Other operant principles have been employed for classroom management purposes. Morris (1980) has described the use of the Premack principle in classroom settings. This principle simply states that high probability behaviors can be used to reinforce low probability behaviors if the high probability event is made contingent on the performance of the low probability event. For example, recess (a high probability event) can be used to reinforce completing an arithmetic assignment (a low probability event). Morris has described a four-step process for implementing the Premack principle in the classroom. These steps include (1) designing an observation session in which the frequency level of various behaviors can be measured; (2) determining the amount of time the child will be allowed to engage in the high frequency behavior; (3) setting up a contingency program in which the child's access to the high frequency behavior is clearly contingent upon performance of the low frequency behavior; and (4) evaluating whether the procedure is successful and modifying it, if necessary, using some other high frequency behavior. Andrews (1971) describes the use of the Premack principle with verbally aggressive and acting out adolescents. In Andrews' research, these aggressive behaviors were occurring at the rate of 15 to 29 per hour. Andrews observed that when students were given free time, they spent much of that time working with tutors or watching television. During these free-time periods, the incidence of aggressive and unwanted behavior was half that previously reported. In order to implement the Premack principle, the students were asked to delineate 12 behaviors which were considered unacceptable. These behaviors included aggressive and destructive behaviors previously mentioned. A contract was drawn up in which the high probability behavior of meeting with tutors and watching television was made contingent on a decrease in the rate of aggressive behaviors from 15 to 20 per hour to no more than 3 per hour. Andrews' results showed significant success in extinguishing the unwanted behavior patterns.

A review of the literature indicates that differential reinforcement of other behavior (DRO) has been shown to be effective in decreasing a number of inappropriate behaviors (Bear, 1980). These behaviors include aggression, perseverative behaviors, self-injurious behavior, and a plethora of more minor disorders. Bear suggests that DRO is most effective in controlling serious disturbance when used in combination with other behavioral techniques. These techniques include punishment, response cost, time-out, and overcorrection.

Meyers (1980) has described the use of time-out procedures in the classroom. Time-out is especially useful for disruptive and aggressive students. The procedure involves withdrawal of the student from reinforcing stimuli contingent upon some response such as relaxation or calmness. The procedure can be put on a gradient ranging from total withdrawal of the student from the environment to simple removal of adult attention. Meyers details a number of considerations in the use of time-out. The child must be given a verbal explanation of why the time-out is necessary. A warning should be provided indicating that a time-out is imminent. The time-out should be administered in a nonemotional manner and in a location that has zero reinforcement valence. The success of time-out depends upon the regular classroom setting being a reinforcing environment. If this is not the case, time-out will not have the desired effect. Furthermore, the skill with which the instructional staff performs the time-out procedure is critical. Thus, a relatively high degee of behavioral training is necessary to perform this procedure correctly, particularly with emotionally disturbed students.

Modeling has been shown to be effective in modifying distruptive and aggressive behaviors in children and adolescents (Bandura, 1969). For example, children in counseling groups can be asked to discuss and to fantasize about their aggressive behavior. Nonaggressive ways of behaving can then be modeled either by the behavior therapist or by peer models. This technique has been shown to be highly effective in modifying behavior patterns. Fears and phobias have been the focus of some modeling efforts (Graziano, DeGiovanni, & Garcia, 1979). Children are asked to observe a model who is successfully interacting with feared stimuli. In some cases multiple models are used with varying degrees of the feared stimuli. Results have tended to indicate improvement through this modeling procedure.

Undoubtedly, operant techniques will continue to be used in the schools at an ever-increasing rate. The success with which they will be used will depend upon the willingness of educators and psychologists to operationalize behaviors and measure the impact of a given program. Although behavior principles have been used extensively in the learning process in the elementary grades, they have not been employed systematically to change emotionally disturbed behavior. This application will undoubtedly be the next major focus for behavior therapy in the schools. An excellent review of operant techniques applied to educational settings is provided by Sulzer-Azaroff and Mayer (1986).

PARENTING SKILLS

The assumption of behavior therapists in training parents to implement behavioral programs is that children's maladaptive behaviors can best be controlled in the context of family and home. Maladaptive behaviors that developed in the home but are treated in the clinic setting may not change in the home environment. Berkowitz and Graziano (1972) point out that behavior therapists assume that it is important to teach their knowledge and techniques to others, including paraprofessionals. This is considerably discrepant from the attitudes of other more traditional therapists in which the basic technology is a closely held professional secret. Berkowitz and Graziano suggest that, because parents maintain a high degree of contact with their children and have the principal moral and ethical responsibility for their children's behavior, they are also responsible for the child's affective well-being. In this regard, the traditional dyadic model in which a professional provides direct services to the child has been replaced by a three-dimensional model where the behavior therapist is to reduce or weaken dysfunctional behaviors and to set up reinforcement mechanisms for appropriate social behaviors.

Several models of behavioral parent training have been identified. The dyadic model (Patterson & Reed, 1970) examines faulty relationships between the child and primary persons in the home. This model postulates that problems in the home result from ineffective interactions between the child and parents. The parents may be providing little or no positive reinforcement for behavior while the child is providing predominantly negative stimulation to the parents. A reciprocal process occurs in which aversive stimulation provided by the child results in aversive stimulus patterns from the parents. This aversive pattern spirals downward until a family crisis occurs. In the dyadic model, treatment is focused on aiding parents in assessing the behavioral nature of their interactions with their children. Here a number of traditional assessment techniques are used including behavioral observation and checklists. After these data are collected, formal parent training begins. Parents are taught the fundamental principles underlying social learning theory and behavior management. A second model of parent training involves an eclectic approach in which dysfunctional interactions are viewed in terms of the child's entire ecological environment. Although parents are part of this ecology, other groups such as peers and teachers are also involved. In this model, dysfunctional relationships are examined in terms of behavioral interactions among all relevant groups. Factors that may interfere with parent training are examined. For example, in a given family the marriage relationship between husband and wife may be in the process of deteriorating. It will be necessary to deal with this factor in order to deal more effectively with the parent-child interaction pattern. A third model, the social systems model, postulates that a child's misbehavior is representative of conflict elsewhere in the family and that this conflict is often in the marriage relationship between the parents. The social system model is similar to the eclectic model except that it postulates faulty interactions between the parents as the main cause for childhood disturbance. Both the eclectic and social system models require that comprehensive ecological assessments be performed which detail the interactional nature of behaviors among family members. It is from these data that therapeutic behavioral techniques are designed.

A five-point model of behavioral assessment has been designed by Keefe, Kopel, and Gordon (1978) for use with families. This model includes (1) problem identification and delineation, (2) measurement of behavior together with a functional analysis, (3) matching of client treatment to the functional analysis, (4) assessment of progress during ongoing therapy, and (5) long-term assessment of therapy. Keefe et al. believe that this model should be applied in all behavior therapy situations in order to maximize the probability of success. Behavior therapists typically neglect to perform adequate functional analysis of family behavior patterns prior to parent training. This omission results in questionable treatment decisions based on the identification of lower priority issues. For example, it must be determined whether the presence of dysfunctional behavior in a given child is the result of faulty interactions between the parent and the child or faulty interactions between the parents themselves.

Berkowitz and Graziano (1972) have divided structured parent training techniques into respondent-based and operant-based categories. The majority of techniques have focused on operant procedures. Most respondent techniques involve the conditioning of enuretic and encopretic children. Devices such as those described earlier in this chapter are used by parents for control of enuresis. Using operant conditioning, parents have been trained to provide simple extinction of behavior, modeling, and the use of simple shaping procedures. Other programs have trained parents to modify autistic and schizophrenic behavior, aggressive and hyperactive behavior, and socially unacceptable behaviors. Berkowitz and Graziano conclude that research is needed to develop predictive measures of parental success and more specific measures of parental and child behavior change as a result of intervention. Engeln, Knutson, Laughy, and Garlington (1968) describe the use of systematic family programming in behavior therapy. In their case, a 6-year-old boy with extremely aggressive behavior toward other children was treated in a family context. The boy's behavior was so extreme that it left the family isolated from the community and the boy from his peer group. A behavioral program consisting of a number of contracts was devised. It consisted of the following steps:

1. Systematic reinforcement of eye contact and command compliance.
2. Training of the boy's mother in relevant behavioral principles through modeling of the therapist's behavior and through discussion.

3. Training of the mother in reinforcement and extinction techniques regarding her son's behavior.
4. Development of a home-based program of systematic reinforcement for both the boy and his siblings.
5. Use of the Premack principle as a reinforcement technique.

The program resulted in a significant decrease in the boy's unwanted aggressive behavior.

In relation to structured parent training, Gordon, Learner, and Keefe (1979) have summarized the research and drawn a number of conclusions. They feel that in providing formal parent training, written materials and supervision should be the first service provided to parents. Those parents who need additional training should be provided with on-site performance instruction. The preferred training techniques include modeling prompting, shaping, and behavioral rehearsal. Modeling has been found to be especially effective when compared with other, more extensive, behavioral interventions such as behavioral rehearsal and feedback. Gordon et al. conclude that the paucity of behavioral parent training materials requires that behavior therapists use their own clinical judgment in deciding what might or might not work with a given client family. An outline of a basic behavioral parent training program should include at least the following:

1. Measuring and operationally defining behaviors, including instrumentation for observations.
2. Establishing behavioral base lines and making meaningful recordings of behavior (e.g., with graphs, charts).
3. Using various kinds of reinforcement as a means of increasing behavioral probability.
4. Identifying antecedents and consequences in the use of various reinforcement patterns.
5. Using the Premack principle: reinforcing low-rate behaviors with high-rate behaviors.

6. Using techniques for reducing unwanted behaviors: DRO, extinction, negative reinforcement.
7. Understanding the uses and misuses of punishment.
8. Understanding how body language affects behavior.
9. The parent being an appropriate social model for his or her children.
10. Learning how to maintain behaviors once they are established.

This set of ten training steps could easily be converted into ten sessions in a parent training sequence. It is important to note that they form the basic core of knowledge for translating behavior therapy principles into parent training techniques. It would be necessary to provide continuous follow-up in order to ascertain whether these techniques had actually been utilized in the home setting.

FAMILY THERAPY

Behavior therapy does not provide a framework for conducting family therapy in the traditional sense. That is, the behavioral family therapist is not likely to bring an entire family together and work on issues in joint sessions. The behavior therapist is more likely to focus on various interactional or reinforcement patterns that exist in the family unit and occur in the natural setting. Although there is recognition of complex interdependencies in families, the behavior therapist is more prone to treat those specific dysfunctional patterns that appear to be creating most of the difficulties and does not necessarily treat the whole family. In fact, behavioral family therapy can best be described as a combination of behavioral approaches to parenting (described above) and behavioral marital therapy.

Marital relationships may be viewed as interactive dyadic relationships in which there is sufficient potential for mutual reinforcement between marital partners. Marital relationships are satisfactory as long as each partner receives adequate amounts of reinforcement. However, when such reinforcement does not occur, various negative interaction patterns may result. Although these negative patterns may not directly involve the children in a family, marital problems can indirectly affect child behavior.

Hope (1976) has described a multifaceted approach for the treatment of marital problems. The first step in the process involves teaching couples to pinpoint behaviors which they wish to change in each other in order to determine precisely what behaviors are at issue. This teaching may include discrimination training to help an individual distinguish between what behaviors are actually positive and which are really negative. A second facet of behavioral marital therapy is communication skills training. This step includes training in how to listen; how to share in a two-way dialogue; and how to reduce negative, aversive, and sidetracking verbal behaviors. How to reinforce one another or provide "positives" is an important part of the communication training. Couples are asked to practice these skills outside the therapy situation. In the next stage of therapy, couples are taught how to problem solve and negotiate. Problem solving is viewed as progressive and future oriented. Changes in each other's behavior are considered negotiable, and compromises are a necessary component of problem solving. In the final stage, couples, utilizing their new skills in communication, reinforcement, and problem solving, are taught how to develop contingency contracts.

Social learning theory approaches—e.g., the work of Gerald Patterson at the University of Oregon—are probably the best examples of behavioral family applications (Hansen & L'Abate, 1982). Patterson has done numerous empirical studies in family interventions, focusing mostly on changes in child behavior. The family is seen as the center of learning for social behaviors, with the family consisting of a series of mutually interdependent dyads. In the dyad, both individuals (e.g., parent and child) influence the behavior of the other. The interactions in the dyad help determine which behaviors will be developed and which will persist. The social learning approach to family intervention places heavy emphasis on teaching parent behavioral (i.e., operant) principles, making the approach virtually indistinguishable from behavioral parenting approaches. In fact, Hansen and L'Abate (1982) criticize this approach because of this relatively narrow focus. They note that the approach fails to consider the family as a system, focusing almost solely on parenting styles. The approach does not recognize ineffective parenting styles as possibly resulting from a broader family system problem or family pathology. The approach also does not view the family as the client because the child's behavior is at odds with many of the traditionally accepted premises of family therapy.

EFFICACY

Behavior therapy, by virtue of its ties to empirical and scientific psychology, is able to offer vast amounts of data to support its efficacy. The behaviorally oriented journals tend to present relatively well-designed studies that provide evidence of observable, measurable behavior change. Further, behavior therapy provides well-specified descriptions of the various therapeutic procedures and has demonstrated effectiveness with a wide variety of disorders. In fact, when the efficacy literature of behavior therapy is compared with that of other types of therapy, the behavior therapy literature is clearly superior in terms of rigor and demonstrated uses.

Despite this superiority, one must read this literature with a somewhat critical view. Agras, Kazdin, and Wilson (1979) have commented on the status of research in behavior therapy and note a number of areas of concern. Behavior therapy suffers from the lack of good long-term follow-up studies, much as do other approaches. Further, some of the research has studied rather trivial concerns of questionable social significance, while other research studies, in an attempt to be scientific, have narrowly defined target behaviors without consideration of how the behavior change might relate to an individual's total functioning. In a similar vein, some behavioral research has not considered the issue of generalization of behavior change to other settings. In general, while the literature of behavior therapy is extremely impressive and much significant progress has been made, the research is still in a developing state.

Ross (1978) and Kazdin (1980) have reviewed areas in which behavioral approaches have been shown to be effective interventions. Kazdin notes that behavioral techniques have been successfully applied with fear and avoidance reactions, social behavioral problems such as withdrawal and aggression, habit disorders, academic problems, conduct problems, delinquency, autism, childhood schizophrenia, mental retardation, and learning disabilities. Further, within each of those areas, a variety of disorders have been treated with a variety of techniques. Ross also notes a similar set of applications but offers several cautions in viewing the research. The lack of follow-up data is also a problem with child behavior therapy research, because children are followed only for a brief period after treatment. A related problem is the fact that most research is focused on treatment of a single disorder or problem. In reality, many children present complex, multiple problems. The research generally has not dealt with the more complex problems; thus little is known about the effectiveness of behavior therapy with children with multiple problems. Still, despite limitations in the research, child behavior therapy presents one of the most comprehensive research bases on the psychological treatment of the child.

In the area of cognitive behavior therapy, Meador and Ollendick (1984) have reviewed the literature on efficacy. Generally they have found that interventions with hyperactive/impulsive children have met with a degree of success. Cognitive therapies have also been shown to be effective in modifying a variety of academic and classroom-relevant behaviors with nonclinical children. Evidence pertaining to the effectiveness of cognitive behavior therapy in clinical samples is less common (e.g, institutionalized, anxiety disorders, or schizophrenics). McAdam (1986) presents a review of the research applying cognitive behavior therapy to adolescents, arguing that cognitive behavior therapy has been more successful with this group than with younger children both in clinical and nonclinical populations.

Because it would be impossible even to begin to review all the research literature in child behavior therapy in this context, a review of behavioral treatments for school phobia will be presented as an example of the efficacy literature. School phobia has been treated with a variety of techniques. It appears to have multiple behavioral explanations from a theoretical standpoint, and behavior therapy has been relatively successful in treating it.

A number of desensitization and counterconditioning techniques have been successfully employed to treat school phobia.

These techniques include systematic desensitization, implosive therapy, in vivo desensitization, emotive imagery, and anxiety-reducing stories. Lazarus (1960) described the application of systematic desensitization with a 9-year-old school-phobic girl. A seven-item hierarchy, based on the theme of separation from the mother, was administered to the girl in five treatment sessions over a 10-day period. At the conclusion of these sessions, the girl voluntarily returned to school. Miller (1972) reported a case study of a 10-year-old school-phobic boy who also displayed separation anxiety and fear of death. Relaxation training was followed by systematic desensitizaton, with reinforcement provided for participating in treatment. Because the boy reported the fear of death at bedtime, the therapist administered relaxation procedures over the telephone just before the child went to bed. Systematic desensitization was followed by in vivo desensitization. A final part of the training was anxiety management training, i.e., teaching the boy to relax when he experienced anxiety. This combined treatment took 6 weeks and resulted in the boy's return to school and elimination of the boy's fear of death.

Lazarus, Davison, and Polefka (1965) employed in vivo desensitization to treat a 9-year-old school-phobic boy. Because of the boy's inarticulate and acquiescent response style, an initial attempt at systematic desensitization was abandoned. The in vivo treatment involved sixteen steps progressing from walking to school with the therapist on a Sunday afternoon to independent re-entry into the classroom. Token reinforcement was also utilized to maintain attendance in this successful intervention. Garvey and Hegrenes (1966) also report a case study using in vivo desensitization. They began by having the subject simply ride to school and place his foot on the curb, with a gradual build up to full resumption of class attendance. Van der Ploeg (1975) interspersed stories of a pleasant sailing experience with discussions of typical school scenes as part of treatment for a 14-year-old school-phobic boy. Successful applications of implosive therapy (Smith & Sharpe, 1970) and emotive imagery (Lazarus & Abramowitz, 1962) have also been reported. Implosive therapy, based on a respondent extinction model, involves high-intensity presentations of the anxiety-provoking stimuli. Emotive imagery involves the visualization of anxiety-producing scenes, with imagined successful outcomes.

Reinforcement-based programs have also been used successfully. Hersen (1970), noting that staying away from school may actually be reinforced at home, has used differential reinforcement of successive approximations of returning to school with positive reinforcement for school attendance. Tahmisian and McReynolds (1971) were unsuccessful in treating a school-phobic 13-year-old with systematic desensitization. They then developed a shaping program in which school-approach behaviors were reinforced with privileges, resulting in a return to full-time school attendance.

Kennedy (1965), using an approach described as consistent with Wolpe's approach, involved paid referral, parent involvement, removal of secondary gains in the home, and the abrupt desensitization approach of forced attendance. Kennedy reported successful treatment of 50 cases of what he called Type I school phobia, a nonchronic, neurotic maladjustment, usually seen in younger children and discussed in the school phobia section above. Stedman (1976) reported a case study that involved behavioral family counseling, systematic desensitization, and an operant contingency contracting program to treat a 9-year-old school-phobic girl.

Although most of the reported efficacy literature is case study in nature, it does seem that school phobia responds positively to a variety of behavioral interventions. Both operant and respondent techniques have been successfully applied, often in combination. Prout and Harvey (1978), in a review of the application of desensitization procedures for school-related problems, found that approximately 80% of the studies reported the use of a combination of techniques. The research literature would appear to support a multimodal behavioral assessment and intervention.

CONCLUSIONS

Behavior therapy has been utilized with a wide variety of populations in institutional settings. It is applicable equally with children, adolescents, and adults and is perhaps the most widely used therapy with children. Prior to the development of behavior therapy, anxiety disorders and phobic reactions were difficult and sometimes impossible to treat. The pioneering work of behaviorists such as Wolpe clearly established the ability of psychologists to condition autonomic behaviors. From the standpoint of dealing with some of the more complex anxiety-related disorders, it is this feature of behavior therapy that has produced its robust success.

In school settings, school phobia and other behavior disorders have proved to be highly susceptible to behavior therapy. The treatment of enuresis in young children has been virtually revolutionalized by the work of Foxx and Azrin (1973a, 1973b). In addition, almost every classroom teacher in the United States has been exposed to and has attempted to use various behavior learning principles. Techniques such as precision teaching have been utilized in the classroom in order to maximize learning and affective harmony.

With the development of cognitive behavior therapy, new applications with adolescents have been made possible. Prior to cognitive behavior therapy, the application of operant principles with cognitively sophisticated adolescents and adults was questionable. It was felt that these principles did not attune themselves to developmental changes in cognition in adolescence and adulthood. Cognitive behavior modification addresses itself directly to internal thought patterns and their modification. Thus, the first step in linking operant theory to cognitive development has been made. The utilization of social learning theory principles with children and adolescents has also aided movement in this direction.

The efficacy research in behavior therapy is substantial and diverse. It tends to indicate that behavior therapy is successful in a large variety of settings, especially those where the behaviors to be changed are well operationalized. Future research in behavior therapy will need to focus on the behavioral assessment of ecologically complex environments and the measurement of behaviors derived from these assessments. In addition, further work will be needed to relate learning in adolescence and adulthood to the methodology currently available in behavior therapy. Achieving this goal will undoubtedly mean the development of new methodology which will improve efficiency of treatment, particularly with more complex psychotic disorders.

CASE STUDY

Client

Jimmy, age 13, was referred for behavioral treatment following a comprehensive behavioral, medical, psychological, and educational evaluation at a children's diagnostic center. Jimmy consistently tested in the upper ranges of the mildly mentally retarded, or educable mentally retarded range (e.g., high 60s) and had been involved in special education programs throughout his entire educational career. At the time of referral, he was in a junior high school educable mentally retarded class. Although Jimmy was a relatively strong student academically, attempts at mainstreaming and other integration into regular school activities were unsuccessful because of behavior difficulties.

The presenting problems included extreme impulsiveness, socially inappropriate behaviors, and noncompliance. The school and home reports were relatively consistent with regard to these problems, although the noncompliance appeared to be more of a problem at home. These problems were long-standing, with Jimmy's parents initiating the first of a series of mental health referrals at age 6. A variety of psychotropic medications (according to reports, eight different drugs had been attempted), loosely structured parent counseling, and individual play therapy had not yielded significant positive changes.

The initial evaluation indicated that there was a significant anxiety component contributing to the behavior difficulties. Although it was felt that some of the impulsiveness was developmental or constitutional in nature, a generalized anxiety response seemed to exacerbate this condition and contributed to the inappropriate social responses and noncompliance. Further, the initial evaluation indicated that both parents, particularly the mother, were experiencing considerable stress and frustration related to management difficulties in the home.

Behavioral Assessment

Prior to the beginning of treatment, behavioral data were collected over a 2-week period to specify goals and concerns further. Based on initial behavioral interview data from both parents and teachers, an individualized behavior rating form was constructed. This form asked the parents and teachers to rate on a daily basis the severity of several problem behaviors. Using the A-B-C format (i.e., *A*ntecedent-*B*ehavior-Consequence), parents and teachers were also asked to provide daily anecdotal reports on desirable and undesirable behaviors they observed in the two settings. Jimmy was observed twice at school by the therapist and was interviewed in an attempt to determine the generality or specificity of the anxiety.

These assessments led to a number of conclusions. No specific source of anxiety could be identified, and it appeared that the anxiety was relatively generalized across a variety of social situations in both settings. The social inappropriateness and impulsiveness were problems in both settings but seemed to increase in group situations or in situations where large numbers of people were present. For example, Jimmy's behavior became more problematic in the school cafeteria and also at large family gatherings in the home. The assessment also confirmed that noncompliance was essentially a problem at home and not at school.

Treatment Program

A multimodal behavioral treatment program evolved over a period of several months. The program, which included periodic assessment of the problem behavior, had the following components:

1. Relaxation training.
2. Individual behavioral counseling with Jimmy.
3. Behavioral parent counseling.
4. Behavioral programming in the home.
5. Referral to a community agency that was conducting social skills groups for mildly retarded adolescents.

The initial phase of treatment focused on the relaxation training. The goal of the relaxation training was to reduce the level of general anxiety based on the hypothesis that this would result in a reduction in impulsiveness and other apparently anxiety-related behaviors. Although relaxation programs for children are available, the relaxation script that was used in this case was a slightly modified version of a muscle relaxation script used with normal adults. The instructions were essentially the same with only modification of the vocabulary so that it was appropriate for Jimmy's cognitive level. Jimmy was initially trained in a clinic setting with his parents observing through a two-way mirror. The parents were then instructed in the procedures and began to administer them to Jimmy at home on a daily or twice-daily basis. The therapist eventually tape-recorded the instructions, and Jimmy was able to use the tape at home. The final part of the training involved instructing Jimmy on how to use the relaxation techniques in stressful situations. Using key words for the script (e.g., "calm down") or slightly tensing certain muscle groups were used to cope with stress. From Jimmy's verbal report, he was able to use these techniques at various times.

The individual behavioral counseling sessions with Jimmy focused on discussions of various situations in which he encountered difficulty. Jimmy was shown ways in which his responses might be maintaining poor relationships with others. Sessions also centered on alternative ways of responding and provided behavioral rehearsal of the alternative response. For example, Jimmy complained about a boy at school who always called him "pumpkin face." Jimmy's typical response was to get upset, make various verbal threats, and usually go running off screaming, apparently much to the amusement of the other students. Initially, Jimmy was shown how the goal of the other boy's teasing might be to get Jimmy upset. A simplified explanation of reinforcement was provided, showing Jimmy how his getting upset might contribute to maintaining the other boy's teasing. It is interesting to note that the example most useful in conveying this concept was showing Jimmy how some of his own behaviors had a goal of getting his parents upset. It was decided in this situation to utilize an extinction procedure by teaching Jimmy to ignore the teasing. In the behavioral rehearsal, the therapist played a rather persistent teaser with Jimmy following instructions on how to ignore and how not to react to the teasing. Jimmy's "new" response was to not respond verbally to the teasing, to maintain a calm disposition, and, if the teasing persisted, to walk quietly away from the situation. Anecdotal reports from the teachers indicated that Jimmy was able to employ the new behaviors in situations where he had been teased in the past, and, more important, the teasing from the other boy ceased to be a problem.

The parent counseling and behavioral programming in the home were simultaneous activities. The parents were asked to read Patterson's (1976) *Living with Children* at the beginning of treatment. (This book is one of several books written for parents that explain basic behavioral concepts and how they can be applied with children.) This book provided the parents with some insight into how their responses to Jimmy's behaviors might be contributing to the maintenance of his problem behaviors. In particular, Jimmy's mother realized that her "yelling" was not promoting behavior change and was probably contributing to the maintenance of certain problem behaviors. After a brief base line, in which Jimmy's mother was allowed to yell normally, Jimmy's mother was instructed not to yell at him for a period of 2 weeks. She was instructed to provide corrective feedback in a calm voice and in a positive manner. This action resulted in a gradual decline of the specific problem behaviors over the 2-week period, with Jimmy reporting positively in the individual sessions that "Mom's acting different." During this period, a token point program was also initiated at home to deal with noncompliance. Jimmy's progress was monitored on a chart on his bedroom wall. Points were awarded for successful completion of a variety of household tasks and chores (e.g., doing dishes, cleaning room, doing homework), with small rewards available daily from a "grab bag." A larger reward (e.g., going to a movie, going out for a pizza) was available at the end of each week if Jimmy met a specified weekly goal.

The social skills training, conducted by another community agency, consisted of a series of small group sessions. Other group members were of similar age and also students of special education classes. Sessions focused on discussions of various common social situations and the appropriate behaviors expected for those situations. Group members then took turns rehearsing the appropriate behaviors and providing feedback to one another. Typical role plays included introducing oneself, asking for help, and saying no to a peer.

Evaluation

Improvements were seen on all measures administered prior to the beginning of treatment. Additional data (e.g., noncompliance) taken during treatment also showed positive behavior changes. In general, although Jimmy still displayed problem behaviors at times, these behaviors had been reduced to a more manageable and tolerable level. On the affective side, Jimmy also expressed more satisfaction and happiness with his own situation. His parents reported considerably less frustration and had more confidence in their ability to deal with him.

ANNOTATED BIBLIOGRAPHY

Gelfand, D. M., & Hartman, D. T. (1984). *Child behavior analysis and therapy* (2nd ed.). New York: Pergamon.

This volume is a thorough overview of behavior analysis applied to children. A wide variety of clinical applications are discussed. The book is highly operant in nature. An excellent array of behavioral interventions for child and adolescent problems is provided.

Hughes, J. M. (1988). *Cognitive behavior therapy with children in the schools.* New York: Pergamon.

This volume provides an overview of cognitive behavior assessment and intervention. Although the volume is school focused, it provides a review of cognitive behavioral interventions with a variety of child disorders including both internalizing and externalizing problems. It also provides guidelines for using cognitive behavioral approaches in the prevention and consultation framework.

Ollendick, T. H., & Cerny, J. A. (1981). *Clinical behavior therapy with children.* New York: Plenum Press.

This book provides a comprehensive overview of behavior therapy techniques for use with children. It includes coverage of desensitization, modeling, and operant and cognitive techniques. This book probably provides the best overview of techniques for those who use an eclectic behavioral approach.

Ross, A. O. (1981). *Child behavior therapy: Principles, procedures, and empirical basis.* New York: John Wiley & Sons.

This book, by one of the leading authorities on children's behavior disorders and behavior therapy with children, provides clinical reviews of behavioral interventions for a variety of childhood psychological problems. Interventions are classified by treatment of behavioral deficits (e.g., social, language, academic or attention) or behavioral excesses (e.g., aggression, disruptive behavior, fears). Although other cognitive and respondent techniques are included, the emphasis in this book is on operant approaches for specific problems or disorders.

Spiegler, M. D. (1983). *Contemporary behavior therapy.* Palo Alto, CA: Mayfield.
This volume is a general review of behavior therapy concepts and procedures. It deals with a variety of interventions, including consequential therapies, substitution behavior therapies, token economies, modeling therapies, and self-control therapies. The book is oriented toward specific interventions and provides numerous detailed case studies.

Sulzer-Azaroff, B., & Mayer, G. R. (1986). *Achieving educational excellence: Using behavioral strategies.* New York: Holt, Rinehart & Winston.
This book is a comprehensive overview of the application of operant methodology with children. It provides thorough explanations of various techniques and numerous examples and suggestions for developing interventions. This book would be especially useful to those in educational settings.

REFERENCES

Agras, W. S., Kazdin, A. E., & Wilson, G. T. (1979). *Behavior therapy: Toward an applied clinical science.* San Francisco: W. H. Freeman.

Andrews, H. B. (1971). The systematic use of the Premack principle in modifying classroom behavior. *Child Study Journal, 2,* 74-79.

Bandura, A. (1969). *Principles of behavior modification.* New York: Holt, Rinehart & Winston.

Bandura, A. (1973). *Aggression: A social learning analysis.* Englewood Cliffs, NJ: Prentice-Hall.

Bandura, A. (1977). *Social learning theory.* Englewood Cliffs, NJ: Prentice-Hall.

Bandura, A., Ross, D., & Ross, S. A. (1963). Vicarious reinforcement and imitative learning. *Journal of Abnormal and Social Psychology, 67,* 601-607.

Bandura, A., & Walters, R. H. (1963). *Social learning and personality development.* New York: Holt, Rinehart & Winston.

Bear, G. G. (1980). Differential reinforcement of other behavior. In *Behavioral strategies for psychological intervention.* Des Moines, IA: Iowa Department of Education.

Beck, A. T., Rush, A. J., Shaw, B. F., & Emery, G. (1979). *Cognitive therapy of depression.* New York: Guilford Press.

Berkowitz, B. P., & Graziano, A. M. (1972). Training parents as behavior therapists: A review. *Behavior Research and Therapy, 10,* 297-317.

Boyd, L. A. (1980). Emotive imagery in the behavioral management of adolescent school phobia: A case approach. *School Psychology Review, 9*(2), 186-189.

Brawley, E. R., Harris, F. R., Allen, E., Fleming, R. S., & Peterson, R. F. (1973). Behavior modification of an autistic child. In J. M. Stedman, W. G. Patton, & K. F. Walton (Eds.), *Clinical studies in behavior therapy with children, adolescents, and their families.* Springfield, IL: Charles C. Thomas.

Brown, B., & Doolan, M. (1983). Behavioral treatment of faecal soiling: A case study. *Behavioral Psychotherapy, 11*(1), 18-24.

Brown, J. H., & Brown, C. S. (1977). *Systematic counseling*. Champaign, IL: Research Press.

Clarizio, H. (1985). Cognitive-behavioral treatment of childhood depression. *Psychology in the Schools, 22*(3), 308-322.

Cotugno, A. J. (1987). Cognitive control therapy in the treatment of an 8-year-old enuretic boy. *Journal of Child and Adolescent Psychotherapy, 4*(2), 101-106.

Crisp, A. H. (1984). The psychopathology of anorexia nervosa: Getting the "heat" out of the system. In A. J. Stunkard & E. P. Stellar (Eds.), *Eating and its disorders*. New York: Raven Press.

Davidson, W. S., & Seidman, E. (1975). Studies of behavior modification and juvenile delinquency: A review, methodological critique, and social perspective. In A. M. Graziano (Ed.), *Behavior therapy with children* (2nd ed.). Chicago: Aldine.

DiGiuseppe, R. (1986). Cognitive therapy for childhood depression. *Journal of Psychotherapy and the Family, 2*(3-4), 153-172.

Dollard, J., & Miller, N. E. (1950). *Personality and psychotherapy*. New York: McGraw-Hill.

Engeln, R., Knutson, J., Laughy, L., & Garlington, W. (1968). Behavior modification techniques applied to a family unit: A case study. *Journal of Child Psychology and Psychiatry, 9*, 245-252.

Erwin, E. (1980). *Behavior therapy: Scientific, philosophical, and moral foundations*. Cambridge, UK: Cambridge University Press.

Etzel, B. C., & Gerwirtz, J. L. (1967). Experimental modification of caretaker-maintained high rate operant crying in a 20-week-old infant: Extinction of crying with reinforcement of eye contact and smiling. *Journal of Experimental Child Psychology, 5*, 363-377.

Eysenck, J. J. (1964). *Crime and personality*. London: Routledge and Kegan-Paul.

Fairburn, C. G. (1984). Bulimia: Its epidemiology and management. In A. J. Stunkard & E. P. Stellar (Eds.), *Eating and its disorders*. New York: Raven Press.

Ferster, C. B. (1961). Positive reinforcement and behavioral deficits of autistic children. *Child Development, 332*, 437-456.

Ferster, C. B., & DeMyer, M. K. (1962) A method for the experimental analysis of the behavior of autistic children. *American Journal of Orthopsychiatry, 32*, 89-98.

Fox, J. E., & Houston, B. K. (1983). Distinguishing between cognitive and somatic trait and state anxiety in children. *Journal of Personality and Social Psychology, 45*, 862-870.

Foxx, R. M., & Azrin, N. H. (1973a). *Behavior research therapy* (Vol. 2). New York: Pergamon Press.

Foxx, R. M., & Azrin, N.H. (1973b). The elimination of autistic self-stimulatory behavior by overcorrection. *Journal of Applied Behavior Analysis, 6*, 1-14.

Frankel, F., & Simmons, J. Q. (1985). Behavioral treatment approaches to pathological unsocialized physical aggression in young children. *Journal of Child Psychology and Psychiatry and Allied Disciplines, 26*(4), 525-551.

Garvey, W. P., & Hegrenes, J., Jr. (1966). Desensitization techniques in the treatment of school phobia. *American Journal of Orthopsychiatry, 36*, 147-152.

Goldstein, A. P., Sprafkin, R. P., Gershaw, N. J., & Klein, P. (1980). *Skillstreaming the adolescent.* Champaign, IL: Research Press.

Gordon, S. B., Learner, L. I., & Keefe, F. (1979). Responsive parenting: An approach to training parents of problem children. *American Journal of Community Psychology, 7,* 45-56.

Gottman, J. M., & Leiblum, S. R. (1974). *How to do psychotherapy and how to evaluate it.* New York: Holt, Rinehart & Winston.

Graziano, A. M. (Ed.). (1975). *Behavior therapy with children* (2nd ed.). Chicago: Aldine.

Graziano, A. M., DeGiovanni, I. S., & Garcia, K. A. (1979). Behavioral treatment of children's fears: A review. *Psychological Bulletin, 86,* 804-830.

Gresham, F. M. (1980). Modeling based interventions with children. In *Behavioral strategies for psychological intervention.* Des Moines, IA: Iowa Department of Public Instruction.

Gresham, F. M., & Lemanek, K. L. (1983). Social skills: A review of cognitive-behavioral training procedures with children. *Journal of Applied Developmental Psychology, 4*(3), 239-261.

Hansen, J. C., & L'Abate, L. (1982). *Approaches to family therapy.* New York: Macmillan.

Hersen, M. (1970). Behavior modification approach to a school-phobic case. *Journal of Clinical Psychology, 20,* 395-402.

Hope, H. (1976). Behavioral treatment of marital problems. In W. E. Craighead, A. E. Kazdin, & M. J. Mahoney (Eds.), *Behavior modification: Principles, issues, and applications.* Boston: Houghton Mifflin.

Houts, A. C., Liebert, R. M., & Padawer, W. (1983). A delivery system for the treatment of primary enuresis. *Journal of Abnormal Child Psychology, 11*(4), 513-519.

Jones, M. C. (1924). The elimination of children's fears. *Journal of Experimental Psychology, 7,* 383-390.

Kanner, L. (1945). Autistic disturbances of affective contact. *The Nervous Child, 2,* 217-250.

Kanfer, F. H., & Goldstein, A. P. (1980). *Helping people change* (2nd ed.). New York: Pergamon Press.

Kazdin, A. E. (1979). Advances in child behavior therapy: Applications and implications. *American Psychologist, 34,* 981-987.

Kazdin, A. E. (1980). *Behavior modification in applied settings* (2nd ed.). Homewood, IL: Dorsey Press.

Kazdin, A. E., Esveldt-Dawson, K., & Matson, J. L. (1983). The effects of instructional set on social skills performance among psychiatric inpatient children. *Behavior Therapy, 14*(3), 413-423.

Keat, D. B. (1979). *Multimodal therapy with children.* New York: Pergamon Press.

Keefe, F. S., Kopel, S. A., & Gordon, S. B. (1978). *A practical guide to behavioral assessment.* New York: Springer.

Kennedy, W. A. (1965). School phobia: Rapid treatment of fifty cases. *Journal of Abnormal Psychology, 70,* 285-289.

Kennedy, W. A. (1971). *Child psychology.* Englewood Cliffs, NJ: Prentice-Hall.

Kettlewell, P. W., & Kausch, D. F. (1983). The generalization of the effects of a cognitive-behavioral treatment program for aggressive children. *Journal of Abnormal Child Psychology, 11*(1), 101-114.

Kimmel, H. D., & Kimmel, E. (1973). An instrumental conditioning method for the treatment of enuresis. In J. M. Stedman, W. F. Patterson, & K. F. Walton (Eds.), *Clinical studies in behavior therapy with children, adolescents, and their families.* Springfield, IL: Charles C. Thomas.

Krumboltz, J. D., & Thoreson, C. E. (Eds.). (1969). *Behavioral counseling: Cases and techniques.* New York: Holt, Rinehart & Winston.

Krumboltz, J. D., & Thoreson, C. E. (Eds.). (1976). *Counseling methods.* New York: Holt, Rinehart & Winston.

Lansky, D., & Vance, M. A. (1983). School-based intervention for adolescent obesity: Analysis of treatment, randomly selected control, and self-selected control subjects. *Journal of Consulting and Clinical Psychology, 51*(1), 147-148.

Lazarus, A. A. (1960). The elimination of children's phobias by deconditioning. In H. J. Eysenck (Ed.), *Behavior therapy and the neuroses.* New York: Pergamon Press.

Lazarus, A. A. (1976). *Multimodal behavior therapy.* New York: Springer.

Lazarus, A. A., & Abramowitz, A. (1962). The use of "emotive imagery" in the treatment of children's phobias. *Journal of Mental Science, 108,* 191-195.

Lazarus, A. A., Davison, G., & Polefka, D. (1965). Classical and operant factors in treatment of a school phobia. *Journal of Abnormal Psychology, 70,* 225-229.

Libert, J. M., & Lewinsohn, P. M. (1973). Concept of social skill with special reference to the behavior of depressed persons. *Journal of Consulting and Clinical Psychology, 40,* 304-312.

Lindsley, O. R. (1968). *Operant behavior management: Background and procedures.* Brecksville, OH: Brecksville Ohio Institute.

Lindsley, O. R. (1972). From Skinner to precision teaching: The child knows best. In J. B. Jordon & L. S. Robbins (Eds.), *Let's try doing something else kind of thing: Behavioral principles and the exceptional child.* Arlington, VA: Council for Exceptional Children.

Lovass, O. I., Koegel, R., Simmons, J. O., & Long, J. S. (1973). Some generalizations and follow-up measures on autistic children in behavior therapy. *Journal of Applied Behavior Analysis, 6,* 131-166.

Lowenstein, L. F. (1982). The treatment of extreme shyness in maladjusted children by implosive, counseling and conditioning approaches. *Acta Psychiatrica Scandinavica, 66*(3), 173-189.

Mahoney, M. J. (1974). *Cognitive and behavior modification.* Cambridge, MA: Ballinger.

McAdam, E. K. (1986). Cognitive behavior therapy and its application with adolescents. *Journal of Adolescence, 9*(1), 1-15.

Meador, A. E., & Ollendick, T. H. (1984). Cognitive behavior therapy with children: An evaluation of its efficacy and clinical utility. *Child and Family Behavior Therapy, 6*(3), 25-44.

Meichenbaum, D. H. (1977). *Cognitive-behavior modification.* New York: Plenum Press.

Meyers, J. (1980). Time-out: Guidelines for the school psychologist. In *Behavioral strategies for psychological intervention.* Des Moines, IA: Iowa Department of Public Instruction.

Miller, P. M. (1972). The use of visual imagery and muscle relaxation in the counter-conditioning of a phobic child: A case study. *Journal of Nervous and Mental Diseases, 154,* 457-460.

Morris, R. (1980). The Premack principle: How it can be applied to change behavior in educational settings. In *Behavioral strategies of psychological intervention.* Des Moines, IA: Iowa Department of Public Instruction.

Mowrer, O. H. (1947). On the dual nature of learning: A reinterpretation of conditioning and problem solving. *Harvard Educational Review, 17,* 102-148.

Mowrer, O. H., & Mowrer, W. M. (1938). Enuresis: A method of its study and treatment. *American Journal of Orthopsychiatry, 8,* 436-469.

Neale, D. H. (1973). Behavior therapy and encopresis in children. In J. M. Stedman, W. F. Patton, & K. F. Walton (Eds.), *Clinical studies in behavior therapy with children, adolescents, and their families.* Springfield, IL: Charles C. Thomas.

O'Brien, S., Ross, L. V., & Christophersen, E. R. (1986). Primary encopresis: Evaluation and treatment. *Journal of Applied Behavior Analysis, 19*(2), 137-145.

Ollendick, T. H. (1983). Reliability and validity of the Children's Fear Survey Schedule-Revised. *Behavior Research and Therapy, 21,* 685-692.

Ollendick, T. H., & Cerny, J. A. (1981). *Clinical behavior therapy with children.* New York: Plenum Press.

O'Mara, M. A., & Graziano, A. N. (1974). *Self monitoring by children to reduce fear of the dark.* Unpublished manuscript, State University of New York-Buffalo.

Patterson, G. R. (1976). *Living with children.* Champaign, IL: Research Press.

Patterson, G. R., & Reed, J. (1970). Reciprocity and coercion: Two facets of social systems. In C. Neuringer & J. Michaels (Eds.), *Behavioral modification in clinical psychology.* New York: Appleton-Century-Crofts.

Phillips, L., Phillips, E. A., Wolf, M. M., & Fixsen, D. L. (1975). Achievement Place: Development of the elected manager system. In A. M. Graziano (Ed.), *Behavior therapy with children* (2nd ed.). Chicago: Aldine.

Prout, H. T., & Harvey, J. R. (1978). Applications of densensitization procedures for school-related problems: A review. *Psychology in the Schools, 15,* 533-541.

Reynolds, C. R., & Paget, K. D. (1983). National normative and reliability data for the Revised Children's Manifest Anxiety Scale. *School Psychology Review, 12*(3), 324-335.

Rhine, W. R., & Spaner, S. D. (1983). The structure of evaluating anxiety among children differing in socioeconomic status, ethnicity, and sex. *Journal of Psychology, 115,* 145-158.

Rimm, D. C., & Masters, J. C. (1979). *Behavior therapy: Techniques and empirical findings* (2nd ed.). New York: Academic Press.

Rose, S. D. (1972). *Treating children in groups.* San Francisco: Jossey-Bass.
Ross, A. O. (1978). Behavior therapy with children. In S. L. Garfield & A. E. Bergin (Eds.), *Handbook of psychotherapy and behavior change* (2nd ed.). New York: John Wiley & Sons.
Ross, A. O. (1980). *Psychological disorders of children.* New York: McGraw-Hill.
Saylor, C. F., Benson, B., & Einhaus, L. (1985). Evaluation of an anger management program for aggressive boys in inpatient treatment. *Journal of Child and Adolescent Psychotherapy, 2*(1), 5-15.
Schacter, S. (1971). Some extraordinary facts about obese humans and rats. *American Psychologist, 26,* 129-144.
Skinner, B. F. (1953). *Science and human behavior.* New York: Macmillan.
Smith, R. G., & Sharpe, T. M. (1970). Treatment of school phobia with implosive therapy. *Journal of Consulting and Clinical Psychology, 35,* 239-243.
Stedman, J. M. (1976). Family counseling with a school-phobic child. In J. D. Krumboltz & C. E. Thoreson (Eds.), *Counseling methods.* New York: Holt, Rinehart & Winston.
Strain, P. S., Shores, R. E., & Timm, M. A. (1977). Effects of peer social imitations on the behavior of withdrawn preschool children. *Journal of Applied Behavior Analysis, 10,* 289-298.
Stuart, R. B. (1973). Behavioral contracting within the families of delinquents. In J. M. Stedman, W. F. Patton, & K. F. Walton (Eds.), *Clinical studies in behavior therapy with children, adolescents, and their families.* Springfield, IL: Charles C. Thomas.
Sulzer-Azaroff, B., & Mayer, G. R. (1986). *Achieving educational excellence: Using behavioral strategies.* New York: Holt, Rinehart & Winston.
Sulzer-Azaroff, B., & Reese, E. P. (1982). *Applying behavior analysis: A program for developing professional competence.* New York: Holt, Rinehart & Winston.
Sutherland, E., & Cressey, D. (1970). *Criminology.* Philadelphia, PA: Lippincott.
Tahmisian, J. A., & McReynolds, W. T. (1971). Use of parents as behavioral engineers in the treatment of a school-phobic girl. *Journal of Counseling Psychology, 18,* 225-228.
Trueman, D. (1984). What are the characteristics of school phobic children? *Psychological Reports, 54,* 191-202.
Van der Ploeg, H. M. (1975). Treatment of frequency of urination by stories competing with anxiety. *Journal of Behavior Therapy and Experimental Psychiatry, 6,* 165-166.
Walker, C. E., Hedberg, A. G., Clement, P. W., & Wright, L. (1981). *Clinical procedures for behavior therapy.* Englewood Cliffs, NJ: Prentice-Hall.
Watson, J. B., & Raynor, R. (1920). Conditioned emotional reactions. *Journal of Experimental Psychology, 3,* 1-14.
Webster, C. C. (1980). The characteristics of autism. In C. D. Webster, M. M. Konstantareas, J. Oxman, & J. E. Mack (Eds.), *Autism: New directions in research and education.* New York: Pergamon Press.
Weiner, I. B. (1973). Behavior therapy in obsessive-compulsive neurosis: Treatment of an adolescent boy. In J. M. Stedman, W. F. Patton, & K. F. Walton

(Eds.), *Clinical studies in behavior therapy with children, adolescents, and their families.* Springfield, IL: Charles C. Thomas.

Weisberg, P. (1963). Social and non-social conditioning of infant vocalizations. *Child Development, 34,* 177-388.

Wish, P. A., Hasazi, J. E., & Jurgela, A. R. (1975). Automated direct deconditioning of childhood phobia. In A. M. Graziano (Ed.), *Behavior therapy with children* (2nd ed.). Chicago: Aldine.

Wolpe, J. (1958). *Psychotherapy by reciprocal inhibition.* Stanford, CA: Stanford University Press.

Wright, J., & James, R. (1974). *A behavioral approach to preventing delinquency.* Springfield, IL: Charles C. Thomas.

Chapter 7

Rational-Emotive Approaches

Russell M. Grieger, Ph.D.
John D. Boyd, Ph.D.

INTRODUCTION

Rational-emotive therapy (RET), a system of psychotherapy orginally founded by Albert Ellis in the 1950s, continues to be developed and expanded by him and many others. RET holds that it is the unique ways that people think about and evaluate their experiences, rather than the actual experiences themselves, that cause their emotional and behavioral reactions. Thus, when youngsters experience emotional difficulties, such as school phobia or clinical depression, it is usually because they hold irrational ideas that create these disturbed states. To prevent emotional disturbance, RET teaches people ideas that facilitate emotional and interpersonal adjustment and shows them how to apply these ideas on an ongoing basis; to alleviate emotional disturbance, RET aids people in identifying, disrupting, and giving up these irrational ideas so that the disturbed states disappear.

History and Status

Rational-emotive therapy traces its roots to the Stoic philosophers, particularly Epictetus and Marcus Aurelius. Their major premise, articulated most succinctly by Epictetus in *The Enchiridion* during the first century A.D., states that "Men are not disturbed by things, but by the view which they take of them." Similarly, several ancient Buddhist and Taoist thinkers emphasized the need to change one's intense feelings by changing one's thinking. Shakespeare, in *Hamlet,* poignantly made the same observation by writing, "There's nothing either good or bad but thinking makes it so." Latter-day philosophers Spinoza and Bertrand Russell brought these principles to Western civilization.

Rational-emotive therapy is also firmly rooted in modern psychology. Perhaps the most significant modern psychotherapist to set its stage was Alfred Adler. Echoing the motto printed in his first book (1931) on individual psychology, *omnia ex opinione suspensa* (everything depends on opinion), he stated, "No experience is a cause of success or failure. We do not suffer from the shock of our experiences—the so-called trauma—but we make out of them just what suits our purposes. We are self-determined by situations, but we determine ourselves by the meaning we give to experiences." Further, "I am convinced that a person's behavior springs from his ideas" (1964a, p. 64), and, "the individual . . . does not relate himself to the outside world in a predetermined manner, as is often assumed. He relates himself always according to his own interpretations of himself and of his present problem. It is his attitude toward life which determines his relationship to the outside world" (1964b, p. 124).

Other significant individuals who predated RET or who concurrently arrived at psychotherapeutic positions and tactics that echo or overlap RET include the following: Paul Dubois, Jules Dejerine, Ernest Gaukler, Alexander Herzberg, Andrew Salter, Frederick Thorne, Franz Alexander, John Dollard, Neal Miller Lewis Wolberg, Eric Berne, Jerome Frank, George Kelly, Abraham Low, E. Lakin Phillips, Julian Rotter, and Joseph Wolpe (Ellis, 1979).

It was Albert Ellis (1957a, 1957b, 1962a, 1971, 1973), however, who founded and primarily developed RET and who directly paved the way for a whole host of other forms of cognitive behavior therapies. Ellis practiced classical psychoanalysis in the late 1940s and early 1950s when he observed that his clients rarely demonstrated elegant or long-lasting benefits from the insights they gained into their early childhood experiences (1962b, 1979). For even when their painful memories were brought to light through the traditional methods of free association, dream analysis, and the exploration of the transference relationship, clients did not entirely get over their symptoms and, in fact, tended to re-create similar problems about other experiences.

Discouraged by these observations, Ellis gravitated toward the thinking of Epictetus and Adler. First, he realized that all people develop and operate on theories (i.e., ideas, beliefs) about themselves and their world. He further observed that emotionally disturbed states are closely associated with absolute, dogmatic beliefs and highly negative self-evaluations. He also realized that people easily acquire such beliefs and actively perpetuate their own disturbance by re-indoctrinating themselves with these ideas despite the overwhelming evidence of their lunacy. Finally, Ellis noted that people rarely would give up their strongly held, disturbance-producing beliefs by more nondirective, relationship, or interpretive-oriented therapies; they would simply say the right things and continue to act and feel the same old ways.

Armed with these discoveries, Ellis developed Rational-Emotive Therapy (1962b). RET is an active-directive, multimodal, philosophic, didactic, persuasive, and highly—though not exclusively—cognitive form of psychotherapy. Its major purpose is to help people rid themselves of emotional disturbance by ridding themselves of the irrational ideas that create these disturbances.

Since the birth of RET in the 1950s, a whole generation of cognitive therapists has emerged, including many avowed RETers and other cognitive behavior therapists who borrow from and use a great deal of RET. Some of the more notable of these people include Ben Ard, James Bard, Aaron Beck, Raymond DiGiuseppe, Edward Garcia, Robert Harper, Paul Hauck, William Knaus, Arnold Lazarus, Michael Mahoney, Maxie C. Maultsby, Jr., Donald Meichenbaum, Richard Wessler, Janet Wolfe, and Howard Young.

Since the beginning of RET more than a quarter century ago, it has undergone quite a few significant developments and has established itself, it is certainly fair to say, as the foremost member of the cognitive behavior therapy movement. Hundreds of psychotherapists identify themselves as RET therapists, and perhaps thousands more borrow substantially from RET in their practice. Literally hundreds of papers and scores of texts have been published that, in large part or in their entirety, focus on the theory and practice of RET.

Perhaps more relevant, RET fares quite well in the experimental literature. We will discuss the findings regarding the efficacy of RET a little later. Suffice it to say that this literature is highly supportive of RET's effectiveness. For the present, however, experimental studies which test the major tenets of RET's theory of personality derived mostly from clinical, social and experimental psychology research, are legion and overwhelmingly supportive (Ellis, 1977a). Close to one thousand of these studies are presented in summary form in a paper by Albert Ellis, "Research Data That Support the Clinical and Personality Hypotheses of RET and Other Modes of Cognitive-Behavior Therapy" (1977a), a comprehensive bibliography of which can be obtained from The Institute for Rational-Emotive Therapy in New York City.

The two principal RET organizations are (1) The Institute for Rational Living, Inc., a nonprofit organization founded in 1959 whose purpose is to teach rational living concepts; and (2) The Institute for Rational-Emotive Therapy, founded in 1968, an RET training organization chartered by the Regents of the University of the State of New York. Both are housed at 45 East 65th Street, New York, NY 10021, and provide an extensive array of lectures, workshops, and training programs, as well as clinical services at low-cost fees.

Most impressive to the practitioner is the vast professional training program offered by The Institute for Rational-Emotive Therapy. With responsibility for the content and conduct of the Institute's training program resting with the International Training Standards and Review Committee, comprehensive training programs are offered at the Primary Certificate, Intermediate Certificate, Associate Fellow, and Fellow levels.

In addition to the parent Institute in New York City, there also exists an Institute for Rational-Emotive Therapy in Los Angeles and affiliates in Cleveland, San Francisco, Charlottesville, VA, and Denver. Training units at the University of Kentucky, Hofstra University, Pittsburg State University (Kansas), and the Unversity of Virginia provide official training programs that qualify successful participants for the Primary Certificate. Affiliates in Chicago, Clearwater, Minneapolis, and Seattle offer clinical services but do not offer professional training.

OVERVIEW OF THEORY

Basic Theory and Assumptions

Rational-emotive therapy rests on a good many well-defined premises about human personality and about personality change (Ellis, 1977a, 1979, 1980). The major ones, summarized from Albert Ellis' major writings, follow:

1. Human thinking, feeling, and behaving overlap and influence one another. People tend to think, feel, and act simultaneously. Moreover, thinking significantly affects feelings and actions; feelings significantly affect thinking and actions; and actions significantly affect thinking and feeling. When one is changed in some substantial way, the others will very likely change as well.

2. People are uniquely able to think and particularly able to think abstractly. They think chronically, or, in other words, they find it virtually impossible to turn off their thoughts. They, therefore, are chronic constructors of theories about how they, others, and conditions in the world should and should not be. Hence, they rarely act without also thinking, for their acts are grounded both in "rules" about what behavior is expected and on predictions about the outcome of their actions; and they also rarely feel without thinking, for their feelings are usually accompanied by some cognitive appraisal or evaluation of the goodness or badness of the experienced situation.

3. People are powerfully disposed to think self-enhancingly, logically, and rationally; in the process, they make themselves satisfied, actualize their individual potentials, foster their interpersonal relationships, attain their basic goals, and are creative and joyful. Concurrently, they also are powerfully disposed to think irrationally, anti-empirically, and shortsightedly

and, thereby, create for themselves all sorts of unhappiness, thwart their goals, and undercut valued interpersonal attachments. Both dispositions have innate, biological components.

4. The human tendency toward crooked thinking is strongly exacerbated by various social institutions, including the family, organized religion, and the media. Following Piaget and Inhelder (1970), human vulnerability to illogical thinking is greatest during early childhood so that youngsters are particularly susceptible to the self-defeating ideas of their social world.

5. Thinking mediates between experiences and responses such that people's emotional and behavioral reactions result not so much from the experiences directly but from their thoughts about the experiences. This central proposition of RET is captured in the now-famous A-B-C theory, whereby: A, an activating event or experience, does not directly or predominantly cause C, an emotional and/or behavioral consequence; rather B, the person's belief, idea, or attitude about A more significantly causes C.

   Take, for example, a 10-year-old boy whose younger brother wrecks his bicycle (an A, or event). He would variously respond at C depending on what his evaluative thoughts at B are. He could, for instance, think: "Well, that's not too bad—it was an old bike anyway," and would react with basic calmness, although perhaps with some mild degree of frustration. Or, he might take the attitude: "That little jerk! He's always taking my things, I'm going to get him." And he would probably react with anger and act in some hostile manner. Or, he might, again at B, evaluate the event thusly: "That's terrible! I'll never get another bike. Nothing else is any fun." And, thinking this he would probably react with sadness and hurt.

6. People are not limited to thinking about and conceptualizing their experiences in words, phrases, and sentences. They also do so by various pictorial represen-

tations, including images, dreams, and fantasies. Such "pictures" also act as mediators and likewise powerfully influence feelings and behaviors. People differ in their ability to "think" pictorially, with some people powerfully causing their reactions in this manner and others doing so only lightly.

7. Not only do people think about and evaluate outside events, but they also are aware of and think about their own thinking, emotions, behavior, and physiological processes. By this process, they cause themselves to react to their own responses in much the same way as they do to outside events.

8. Because almost all emotional and behavioral responses have a cognitive (e.g., idea or belief) base, what are commonly called emotionally disturbed states also result from the ideas or beliefs people hold. In other words, the main reason why people become and remain chronically and/or frequently anxious, depressed, guilty, angry, procrastinating, and a hundred other symptomatic ways is that they adopt and regularly endorse ideas that logically lead to these assumptions.

   The presence of an emotional disturbance, then, results from people holding dogmatic, unverifiable, and superstitious ideas and continuing to hold them on an ongoing basis. More specifically, emotional disturbance consists of a person endorsing the belief that he or she *must* have some state of affairs or else it would be too *awful* or *terrible to stand.* Holding such absolute life necessities, people endlessly worry about getting them *and* desperately seek after them; when they do get what they want, they worry incessantly about keeping them; and when they do not get what they believe they must have, they become despondent, self-downing, and outraged.

   Take, for example, a sixth-grade girl participating in a spelling bee. If, while standing in line waiting for her turn, she only thought, "I hope I do well, but if I don't it's OK and I'm OK," she would at worst be only slightly apprehensive and she would probably perform to the best of her ability when called upon. But if she were to think something like, "I *must* do well and *must* have my classmates think I'm bright or else I *won't be able to stand it,*" she would experience panic, would be unlikely to perform well, and would feel ashamed and depressed if she indeed did perform poorly. This young lady has made herself disturbed by her beliefs in the necessity of succeeding, by her characterizing not succeeding as awful, and probably by also downing herself for behaving inefficiently.

9. Because of both human nature and the exacerbating training that society offers, people easily adopt and perpetuate their disturbance-producing ideas. Moreover, when people feel upset or view themselves as disturbed, they tend to think about their upset or disturbance in such a way as to feel further upset or disturbed about their disturbance. They, in effect, tend to create emotional problems through the same processes by which they create their original problems.

10. Effective psychotherapy invokes cognitive, emotive, and behavioral change in people. To understand and appreciate a person's disturbed emotional and behavioral reactions, it is important for the therapist to understand the ideas, beliefs, or philosophies a person holds about himself or herself and the world. To help people change the ways they habitually and maladaptively respond, the therapist must help change the way they think and believe. Rational-emotive therapy employs an array of behavioral, emotive, and especially cognitive techniques to help people identify, acknowledge, analyze, and give up their irrational ideas or beliefs. In its most elegant form, RET helps people relinquish absolutistic "musts," helps them accept undesirable realities as nonawful and bearable, and shows them how to stubbornly refuse to rate themselves and others.

Rational-emotive therapy does not possess a theory of human development analogous, say, to the stage theory of psychoanalysis. It does, however, hold a definite view of the development of human psychopathology.

RET differs from most other current systems of psychotherapy by emphasizing the biological underpinnings of human personality (Ellis, 1977a, 1979, 1980). Although acknowledging the impact of experiences on personality development, RET holds that humans are powerfully disposed to think irrationally, to defeat their own ends, and to perpetuate their problems in the face of its stupidity (Ellis, 1976a). And humans are particularly disposed to *demand* that they get what they want and to *condemn* the world, themselves, and others when their wants are thwarted.

Added to this human proclivity toward irrational thinking is the modeling, training, and reinforcing that is rampant in society. Society in general "values" much of what is irrational and has a multitude of forums for socializing its members with these ideas, including organized religion, popular music (Protinsky & Popp, 1978), and television (Grieger & Czajkowski, 1980). In the process, people are heavily propagandized to believe that they must do well and be loved, that others must treat them well, and that the conditions of the world must be good and easy.

VIEW OF PSYCHOPATHOLOGY

Backed by a considerable amount of empirical evidence (Ellis, 1977a), RET asserts that almost all forms of emotional disturbance stem from the holding of magical (i.e., nonsupportable) and absolute beliefs. Endorsing such dogma, disturbed people make themselves frequently miserable; they are self-downing, intolerant of their own and others' errors, aversive to ambiguity and uncertainty, inflexible, lacking in risk-taking, unusually focused on themselves and dependent (Ellis, 1980).

Although a good many other personality theorists (Adler, 1931, 1964a, 1964b; Beck, 1976; Horney, 1965; Kelly, 1955) agree with this basic RET tenet, RET is much more specific by categorizing the major disturbance-producing irrational ideas into three major categories (Ellis, 1977a).

1. *Demandingness.* This is the core of almost all emotional disturbances. Emotional disturbance rarely if ever

results from a person simply wanting, preferring, or desiring something, no matter how strong are their wants; for simply wanting something rarely leads to desperation (i.e., anxiety), and not getting what one wants rarely leads to being destroyed (i.e., depressed, guilty, feelings of worthlessness). To the contrary, emotional disturbance results from people *believing* that they *need* (must or should have) what they want. They, in effect, convince themselves that what is merely desirable is an absolute necessity of life.

Although there are literally hundreds of ideas people can believe to make themselves disturbed, and although people can *must*urbate about all sorts of things, demandingness can be categorized under four major headings, each with several derivatives (Ellis, 1977a, 1979, 1980; Ellis & Abrahms, 1978; Ellis & Grieger, 1977): (1) I *must* do well; (2) I *must* be approved; (3) you *must* do right by me; and (4) the conditions of the world *must* be easy.

Demandingness is illogical and anti-empirical, and hence irrational, on several counts. First, it represents a distortion of reality by confusing a personal preference, or a desirable outcome, with an absolute necessity. The person is saying: "Because I want something and view it as an important ingredient to my well-being, I cannot survive without it." This is tautological malarkey, creating urgency and life- and death-ness when only a preference is real. Second, demandingness casts a black/white, either/or connotation on circumstances that most often have many shades of gray to them. For it, in effect, says, "I must do perfectly well or else I've totally failed; I must have total approval or I'm totally disappointed; you must be thoroughly appropriate or you're thoroughly inappropriate; and conditions must be all easy or else they're all rotten." Clearly, one can do poorly in something without doing the thing totally wrong, or do poorly in some things while doing well in others, and likewise with other forms of demandingness.

A third irrational underpinning to demandingness is that it is, at the core, grandiose. Underneath the notion of "I must have it" is the assumption that "I am special, and, because I am special, I deserve to get what I want." But no one is special in the sense that he or she is immune from the slings and arrows of everyday living—all people fall under the law of nature that everyone receives some degree or another of frustration and hardship. The irrational thought, however, is, "Because *I* want it, *I* should get it!"

2. *Awfulizing.* Awfulizing is a second major way that people disturb themselves and is a logical derivative from the basic irrational *musts* described above. For it follows that if something *must* be a certain way, then it is awful, horrible, or terrible when it is not. But, again, awfulizing is illogical on a number of scores. First, it means more than unfortunate, bad, or even really bad. It means totally or 100% bad. But nothing can be 100% bad; and most things to which people unthinkingly assign a score of 100% bad are, upon reflection, considerably less than that bad. When held against a criterion where "awful" is represented by dying a slow, painful death of cancer, such things as failing a test, losing a girlfriend, having an unjust amount of homework, and so on hardly rank.

   Second, "awful" also falsely connotes that the whole world—everything—is bad because some thing in life is bad. It connotes, in other words, that every aspect of life is negative when one or two things go wrong. But, again, this is very rarely the case. Third, the concept of "awful" falsely suggests that the undesirable things in life are unstandable or unbearable, a premise that is patently absurd because people always bear adversity—they just bear it with some degree of pain or discomfort. Finally, awfulizing swings full circle and connotes that because something is bad or undesirable, it should not exist. And here we are back to where we started, ready to start the whole process over again.

TABLE 1: CHILDHOOD EMOTIONAL PROBLEMS

	Manifestations		
Problem	Behavioral	Emotional	Irrational Ideas
1. Withdrawal, avoidance	Avoidance of people and tasks Shyness Dependency	Anxiety and fears Feelings of inferiority Depression (secondarily)	I must do well and be approved of. I must avoid getting noticed at all costs, because if I try, I will fail and be disapproved of. That would be terrible and I would be worthless. So long as I can be left alone and nothing is demanded of me, my worthlessness will not be obvious and I won't feel worthless.
2. Perfectionism	Compulsiveness Overachieving Overdriving to excel	Feeling OK when he or she succeeds Anxiety before performance Depression, guilt, self-downing when he or she fails	I must do well in order to get attention and be approved of or else I will be lost and worthless. I must always do my very best. My performance at school and everywhere else should always be competent. It's terrible to do poorly and doing poorly shows what an incompetent person I am. If I don't totally and always do well, then I'm totally and always a failure.
3. Attention seeking	Being the model child, cute, charming Being the class clown, showing off, pest Shyness, helplessness, dependency	Anxiety Feelings of inferiority Depression (secondarily)	I must be noticed at all costs or else I am lost and worthless. I must be loved and approved of, all the time. It's awful to be unnoticed or unacknowledged.
4. Power struggling	Disobedience Stubbornness Not cooperating Argumentativeness "Smart-mouthing" Hostility toward students who do not agree	Anger Jealousy	The only way I can feel like somebody is to defy pressure and do what I want. I must win, because if I don't I am a loser. People must acknowledge that I am right. I must be on top. People should give me attention and approval by making me No. 1.

Table 1 (Continued)

	Manifestations		
Problem	Behavioral	Emotional	Irrational Ideas
5. Revenge seeking	Bullying Stealing Violence "Viciousness"	Anger Resentment Jealousy	People should/ought/must do right by me. People who do wrong by me are wicked and blameworthy and deserve to be punished and to suffer. Those who do not give me attention deserve to be hurt. Those who get the attention *I* want, deserve to be hurt. I must feel significant, and the only way I can feel significant is to hurt others as much as I feel hurt.
6. Depression	Lethargic behavior Excessive sleeping Significant loss or increase of appetite Withdrawing Excessive daydreaming Verbal expressions of helplessness & hopelessness	Guilt Depression	I did a bad thing and I'm a bad person for having done it. I must be totally competent and loved, or else I'm worthless. This is a hassle; it's too much of a hassle; I can't stand it. Poor me.
7. Procrastination	Laziness Sloppiness Self-indulgence Grousing and griping Not doing assignments	Frustration Self-pity Resentment	I shouldn't have to work so hard to get things done. I can't stand to do these boring things necessary to reach some goal. It's too hard and it takes too much work. I can't stand to delay pleasure. Because I don't like it and it's not fair, I shouldn't have to do it. It's easier and better to take one's pleasures now rather than deny oneself and get pleasure later.

3. *Self-rating.* Self-rating is directly or indirectly involved in almost all forms of emotional disturbance. Again a logical derivative of demandingness, it refers to the almost universal, but illogical, philosophy of rating oneself (or others) as good or bad for doing or not doing what "should" have been done.

   Now, why is self-rating irrational? Is it not appropriate for people to rate or evaluate themselves? Is it not proper for parents, educators, and child mental health professionals to help youngsters rate themselves as good—in other words, hold high self-esteem? The answer to these last two questions is an emphatic NO! First, the self-rating response represents a gross overgeneralization. If I say I am a bad person, I mean that I am thoroughly rotten in everything; contrarily, if I say that I am a good person, I mean that I am thoroughly good. Neither of these can be true, for I am too complex and multifaceted to behave always in either a good or bad manner. At best I can say only that I am a person who is sometimes good and sometimes bad.

   Self-rating is also illogical in communicating a fatalism about the future. For if I am a bad person, there is an implication that I have to go on forever behaving in the bad ways that I now do. But each human being is amazingly adaptable and trainable and hence able to unlearn old ways of acting and learn new ways.

Having taken some pains to describe the three main themes of emotional disturbance, we now present some of the more common forms of childhood emotional disturbance. Table 1 lists these, along with their typical behavioral and emotional manifestations and the irrational attitudes behind them.

General Therapeutic Goals and Techniques

Because rational-emotive therapy states that emotional disturbance is "caused" by the irrational ideas that a person holds, its major thrust is to induce people to give up those ideas. In so doing, it has distinct goals, processes, and techniques.

GOALS. RET makes a fundamental distinction between elegant and inelegant goals for clients. *Inelegant goals* are tantamount to symptom removal. To pursue this end the RET therapist directly teaches clients appropriate behaviors and teaches, conditions, and indoctrinates them with irrational beliefs and coping statements that will help them function more effectively (Ellis, 1977a, 1979, 1980; Grieger & Boyd, 1980). In this process, there is little effort directed toward achieving insights into the philosophic errors of the irrational beliefs or making independent choices of new philosophies.

Elegant goals in RET stress "the achievement of a profound cognitive or philosophic change in clients' basic assumptions, especially their absolutistic, demanding, irrational ways of viewing themselves, others, and the world" (Ellis, 1977b, pp. 34-35). Elegant goals include teaching clients how to recognize and scientifically dispute their irrational ideas and behavior so that they have skills to solve future emotional problems creatively on their own. Elegant change, then, is movement to less disturbability through a cognitive-emotive-behavioral re-education in which clients understand the errors in their fundamental assumptions and adopt philosophies that make logical, empirical, and practical sense. The final goal is a greater degree of human freedom unencumbered by absolute laws or "musts" that limit a person's choices and prompt compulsive, rigid behavior.

With higher value placed on elegant goals, it is nevertheless recognized that not all clients are capable of elegant change. The young child, the less intelligent, the psychotic, and the severely depressed person (at least temporarily) are prime examples. For these people it is important to set realistic goals, probably inelegant ones. However, it is vitally important to consider whether each and every client can attain elegant goals and to be very careful not to sell him or her short with inelegant change if elegant goals are attainable (Grieger & Boyd, 1980).

PROCESSES. At first blush it often seems that RET therapists behave in a very disorganized fashion. In reality, RET is a craft consisting of highly developed and refined skills that generally evolve in an orderly fashion through four somewhat overlapping, yet distinct, stages (Grieger & Boyd, 1980).

Rational-emotive therapists typically spend very little time when first seeing a client in taking a lengthy history or establishing a therapeutic alliance. Rather, the RET therapist quickly begins *Rational-Emotive Psychodiagnosis and Goal Directing.* This first stage of RET consists of several things: (1) conceptually separating environmental concerns or problems in living (A problems) from emotional and/or behavioral problems (C problems); (2) ascertaining the irrational beliefs that create the emotional disturbance; (3) determining whether or not the client is disturbed about the original disturbance or, in other words, has developed a problem about the emotional problem itself; and (4) directing the client to focus on the emotional and/or behavioral problem as the prime arena for therapy, rather than the external or environmental problem.

In the second stage of RET, *Rational-Emotive Insight and Goal Setting,* the client is helped to acknowledge maladaptive feelings and behaviors, to assume full responsibility for them as self-created, and to look for, find, and genuinely acknowledge the cognitive source of their symptoms. In doing this, the RET therapist teaches six basic insights: (1) that maladaptive feelings and behaviors do exist (a C problem as well as perhaps an A problem); (2) that through their own thinking and believing they cause their emotional disturbance, or C problem; (3) that they can accept themselves even though they have foolishly created their emotional problems; (4) that their disturbance is caused by specific irrational ideas, which they acknowledge and appreciate; (5) that it is acceptable and highly desirable to check out the validity of their beliefs; and (6) that they can give up their irrational beliefs and can adopt new ones that will make them function more effectively and happily in the future. Following the successful induction of these insights, specific therapeutic goals—either elegant or inelegant—are agreed upon.

The third stage, *Rational-Emotive Working Through,* is the heart and soul of RET. It is at this stage that the therapist expends the most time and energy. Through a whole host of cognitive, behavioral, and emotive techniques, the RET therapist helps clients actively dispute their irrational beliefs in order to see the foolishness of them clearly and repeatedly and thereby give them up. The therapist assists the client to *debate* against the irrational belief in order to see its phoniness; to *discriminate* rational wants or preferences from irrational demands, undesirable outcomes from awful, horrible, or terrible ones, and bad acts or behaviors from bad people; and to *define* terms precisely until overgeneralizations, absolute propositions, and other cognitive distortions are seen as fallacious (Ellis, 1977a). Throughout this process, the therapist encourages the client to find alternative ideas that withstand the same disputational process and lead to healthier functioning.

Rational-Emotive Re-education is the fourth and final stage in RET. The therapist's purpose at this point is to habituate the client to think in the new, rational ways or to come to automatically believe the new ideas.

TECHNIQUES. With the foregoing process in mind, we will now briefly describe the *hows* and *whats* of RET. First, how or in what manner does the RET therapist proceed? In several distinct ways, although we caution the reader not to view these as dogmatic, RET is applied as flexibly as particular needs of different clients dictate and differently by therapists with different personality styles. In the main, however, RET does advocate the following *hows* (Ellis, 1973, 1977a; Grieger & Boyd, 1980):

1. Because it is assumed that people easily get disturbed and tend to reindoctrinate themselves with their irrational ideas, RETers believe an active, directive approach is more effective in intercepting the self-disturbing process. The RET therapist consequently does a great deal of explaining, particularly in the early stages of therapy when the client is relatively ignorant; goes right to the heart of the problem; and probes, challenges, persuades, cajoles, exhorts, and sometimes even argues with the client in order to help break up the ongoing irrational process.

2. Because emotional problems are basically attitudinal or ideological, the RET therapist is unusually didactic and philosophical. There is a constant attempt to show clients the philosophic dynamic of their problems, to teach them rational ideas, and to show them logical-empirical modes of inquiry.

3. Again, because clients find it easy to be disturbed, and because they tend to be habituated to thinking and believing their irrational, disturbance-producing ideas, the RET therapist is persistent and repetitive, particularly with children. Although backing off of some clients may be necessary, the therapist generally keeps after them, knowing that frequent and repeated working through is necessary.
4. Because RET holds that clients are disturbed by holding beliefs that are irrational, no matter what their life history may be, the RET therapist focuses on the here and now. Clients are strongly encouraged to be self-aware, i.e., to catch themselves thinking and acting on irrational beliefs and immediately work them through.

The *whats* of RET are many and involve a comprehensive, multimodal, cognitive-emotive-behavioral array of therapeutic techniques (Ellis, 1962, 1973, 1977a, 1979; Grieger & Boyd, 1980). RET is first and foremost a highly *cognitive* therapy whose main thrusts are to get clients to give up their demandingness, awfulizing, and self-rating and to teach them how to think scientifically and logically about the validity of their own thinking. It does so through didactic teaching and persuasion, information giving, the consideration of alternatives, and a whole host of other cognitive techniques. But it mainly does so through a rigorous and thorough disputation (via discussion, Socratic questioning, and empirical analysis) of the validity and practicality of holding these views. In short, disputation in RET consists of first holding each idea or assumption up as a hypothesis to be tested and then energetically challenging and questioning until it is shown to be untenable.

In its *emotive* aspects, RET tries to help clients change their irrational ideas by dramatizing these ideas in such a way as to show their phoniness (Ellis, 1979). Thus, the RET therapist invokes humor a great deal, poking fun at the client's ideas but never at him or her. The therapist exaggerates clients' irrational beliefs to the point of absurdity in order to highlight their lack of validity. The therapist may employ role playing designed so that the client can be shown the negative effects of the irrational thinking and acting. And the RET therapist strongly encourages clients to do embarrassing, self-disclosing, sometimes shameful things in order to prove to themselves concretely that they need not die from the wayward looks of others.

The *behavioral* aspects of RET rest on the premise that an effective means of cognitive change is through behavioral change. In other words, getting a client to behave in a way that contradicts irrational ideas often serves to eradicate the ideas. Consequently, RETers assign clients written disputational homework, encourage them to do the things they are afraid of doing, assign them risky (though not dangerous) things to do, tell them to fail at things purposely, and engage in many other creative things, all to change their cognitions.

To sum, RET is a highly comprehensive system of psychotherapy populated with many techniques and aspects and generally following an orderly sequence of stages. Its goals are both elegant (a philosophic re-education) and inelegant (symptom removal); more value is given to elegant goals, goals that are striven for unless circumstances dictate otherwise, unless client characteristics, such as age, argue for inelegant goals.

INDIVIDUAL PSYCHOTHERAPY WITH CHILDREN

RET began as a therapy for adults, but shortly thereafter, Ellis applied his theory to therapeutic work with children. These efforts were consummated in The Living School, an educational facility within The Institute for Rational-Emotive Therapy which offered programs and services to emotionally disturbed children in the 1960s and 1970s. From these pioneering experiences, the concept and guidelines for applications of RET with children were begun.

Rational-emotive therapy is appropriate with children who have almost all types of emotional disorder, i.e., problems in living and experiencing that have a psychological rather than an organic basis. As with adults, RET is also appropriate for youngsters who develop emotional problems about other non-psychologically based problems, such as dyslexia.

Before explaining RET methods for children, however, it is appropriate to overview some of the psychological characteristics of youngsters that dictate treatment modalities. Rational-emotive methods differ for the three major client groups—children (ages 3 to 12), adolescents (ages 12 to 18), and adults; and children in particular require special considerations so that services are compatible with their level of maturation in the cognitive-emotional-behavioral domains. When doing RET with children, it is particularly important to consider certain psychological characteristics of children:

1. Tendency to be resistive because of nonvolunteer status.
2. Low capacity for verbal therapy.
3. Necessity of involvement of parents.
4. Childish emotions, behaviors, and word changes.
5. Limited cognitive development.

Techniques

While acknowledging that RET with children is idiosyncratic in some ways, we note that it still follows the orderly process described above (Grieger & Boyd, 1980). In *RET Psychodiagnosis*—the first stage for children—the RET therapist first tries to overcome children's resistance and their low verbal capacity by following three suggestions offered by DiGiuseppe (1981): (1) don't be all business, (2) always be honest with the child, and (3) go easily and carefully with questions. The beginning of therapy is a time for building rapport rather than immediately entering an investigation of the problem; talking about the child's interests and games and nonintrusive conversation are good techniques for gaining trust and acceptance.

As the RET therapist is establishing a working relationship with the child, an assessment task can also begin. The authors recommend a *psychosituational assessment* strategy (Bersoff & Grieger, 1971), which gathers and interprets information about the child's problem behaviors, the environments and situations in which they occur, and the attitudes, expectations, and emotions of the child and influential others in the problem situations.

The psychosituational strategy begins with the therapist interviewing the referring agents (e.g., parent or teacher) and converting their complaints into child behaviors; the frequency, intensity, and duration of these behaviors; and the situations in which they arise. As the referring parties offer this information, the therapist listens for and asks about their attitudes toward and expectations of the child, noting both rational and irrational ideation. The picture is then firmed up with a similar interview with the child, which may confirm, refute, or enrich the material already collected. The rational-emotive psychodiagnosis is then composed of a categorization of the child's and referring adults' problems into a host of A-B-C sequences. Throughout all of this an attempt is made to distinguish emotional-behavioral problems in the child and adults (B-C problems) from practical problems and developmental problems (A problems).

The verbal or written explanation of this assessment is called a *psychodiagnosis paper,* that is, a diagnostic statement that separates emotional-behavioral problems from practical-developmental problems for each of the parties involved. Its purpose is to point each party toward the goal of first solving the emotional-behavioral components and only secondarily solving practical problems. A brief excerpt from a recent session is offered to illustrate these points. In this instance, problems were identified but not delineated in A-B-C terms.

> *Therapist:* After talking to all three of you, I think I have a clear picture of your concerns. Mrs. Jones [divorced mother of two children], you are angry and disgusted with the kids because of their frequent fighting. Sometimes you feel overwhelmed by their behavior, nothing you do seems to help them stop their fighting, you'd like to pick up some discipline methods that work, and you particularly want to calm down because your stress level seems to be up. So, we have two goals: dealing with your emotional stress, and learning some effective disciplining methods.
>
> Jill, you are also a bit unhappy, or so I gathered from what you said. You seem to find yourself continually battling with Jack and in conflict with your mother because of this fighting. Worse yet, the conflict between you and Mom sets you up for arguments and misunderstandings about other matters, like dating, money, helping out around the house, etc. I don't think either of you knows how much the

> other wants to be closer, and these conflicts are keeping you apart.
>
> Jack, we had a great chat. I sure appreciate how honest you were about your feelings. It's been tough since Dad moved away, but you're hanging in there! I'd like to help you deal with some of those tough feelings, and together I think we can also work on getting along better with your teacher at school [a male whom Jack resents and defies].
>
> How does my understanding of things fit with yours? Tell me if I'm off track [confirmation from clients]. If there is anything I've overlooked that needs discussion . . . [pause] OK, you can of course bring up anything you want later on as we work on these concerns.
>
> Mrs. Jones, let's you and I get together next week to work on your goals. I'd like to see Jack and Jill for individual sessions also, and then probably the week after that we can get together to help you establish a strategy for dealing with the fighting.

Children are not as intellectually and emotionally capable of gaining *Rational-Emotive Insight*, the second stage in RET, as are adults. To gain full measure of insight one must be able to conceptualize behavioral and emotional alternatives, be able to predict the consequences of one's actions as well as those of alternative actions, and be able to view oneself objectively as an observer, noting one's own thoughts and feelings in relation to events. Children typically lack these notions, much less an awareness and appreciation of their irrational thoughts. A first step in RET insight with children is to teach them these basic skills, as well as to help them become aware of their irrational ideas.

Initially in the insight process we have found it very productive to have youngsters role-play different emotional reactions to the troublesome event in their lives. This helps them understand that there are different ways to feel and act. We first demonstrate alternative responses to the event for them and then have them do this. Once they see that other, less disturbed responses exist, we then help them explore the consequences their disturbed behaviors and feelings provide for them. This activity is designed to motivate them to put energy into changing. Virtually any technique to accomplish this is acceptable within the RET framework, including list making, role playing, observing other children, puppet play, use of games, and so on.

Finally, in RET insight, an attempt is made to show children that, by thinking in particular ways, *they* are causing the disturbed feelings and behaviors. Again, role playing can be used to accomplish this, and it is also advisable to help the youngster again see the negative consequences of thinking the thoughts and behaving in ways that are consistent with these thoughts. An 8-year-old client, for instance, was recently taught to label as "fit thoughts" certain of his thoughts that led to temper tantrums and subsequent punishment; these were contrasted with "level one" thoughts, or thoughts that led to appropriate behaviors required to gain a certain status in an operant program at his school.

Once children gain these insights, they are ready for *Working Through and Skill Training,* the third stage. As opposed to adults, they are rarely capable of a philosophic understanding of the illogic in their thinking (i.e., elegant change). Rather, because of their mental immaturity, they require a concrete reeducation of their false assumptions, inferences, and evaluations. Goals in this stage, therefore, are to teach the youngster more appropriate, rational attitudes, positive emotional responses, and constructive behavior (Boyd, 1980).

Central to "working through" with children is the method of rational self-instruction and coping, and it deserves special mention. It consists simply of constructing a rational self-talk dialogue which the child can practice at various times and can use when confronted with the problem situation. The rational beliefs are put in the child's language and practiced through imagery, role playing with the therapist, and rehearsal with other adults, among other methods. With young children this practice is most effective if it follows Meichenbaum's (1977) guidelines for teaching verbal self-instructions.

It is also at the "working through" stage where the RET therapist attempts to apply a complete, psychosituational set of strategies to "drown out" the child's old irrationalities and habituate the new rational ideation. Techniques in the "working through" stage are aimed at helping the youngster put into successful practice a rational A-B-C sequence which replaces the problematic A-B-Cs. Some of the common "working through" techniques are listed here and briefly explained.

INTERPERSONAL SKILLS TRAINING. When youngsters lack the interpersonal skills that normally accompany the rational beliefs they are learning, the skills are taught in RET. Some emotional education may also be needed, thus enabling the youngster to build and practice a rational A-B-C sequence. As RET enters The "working through" stage, the therapist should check to be sure the requisite skills are in the child's repertoire.

HOMEWORK ASSIGNMENTS. Some "working through" experiences can be orchestrated within therapy, but many of them take place at home and school through homework assignments whereby the youngster faces problems and practices progressive gradations of rational responses. Adults must set up such experiences for young children, but older children can handle them on their own if the assignment is clear, if it is within their ability to accomplish, and if adequate motivation is present.

STRUCTURED SITUATIONS. Intervention can include manipulation of the As by requesting and instructing teachers and parents to arrange situations that give the child an opportunity to use newly developed skills. The child may or may not be privy to this planning.

WRITTEN HOMEWORK. Young children benefit from writing and reciting rational beliefs and completing simple A-B-C fill-in-the-blank exercises. Older youngsters can complete uncomplicated rational self-analysis exercises.

PARENTS. Parents may require RET themselves (see later section). But the reading and/or discussing of the stories in Waters' (1980) parenting pamphlets is an excellent "working through" and insight aid. Parents can also be taught to teach rational ideas and help youngsters practice them.

RATIONAL-EMOTIVE IMAGERY. Youngsters can practice desirable A-B-C sequences via imagery in therapy, and older children can use this technique outside therapy.

OPERANT CONDITIONING. Parents and teachers can be taught to reinforce rational behavior and to withdraw their unintentional rewarding of maladaptive responses.

ROLE PLAYING. Youngsters can practice rational A-B-Cs with the therapist.

EVALUATING SUCCESS. A key difference between "patient" and "nonpatient" clients is that the former overlook their success, focus on their failures, and downplay themselves for their misperceived incompetence. It is critical that the therapist thwart this cognitive syndrome and reinforce the youngster for small therapeutic gains. Eventually the child is taught self-reinforcement skills and self-acceptance ideas.

Success in the "working through" stage of RET means that the client is doing well with those situation-specific problems on which therapy has focused. A final stage in the RET process, *Generalized Learning,* is to generalize therapeutic learning beyond a few specific problems to similar problems in other situations, to different problems, and to the child's view of self. Young children's generalization ability is slim, and attempts to generalize may even weaken the basic learning. But with older youngsters (10 years and above) the therapist can "test the waters" and do as much generalizing as possible. In the previously used case example, generalization would take the form of the boy first managing anger and hostile behavior toward his sister, then toward his classmates, and on to his anger and resistance toward authority figures (father and male teacher). Finally, the boy would be helped toward gaining a broad perspective of his characteristic ways of dealing with anger and of what he could do in the future to continue using and developing rational means of handling anger. With this done, RET would terminate if no other problems had surfaced during the four stages.

INDIVIDUAL PSYCHOTHERAPY WITH ADOLESCENTS

As with children, RET is appropriately used with adolescents who present problems anywhere in the gamut of psychological problems, including conduct, anxiety, eating, affective, somatoform, psychosexual, and adjustment disorders. In addition, RET is appropriate for those developmentally "normal" problems adolescents face such as rebelliousness, concrete and inflexible ideation processes, excessive concerns about peer approval, sexuality and guilt about sexuality, autonomy-dependence conflicts, and the like. This latter set of issues may be therapy targets themselves, may simply be As (in the A-B-C sequence) about which adolescents develop emotional problems, or may simply be factors to consider when shaping the therapy process.

Techniques

Although effective RET with adolescents means taking the client through RET's four stages, in doing so, the therapist had better be sensitive to some unique adolescent features. First, the adolescent's "natural" oppositional tendencies make the establishment of a therapeutic alliance particularly important. Succeeding to this end means initially allowing the adolescent to define the problem, even if greater problems lie elsewhere. It means withholding a problem *diagnosis* and conceptualization lest the adolescent become defensive and prematurely abort the process. It may mean temporarily going along with the adolescent's irrational beliefs, labile affect, and outrageous behavior, so as not to play into adolescent-adult power struggle patterns. And it means a good deal of chatter for an extended period of time until the adolescent feels comfortable enough to address issues and hear feedback.

For adolescents, *Rational-Emotive Insight and Education,* the second stage, serves the dual purpose of knowledge acquisition and capturing the interest of the adolescent. A standard motivational procedure is to help adolescents see that they can control their feelings and behave so as to get the things out of life they desire. Being careful not to play a parental role, the RET therapist in essence appeals to the typical adolescent concern of powerlessness and the push toward autonomy, power, and independence. For instance, while covertly believing an 11-year-old boy's desperate attempts to keep his recently divorced mother from dating were out of bounds, a great deal of time was spent convincing the youngster he could feel differently from the way he did, that it was in his best interest to feel differently, and that he could still act upset while calmly figuring out how to manipulate his mother. Seeing that he could both still "win" with her *and* control himself as well, he willingly worked on changing his irrational thinking.

Once the adolescent learns to value self-change, a host of learning aids, such as reading material, models, pictures and charts, and excercises, can be effectively used to teach the A-B-Cs and to identify irrational beliefs.

Skill training is often an important adjunct to the insight stage. Adolescents are more likely to incorporate rational beliefs and emotions into their personalities during the upcoming stages if they have the skill behaviors that accompany the outcomes.

The essential differences between the second stage of RET with children and with adolescents, then, are that the latter can benefit from insights and the dialogue of therapy is more interactional. Adolescents can be partners as well as learners; that is, they have the ability to be more responsible than children for their behavior, and they assume more and more of this responsibility as RET progresses.

Working Through, the third stage, can be used with adolescents on the same elegant level as used with most adults, but inelegant working through is also accepted and reinforced where appropriate. A combination of inelegant and elegant working through is portrayed in the interchange that follows.

> *Client:* I'm seeing it now. . . . I really got upset over losing her approval and put myself down, but that's just a crazy way to think. [Client parrots what he's learned.]
>
> *Therapist:* What's crazy about thinking you *must* get her to think you are a very neat guy? [Therapist forces client to dispute.]
>
> *Client:* Well, because she likes to change boyfriends. I'm not the first guy she's dropped. [Concrete reasoning.]

Therapist: Yes, but doesn't her rejection prove you aren't worth much as a boyfriend, or a person? [Playing devil's advocate.]

Client: No! My worth doesn't depend on her approval. It'd be nice to have her as a girlfriend, but I don't need her or any girl to be an OK person. [Elegant disputing.]

Therapist: But won't it be unbearable to go to dances without her, maybe see her with another guy?

Client: Yeah, it's going to be. . . . I'll feel lousy, but I can stand it. I'll try to think about the things we've talked about; that will help. [Elegant disputing and application of rational self-talk.]

Success in the "working through" stage is reached when the adolescent is having regular success with tough homework assignments, has overcome most symptoms, and has established adaptive modes of dealing with target situations. *Rational-Emotive Re-education,* the fourth stage, follows and is the same as for adults. Using the gamut of techniques described in Grieger and Boyd (1980), its aim is to generalize learnings and to ingrain or habituate in clients the rational ideas they have acquired and their emotional-behavioral contingencies.

In summary, successful RET with adolescents involves, on the part of the therapist, devoting appropriate attention to their special characteristics and issues and helping them utilize their emerging cognitive capacity to think objectively, doing both throughout the four stages of RET. As Young (1975) emphasizes, therapists may be forced to make major concessions in their usual therapy styles and to settle for inelegant gains. But these alterations are sometimes both necessary and in the adolescent's interest, and the "rational" therapist maintains ideal hopes but realistic expectations and goals.

GROUP PROCEDURES WITH CHILDREN AND ADOLESCENTS

There are two group RET methods for therapeutic work with youngsters: *Rational-Emotive Education* (REE) and *Rational-Emotive*

Group Therapy. In this section, we will present an overview of rational-emotive group therapy, and REE will be covered as a separate classroom/educational application.

Rational-emotive group procedures can be used to tackle, again, the various emotional disturbances presented by youngsters. It can also be used in the context of classroom problem-solving meetings (Glasser, 1969), developmental groups (Duncan & Gumaer, 1980), and the like. The authors, however, advocate using group RET with middle school youngsters and adolescents but advise against using it with younger children, those below the ages of 10 to 12 (Boyd & Grieger, 1980). Group therapy requires more verbal interchange among members than children can offer, and children lack the cognitive capacity to deduce, induce, and think abstractly about themselves and their problems as done by group therapy participants.

Rational-emotive group therapy with youngsters consists of a flexible framework within which the therapist has wide latitude to tailor the group process to fit the group. Rational-emotive therapy is not imposed on the group; instead, a group atmosphere and camaraderie are developed which are conducive to learning and problem solving, and rational-emotive techniques are infused into the group process. The stepwise procedures would follow a sequence like this:

Sessions 1-2: Group rapport is established and guidelines are set for members' in-group behavior. Everyone is encouraged to talk, and individual's concerns and problems are identified. The group's purpose and goals are discussed and agreed upon.

Sessions 3-4: Discussion of individuals' concerns and problems continues, and the leader introduces the A-B-C theory and uses it to help members understand their problems. This is an educational and insight stage of RET.

Sessions 5-6: Alternative, rational ways of thinking, feeling, and acting are explored, and same-aged models, via case studies, tapes, and stories, are used to engender motivation and the beginnings of a new response sequence.

Sessions 7-10: Members are encouraged to "work through" at least one problem using methods and techniques offered by the therapist and others presented by group members. Methodology employed consists of techniques previously mentioned in the "working through" stage of RET.

Sessions 11-12: Members' gains are reinforced and generalized to other concerns. Learnings are reviewed, future plans are discussed, and the therapist makes a warm termination.

Techniques

This stepwise sequence involves two kinds of technique: (1) the expertise needed to do any kind of therapy with youngsters, and (2) the RET techniques mentioned earlier. A common roadblock to effective group RET is that the group process or rapport is below par, making it necessary for the leader to sacrifice RET methods and concentrate on keeping the group together. In such cases the therapist tries to help the group reach as high an outcome as possible. The lowest outcome is simply a successful group process where members learn to interact in a mature fashion, accept and support one another, and gain an awareness of one another's concerns. A better outcome is for members at least to gain RET insights and knowledge of rational ideas, feelings, and behaviors. The optimal goal is, of course, to help members completely work through their most serious problems and learn the RET skills with which they can assault other and future problems.

CLASSROOM AND EDUCATIONAL APPLICATIONS

The application of RET principles and concepts to children in classroom settings is called *Rational-Emotive Education* (REE).

This method was first developed at Ellis' Living School and outlined in a manual by Knaus (1974); recently REE has been widely popularized in the writings of Boyd (1980), Boyd and Grieger (1980), and Vernon (1980); and a review of RET research by DiGiuseppe, Miller, and Trexler (1977) has shown REE to be a most effective method of psychological education.

The purpose of REE is to teach and put into children's practice a set of rational attitudes and behaviors which are pertinent to their developmental problems. Instructional modules focus on topics such as learning how to overcome inferiority feelings, understanding why it's normal and not terrible to make mistakes, raising low frustration tolerance, developing empathic understanding for others, giving up the stereotyping habit, understanding teasing and name-calling, and learning how to handle bullies. Teaching and learning activities for these particular topics are presented in Knaus' (1974) REE manual, but modules can be developed for any problem or psychological issue that deserves therapeutic attention. Within these modules the teacher/counselor plans a set of multimodal learning activities that cognitively, experientially, and behaviorally help children to become aware of irrational and self-defeating methods of dealing with a difficult concern or developmental issue and then teaches them a new attitude, emotion, and behavioral skill sequence.

Methodology in REE does not differ from other forms of psychological education for children, except for a stronger emphasis and more learning exercises on examining one's attitudes, disputing faulty beliefs, and practicing sensible ideas. The key is to involve the children completely in a fun- and action-oriented learning enterprise and to follow the theory of RET in developing and presenting modules.

The outcome of REE is seen not only in more emotionally stable and responsible behavior in the children but also in less teacher stress and in the teacher's modeling of rational behavior. The teaching of REE tends to make the one who teaches more rational! It also enables the teacher or counselor to employ the principles of RET in disciplining children and in dealing with their daily problems.

PARENTING SKILLS

It is fairly widely agreed that the involvement of parents in treatment is an exceptionally important part of psychotherapy with children (Abidin, 1977; Bersoff & Grieger, 1971; Dreikurs, 1964; Patterson & Gullion, 1968; Patterson & Reid, 1973; Ross, 1974). In RET a situation where the parents behave in ways that create, maintain, or exacerbate emotional and/or behavioral problems in their child is a first and most appropriate reason for working with the parents. That is, parents are seen as a crucial element and sometimes even the primary focus of their child's RET when they hold inappropriate expectations for their child and/or exhibit emotional disturbances that prompt debilitating parenting practices.

Noting the vast variety of parenting behaviors, it is possible to abstract four faulty styles of parenting requiring intervention. The *Criticism Trap* (Becker, 1971) is a style in which parents habitually criticize their children—nagging, correcting, reminding, blaming, even ridiculing and directly putting down. The key is that they catch the child being bad and then angrily interact with him or her, rather than catching good behavior and praising or rewarding it. Associated with anxiety, withdrawal, perfectionism, attention getting, procrastination, depression, and low self-esteem in children, this style is reflective of a series of irrational attitudes: (1) children *must* do well (e.g., achieve, be motivated) and behave correctly (e.g., be considerate, quiet); (2) children *must* not question or disagree with their superiors; (3) bad behavior *must* be punished because punishment, blame, and guilt are effective methods of child management; (4) praise spoils children; and (5) a child and his or her behavior are the same (Hauck, 1967).

A second parenting pattern, the *False Positive Trap,* tends to lead to the egocentric, selfish, spoiled child with low frustration tolerance. In this style the parents lavish a great deal of positive affection on their child but do so excessively and indiscriminately. The youngster not only receives praise for doing well but also for misbehaving; and the parents act in ways to make sure that the child rarely if ever experiences frustration. Although often motivated by a great deal of love, people who parent in this way are often rather neurotic and are motivated by unrealistic fears and anxieties. They typically hold one or more of several irrational ideas: (1) it is awful for my child to suffer, and I must see to it that this is prevented; (2) I must always do the right thing by my child; (3) I must always be loved and approved by my child; (4) my self-worth is tied to how well I do as a parent; and (5) it's terrible to have/express anger, and I should never do it, especially to my child.

On a behavioral level, the *Guilt Trap* is very similar to the False Positive Trap in that these parents overly indulge their children with strokes. Contrarily, they may be so depressed and guilt-ridden themselves that they cannot summon the energy to impose rules at all. Either way the child has few if any limits and can easily conclude, by default, that anything and everything he or she does is OK. Again, we see the spoiled child syndrome and perhaps the beginnings of a sociopathic adjustment. The attitudinal problem with these parents is similar to people with guilt: (1) I did a bad thing (as a parent or person) that I *should* not have done; (2) it was horrible to do that; and (3) I'm, therefore, a *bad person* and had better not make further attempts at parenting lest I fail so miserably again.

A final parenting style might be called the *Inconsistency Trap.* In such a pattern, the parents have essentially no game plan for their child at all, inconsistently rewarding and sometimes punishing. Another pattern is to criticize this child strongly while setting no rules or guidelines. It is parenting by whim and variously is backed by such attitudes as: (1) everybody has to make their own decisions; (2) whatever "feels" right as a parent is right; and (3) I'm too weak and helpless to know what is the right thing to do, so I can't possibly make a rather firm decision. Regardless, the result for children is confusion, resentment, and anxiety.

These, then, are four destructive parenting styles that make parent intervention appropriate and useful. Parents are also seen as crucial figures in RET parenting therapy when they themselves find it difficult to adjust to and live with their disturbed or even not-so-disturbed child; that is, when they make themselves emotionally disturbed by their children's presence or behavior (Ellis, Wolfe, & Moseley, 1972). They have low frustration tolerance and require traditional RET.

Techniques in Parent Counseling

RET parent counseling proceeds along the same lines as RET in general, starting with a psychodiagnosis of the problem and moving through parental insight, a working through of the parents' irrational ideas, and finally, to a cognitive-emotive-behavioral re-education. With parents, however, rational-emotive psychodiagnosis and rational-emotive insight pose especially thorny problems for the clinician.

Sometimes parents directly request clinical assistance for themselves in their role as parents. More typically, parental overtures to the clinician result from their concern about their child's behavior and well-being. Usually their concerns have been brewing for a long time and are accompanied by a great deal of worry or upset. In presenting the problem, they most often present the child as having the difficulty and frequently express their concerns in a blaming way.

It is extremely important in such circumstances for the clinician to sort out ownership of the problem, determining to what extent parental feelings, behaviors, and attitudes contribute to the child's problem or actually are the problem. Too often the opinions of parents are accepted as fact without their complaints being checked against reality. As a result the child is managed or fixed in some way, thereby violating the child's rights and ignoring needed parent counseling. In fact, the child may present only an event that elicits disturbed parental reactions; or disturbed parental attitudes and behaviors may actually precipitate problem behaviors in an otherwise healthy child.

In the RET diagnosis of parental pathology, the authors recommend beginning with a psychosituational assessment (Bersoff & Grieger, 1971; Grieger & Abidin, 1972). This assessment refers to a detailed analysis (through both interview and observation) of the child's alleged problem behaviors as elicited through interaction with the relevant stimulus situations, including the attitudes, emotions, and expectations of the parents. It includes a detailed definition of the child's "problem" behaviors (including frequency, intensity, duration); an explication of the details of the stimulus situation in which the "problem" behaviors occur, particularly the expectations in that situation for the child and the "self-talks" about the child; and uncovering of the immediate contingencies following the child's "problem" behavior, again including the thoughts and feelings about the child at this time; and an exploration of the more ongoing, general patterns of interaction between the parents and the child.

Such an examination carefully delimits the problem for the RET therapist, helping him or her determine what elements of the problem situation belong to the child and which belong to the parents. Perhaps equally as important, it provides the parents an opportunity to check their perceptions and to begin to see that they might harbor inappropriate feelings and attitudes and behave in an unhelpful way toward the child.

Helping parents gain insight (i.e., a full acknowledgment on their part that they indeed own a parenting problem) is the next major hurdle in the RET parent counseling process. Although it is hoped that parents would come to this insight through the psychosituational assessment, parents may still resist acknowledging this for any number of reasons. In these cases, we generally find it better to begin fostering the insights by empathizing with the parents' concerns, thereby undercutting resistance and communicating our respect. But we also recommend pointing out to them that they also seem to have a problem about their child's problem, and that their problem will interfere with efforts at solving the child's problem. In other words, we recommend a direct confrontation at this point, entering through the back door by first aligning with them and offering to change them in order ultimately to change the child. Then, once the parents acknowledge their problem, the typical RET process takes over.

Techniques in Parent Education

Parent education in RET is very similar to the classroom and educational applications of RET to the parents and to the children. For themselves, parents are first taught the basics of RET theory and then to (1) acknowledge that they cannot be perfect and will make mistakes as parents; (2) recognize that their inappropriate feelings and actions are their own making, not caused by their child; (3) look for, find, and acknowledge the irrational beliefs that create these inappropriate responses; (4) actively dispute or think through the validity of their irrational beliefs; (5) act contrary to their irrational beliefs; and (6) practice acting and thinking toward their children in ways that are consistent with sound parental practices.

For their children, RET parent education teaches parents to recognize irrational thinking in their children and to respond in order to intercept it. It also teaches them the basics of rational-emotive education so that they themselves can apply these basics to their children.

At this time there are only two packaged programs on RET for parents. Dr. Richard Abidin (1977) at the University of Virginia has developed a parent education program integrating RET ideas and techniques with behavior modification and communication skills. Dr. Virginia Waters (1980), Supervisor of Children's Services at The Institute for Rational-Emotive Therapy in New York, has written a series of RET-oriented pamphlets for parents on such topics as developing frustration tolerance and overcoming anger. Both of these materials are excellent resources for parents which we highly recommend.

FAMILY THERAPY

The rational-emotive approach to family intervention combines RET's unique techniques of cognitive therapy with relationship methods and skill training derived from such diverse models of family therapy as systems theory (Haley, 1977) and behavior therapy (Patterson & Reid, 1973). Unlike other approaches, however, RET never loses sight of the individual in the family system. It emphasizes, with Levant (1978), the primary fact that individuals bring their own phenomenological perspective to the family. In RET terms, people in family systems are affected mostly by their interpretation and evaluation of what takes place and only indirectly by the family events themselves. Individuals, then, play *the* major role in family dysfunction by overreacting both to the normal frustrations of family life *and* to the abnormal and unrealistic demands of other family members. The others, in turn, react poorly to both the sensible behaviors and the unreasonable demands of the first person, thereby setting in motion conflicts, pathological alignments, mutually self-defeating patterns of interaction, or all of these.

Following Ellis (1976b, 1978a, 1978b, 1978c), these principles can be articulated as follows:

1. All humans have strong innate tendencies to make unrealistic demands on others, to act selfishly, to have low frustration tolerance, and to put down themselves and others. It is, therefore, easy to create and maintain conflicts within family systems.
2. Disturbed family relationships stem primarily from the faulty perceptions family members have and the erroneous evaluations they make of the events within the family system, not mainly from what actually happens in the family. Particularly, disturbed family relationships result primarily when individuals make unrealistic demands on one another and evaluate both the family events and one another in catastrophic (awfulizing) terms, thereby setting in motion disturbed interaction patterns.
3. Once family members begin to think and act in irrational ways toward one another, they tend to lock themselves into doing so and to practice or rehearse these patterns till the patterns become habitual. These self-defeating behaviors are, therefore, resistant to change.
4. In addition to the above, a great deal of family difficulty results from ignorance and misinformation about what to expect in family living.
5. Special hardships, such as low socioeconomic status or the presence of a handicapped child, exert an even greater strain on family systems by making it even easier for family members to think and act crookedly toward one another.
6. Changing the manner in which the members of disturbed families interact will not likely be successful so long as they continue to think about themselves and one another in irrational ways. It is essential for family members to take responsibility for their own behavior, recognize how they create their own negative feelings and actions toward other family members, and work rigorously to change themselves in significant ways in order to effect long-lasting changes in disturbed family patterns.

These principles argue for an active-directive, cognitive-phenomenological approach to family interventions. Accordingly, Rational-Emotive Family Therapy is the treatment of choice in three circumstances: (1) when family dysfunction is caused, maintained, or exacerbated by disturbances in one or more family members, as is usually the case; (2) when ongoing family interactions or individual problems in other family members impede the amelioration of pathology in a particular family member; and (3) when family members can be effective in supporting the increased adaptive behavior on the part of a particular family member.

Techniques

Rational-Emotive Family Therapy has two major goals that may flow consecutively or concurrently. The *first goal* is to change individual family members' patterns of neurotic thinking and perceiving so that they (1) become happier individuals and (2) are free to make sensible, self-actualizing choices for themselves with various family members in appropriate patterns. The *second goal* is to teach families the skills of effective family relating.

The therapeutic modalities employed in RET family therapy are indigenous to RET in general and include all of RET's methods: emotive (shame and risk-attacking exercises, rational-emotive imagery, role playing, and humor), behavioral (activity and written homework, operant conditioning, diversion methods), and especially cognitive. Consistent with RET's cognitive thrust, each family member is encouraged to take full responsibility for his or her own behavior/emotional disturbance, acknowledge the irrational ideas that cause these disturbed overreactions, and actively dispute and argue against the disturbance-producing ideas until they are given up.

All of the above are designed to accomplish RET's first goal in family therapy. The second goal of skill training invokes methods from any and all other schools, including assertiveness training, relaxation training, communication skill training, negotiation skill training, sexual skill training, training in positively reinforcing others, contracting skills, and others.

EFFICACY

Throughout the history of psychotherapy a simple question concerning efficacy has been most difficult to answer: Is psychotherapy effective? That is, does it do what it purports to do? Concerted scientific attempts to answer this question are of recent origin, and VandenBos and Pino (1980) view this work as having passed through four stages. During this same time period, RET was undergoing its birth, growth, and a quest for validation. We think it is illuminating to trace the establishment of RET's efficacy during this time when all of psychotherapy was desperately seeking empirical support.

The first stage (1952-1965) of research on psychotherapy's effectiveness was a bleak one; the psychoanalytic model was in vogue and Eysenck (1952) attracted professional and public attention to the fact that this approach and psychotherapy in general had not produced enough evidence to prove that it was more efficacious than no treatment. During this same time period, RET was born and quickly gained recognition as an innovative, albeit radical, new form of psychotherapy. Ellis (1957a) published his first outcome report, a documentation and analysis of his psychotherapy cases during his transitions from the practice of orthodox psychoanalysis to directive analytical therapy and on to RET. Though empirical validation was not yet attained, Ellis' prolific writing put his theoretical views and self-reported therapy success into view (e.g., Ellis, 1957b, 1957c, 1958a, 1958b, 1962a, 1962b, 1965; Ellis & Harper, 1961a, 1961b).

In the late 1960s, during the second stage, there were a few studies which provided some cautious optimism for the future of psychotherapy. Reviews by Cross (1964) and Dittman (1966) continued to assail the weakness of psychotherapy research, but results from these questionable sources were at least suggestive of the possibility that psychotherapy might show positive effects if better research were done. It was still too early for such research to be provided by RET therapists; the late sixties were a growth phase when Ellis refined his therapy methods, substantiated them with personality hypotheses having theoretical and empirical support from a wide range of sources (see Ellis, 1977a), and continued to publish articles and major texts concerning RET (e.g., Ellis, 1967, 1968, 1969a, 1971; Ellis, Wolfe, & Moseley, 1966). As the 1960s drew to a close, RET was firmly established in a theoretical sense. Its underlying hypotheses were in agreement with those from some earlier personality theories and with the scanty research evidence which existed concerning basic facets of personality functioning, but RET was conspicuously devoid of empirical support for its efficacy.

During the next two stages of psychotherapy research, the early and late 1970s, empirical support for the efficacy of RET came forth, paralleling similar affirmation via research for psychotherapy in general. VandenBos and Pino's (1980) overview of research reviews in the 1970s led to their conclusion that the efficacy of psychotherapy as a generic treatment process was supported. Similarly, the studies which we will cite in the remainder of this section strongly support the effectiveness of RET in resolving a broad array of problems.

Before presenting efficacy research, however, we want to clarify that clear-cut effectiveness is very difficult to establish for RET because it is such a broadly based therapy approach and because many treatments dabble in RET methods rather than apply it thoroughly and intensively. During a lengthy RET case, the therapist may at times employ insight techniques, cognitive restructuring, imagery exercises, behavioral shaping, in vivo homework assignments, and a host of other methods. All of this is RET, yet research rarely focuses on the outcome of a comprehensive treatment; instead it zeroes in on one facet, such as brief cognitive restructuring. Moreover, if a therapist without adequate RET training administers a superficial and so-called RET treatment, should the outcome be considered a legitimate efficacy study?

These and other problems, plus the ever-present opportunity for error in conducting applied research, have slowed and confused the progress toward empirically based efficacy for RET. With these difficulties in mind, we now look at the evidence.

Mahoney's review of RET research in 1974 preceded the bulk of the studies to be conducted in the decade, but he did offer some "preliminary empirical evaluations." Several chapters in his text presented an extensive body of evidence which supported

RET's main tenet: that thoughts and images can induce and maintain painful physiological and emotional distress and maladaptive behavior patterns. Clinical outcomes showing cognitive restructuring to be a viable technique for therapeutically changing pathogenic ideation were also cited via successful case studies by Beck (1970a, 1970b), Davison (1966), Ellis (1957a, 1962b, 1971), Goodman and Maultsby (1974), and Maultsby (1971).

Nine studies on the effects of cognitive restructuring as applied to groups of subjects were presented and evaluated (Baker, 1966; Burkhead, 1966; DiLoreto, 1971; D'Zurilla, Wilson, & Nelson, 1973; Goldfried, Decenteceo, & Weinberg, 1974; Karst & Trexler, 1970; Maes & Heinman, 1970; Montgomery, 1971; Trexler & Karst, 1972). Although the evidence from these studies did not provide conclusive support for RET, and Mahoney withheld a confident judgment, the data were promising. RET was shown to be capable of effecting reductions in several measures of subjectively perceived distress, several physiological manifestations of anxiety, and it proved effective at increasing positive self-statements.

In the mid-1970s, there was a large increase in the amount of RET efficacy research. It would seem that RET was beginning to be taken seriously by the empirical community, and at the same time cognitive-behavioral psychotherapy in general was being endorsed (Mahoney, 1977). A review of RET outcome studies by DiGiuseppe, Miller, and Trexler (1977) did much to advertise the rapid advance of research support for RET. Noncomparative outcome studies demonstrated RET's effectiveness in (1) reducing irrational ideation and anxiety in geriatric clients (Keller, Crooke, & Brookings, 1975), (2) overcoming vulnerability to criticism and rejection (Yu & Schill, 1976), and (3) lowering public speaking anxiety (Straatmeyer & Watkins, 1974; Trexler & Karst, 1972). Numerous studies of "rational-emotive education" supported its ability to improve the emotional-behavioral adjustment of youngsters (Albert, 1972; Brody, 1974; Katz, 1974; Knaus & Bokor, 1975; Warren, Deffenbach, & Broding, 1976).

A number of comparative studies in the mid-1970s tested the relative efficacy of RET and other therapeutic treatments. DiLoreto (1971) found RET to be more effective than systematic desensitization and client-centered therapy for reducing post treatment (three months) behavioral measures of interpersonal anxiety. On two physiological measures of test anxiety in high school students, Maes and Heinman's (1970) study showed RET and desensitization to be more effective than client-centered and no-treatment conditions.

Kanter's (1975) comparison of systematic desensitization, rational restructuring, and the two combined for reducing self-reported anxiety revealed that all treatments were effective, with RET being the best. Cognitive restructuring also proved more efficacious than systematic desensitization for reducing phobia symptomatology in research by Wein, Nelson, and Odom (1975). Finally, in what DiGiuseppe et al. (1977) called the strongest support to date for RET, a study by Molesky and Tosi (1976) found RET more effective than systematic desentization in reducing the irrational attitudes, anxiety, and behavioral symptoms of stuttering. Furthermore, a follow-up evaluation 1 month later showed that these results were maintained.

Though RET has been rather consistent in producing greater therapeutic benefits than most of its competitors, it was effective, though second-best, to modeling/behavioral rehearsal for increasing women's self-reported assertion in a study by Wolfe (1975). Tiegerman (1975) also found assertion training to be more effective for decreasing interpersonal anxiety in college students than RET or a combined treatment. Fixed-role therapy has also equaled RET's effectiveness for reducing speech anxiety in college students (Karst & Trexler, 1970).

Certainly, the RET efficacy research of the mid-1970s can be criticized for methodological failings, as can much of the psychotherapeutic research to date; and one cannot say that RET had at that time achieved a conclusive degree of effectiveness in treating a wide variety of emotional-behavioral problems. But an exhaustive review of 375 psychotherapy outcome studies by Glass and Smith (1976) led them to suggest that RET ranked second among the prominent therapies in terms of effectiveness; systematic desensitization ranked first. By the late 1970s, RET had attained a respectable degree of empirical support, and this support continues to grow.

Recent studies continue to verify the A-B-C theory of RET, i.e., irrational ideation is associated with and tends to cause emotional-behavioral maladjustment (Alden & Safran, 1978; Epstein, Finnegan, & Bythell, 1979; LaPointe & Crandell, 1980; Schill & Scott, 1978; Sutton-Simon & Goldfried, 1979). Successful case studies with multiple dependent measures continue to illustrate RET's effects with a broader set of clinical problems such as anger (Hamberger & Lohr, 1980), irritable colon syndrome (Harrell & Beiman, 1978), and chronic depression (Reardon, Tosi, & Gwynne, 1977). Although these kinds of reports are supportive of RET, straightforward efficacy studies are the most impressive evidence for RET's effectiveness.

In one study, Block (1978) compared the effects of one year of rational-emotive education (REE), a human relations program, and no-treatment control condition upon twelfth-grade students who were prone to failure and misconduct. Participants in REE, at both post treatment and follow-up, had higher grades, fewer incidents of disruptive behavior, and cut class less often.

Zellie, Stone, and Lehr (1980) also employed a rational-emotive treatment with school-age youngsters. They administered a single rational behavior interview to junior high school students referred to the principal's office for disciplinary action. These students thereafter had a lower recidivism rate and were rated higher in proper classroom behavior than disciplinary students in a no-treatment control condition.

In both studies, a rational-emotive treatment was successful in beneficially influencing youngsters' school behavior. This would seem to underscore the versatility of the rational-emotive approach—its applicability and effectiveness with young people (vs. adults) in school settings (vs. therapist's office).

The last few years have also seen RET proper score impressive gains in the efficacy literature. Experimental studies continue to show it to be an effective treatment for socially anxious and nonassertive people (Carmody, 1978; Hammen, Jacobs, Mayol, & Cochran, 1980; Jacobs & Cochran, 1982; Linehan, Goldfried, & Goldfried, 1979; Malkiewich & Merluzzi, 1980), depression (Taylor & Marshall, 1977), and speech anxiety (Glogower, Fremouw, & McCroskey, 1978). Nontraditional treatment successes include weight reduction (Block, 1980) and pain endurance (Beers & Karoly, 1979). In some of the studies RET was contrasted and/or combined with other treatment conditions.

In these instances, the summary findings showed that RET was rarely surpassed in its effects on dependent variables and that it was particularly effective when combined with other treatment modalities.

The space limitations of this chapter have restricted the authors to a brief overview and citation of the foregoing efficacy studies, and readers are encouraged to seek out the references of interest and see the effects of RET for themselves. A final review of a particularly significant study will serve to point the way.

Lipsky, Kassinove, and Miller (1980) have produced a clinical outcome study which is the first one to demonstrate the efficacy of RET with a sample of multisymptomatic applicants to a community mental health center. They examined the comparative effects of a no-treatment condition and four group treatments: RET alone, RET with rational role reversal, RET with rational-emotive imagery, and relaxation training and support. Results showed that RET, particularly with the addition of rational role reversal or rational-emotive imagery, produced significantly better results than the other two groups on measures of rational thinking, anxiety, depression, and neuroticism.

To conclude, the authors suggest that RET has proven itself to be one of the most effective therapeutic treatments in existence today. Certainly, research is needed into the components and ingredients of RET, and in particular more study is needed on RET applications to child populations and problems. But present evidence suggests that RET is a viable therapy for children if it is tailored to their characteristics. Also, future research is likely to demonstrate more extensively the effectiveness of RET with children, as has been done in the last two decades for the adult population.

CONCLUSIONS

A historical view and current appraisal of RET leads one to see how far this approach has come. Begun by Albert Ellis in 1955 as a firm but narrow set of propositions and methods, RET has become one of the major approaches in the field of psychotherapy. Its origins were theoretical and clinical; Ellis was an objective and scientific thinker but not an empirical scientist.

Yet his clinical views were brilliant and farsighted; in fact, they were a forerunner of the cognitive-behavioral mode of intervention which was empirically born and became a prime force in the 1970s. Currently RET stands as the most clinically distinctive, philosophically elegant, and well-developed psychotherapy approach under the broad cognitive-behavioral umbrella. Throughout the United States and several foreign countries there is a large and growing number of clinicians who identify themselves as RETers. In addition, an even greater influence upon the therapeutic community has come about as a multitude of therapists have infused RET theory and techniques into their clinical work without specifically identifying with the approach.

The application of RET to adult populations has been extensive, covering nearly all neurotic and personality disorders. Within the next 10 years, RET with children and adolescents may approach this level. Also, the breadth of techniques employed within the RET framework (e.g., hypnosis, experiential method, diet alteration) is likely to continue increasing; and although this may make RET appear less distinctive, it is the core methods and theoretical emphasis on ideation restructuring that will remain the RET trademark.

Empirical support for RET will continue to accumulate steadily as the clinical efficacy of RET and the body of promising research results are increasingly recognized by the research community. A potential inhibitor, however, is that many researchers may continue to focus on the investigation of cognitive-behavioral therapy in general rather then on RET in particular.

An optimistic future for RET is, therefore, predicted by the authors, particularly regarding clinical applications to the emotional-behavioral problems of children and adolescents. It certainly seems sensible to thwart irrational tendencies at an early age, to guide and facilitate a "rational" process of psychological development, and to help youngsters avoid the emotional pain experienced in the lives of disturbed adults.

CASE STUDY

The case of Billie S. illustrates how RET is applied to youngsters and other members of their families. Mr. S., Billie's father, asked that the therapist help Billie, an 11-year-old boy, work on problems of anger and resentment most often directed toward the father. In an initial interview, Mr. S. specifically defined the problem as Billie's refusal to communicate with him or to engage in activities with him; he related that most overtures were turned down in "a nasty way," whereupon an argument generally ensued. Upon questioning, Mr. S. admitted that his habitual response to this situation was to become angry and actually to initiate the arguments. Further questioning also revealed that Mr. S. typically took anger-inducing attitudes toward Billie when these events occurred, as in: "He should be more responsive. It's terrible for him to be so difficult." He was able to acknowledge these irrational ideas and to see their relation to his anger.

Turning to a more general look at the family picture, Mr. S. shared the fact that he had left his wife and family approximately 18 months before but, because of guilt, had not yet acted on a divorce. When it was suggested to him that perhaps his *demands* for Billie's attention were motivated by guilt, he allowed that this might be true and, with the therapist's help, saw the connection between his guilt-producing thoughts and his conflicts with Billie. In essence, his irrational thinking went something like: "I should never have left my family. I'm a terrible person for having done this. I must, therefore, atone and salvage my self-worth in part by making my son and me have an exceptionally close relationship."

Billie presented quite a different picture. When seen alone, he described his problem as being his mother rather than his father, whom he saw as more of a nuisance. It seemed that his mother had recently started a regular relationship with a man, and Billie had become obsessed with this situation almost to the exclusion of any interest in his father (in turn exacerbating his father's irrational thinking and feeling). Essentially, he had become preoccupied with the idea that his mother's new boyfriend might nudge him out of the picture and that, if this were to happen, it would be *catastrophic* because he *needed* to be primary in her life. Believing these things, he worried incessantly about her whereabouts when he was not with her, angrily lobbied, to all who would listen, against this man and his mother's "unfair" behavior, and hysterically tried to convince her to stop seeing this man.

As is most often the case with disturbed youngsters, all members of the family have some psychopathology. Besides being perplexed about Billie's behavior, Mrs. S. possessed emotional problems of her own which had caused her, over the years, to "train" Billie to become dependent on her and which currently blocked her from setting limits with him over the present issue. For one, she had historically viewed it as *horrible* for Billie to be hurt or upset and had, thereby, made his life virtually problem-free until the marital split-up. For another, she took the attitude that conflicts or hassles are *too difficult to bear,* prompting her to avoid them at all costs and to give in to Billie's slightest whims.

Rational-emotive therapy in this case involved working with each member of the family. As for Mr. S., he needed information to understand what was going on with Billie so as not to personalize Billie's behavior. More elegantly, he also needed to work through the irrational ideas that caused the guilt and also his "ego anger" (Grieger, 1982) so as both to feel better and to act better toward himself and Billie. And he needed advice as to how to respond empathically, yet "therapeutically," when Billie complained about his mother and her boyfriend. Likewise, Mrs. S. required much of the same thing in her therapy, except that interventions were geared toward the particulars of her dysfunctional attitudes and behaviors. Both the content and the process of the work with them followed typical RET lines, intertwining with Billie's therapy.

Because Billie was 11 years old and because he was both very upset and very adamant about holding onto his irrational ideas and behaviors, considerable time was spent establishing a relationship with Billie before any semblance of a working through process took place. The therapist often took Billie to an electronic game room close to the office, talked at length to him about the movies Billie liked, and, most important, took pains not to voice any opinions about the "correctness" of his mother's dating. This last point was crucial to get Billie invested in RET insight, as "working through" required an ally, not an adversary.

Movement in therapy for Billie actually took place on the heels of a particularly angry outburst on his part. Complaining vehemently about his mother's refusal to break an all-day Sunday outing with her boyfriend, Billie and his therapist took part in the following exchange:

Therapist: You know what, Billie? I don't think your mother is going to stop this.

Billie: She'd better! It's not fair and . . .

Therapist: [Interrupting.] Look! I don't know this for a fact and she certainly hasn't told me her intentions. But I really believe she is going to go on seeing Larry for as long as she likes.

Billie: It's not fair!

Therapist: I'm not saying it is. And I'm certainly not saying she is right. But I really hate to see you so upset about all this. I'd really like to help you feel better than you do.

Billie: I don't care. She's wrong and she's going to stop. I hate him.
[A lengthy interchange took place much along the same lines with the therapist empathically but firmly hammering reality home.]

Therapist: Billie, I'm sorry for the way it is. But I don't see where this misery of yours is doing you any good. You sound upset a lot. Isn't that true?

Billie: Yeah.

Therapist: What good does the upset do you? [No response.] Want me to take a guess? [Billie pauses and nods.] I think you want to be upset, because if you stop, you think your mother will take it as OK to keep this up with Larry and you'll lose. What do you think about that?

Billie: [Startled.] I'm not going to lose. She's wrong and . . .

Therapist: [Interrupting.] But I think I have a better idea for you. You can win two ways.

Billie: [Pauses, eyes therapist.] How?

Therapist: You can not be upset and you can still tell your mom you don't want her to see Larry. See, you can still let her know you don't like it and even act upset, but you can stop feeling bad. That way you can feel a lot less miserable, even be happy, and maybe get more of her time too. And even if you don't get that, you can at least feel better. Now what do you think about that?

Billie: [No comment.]

Therapist: Well, let's take a minute and take a look at the advantages and disadvantages of feeling so bad. We know what the big advantage is, but how does it hurt you to be so upset?

At this point, Billie and the therapist listed six major disadvantages of Billie's being upset, and they then contracted to work on Billie's learning to calm down but to retain the option of protesting to his mother if he so desired. Once this contract was made, the therapist, in typical RET fashion, taught Billie the A-B-Cs of emotional reactions and hypothesized what irrational ideas Billie held to get upset. When Billie agreed that he did hold these ideas and that these ideas indeed made him upset, the following took place.

Therapist: So, what can you do to change?

Billie: Change the ideas?

Therapist: Right!

Billie: But she has to change too.

Therapist: Billie, be careful there. As I told you before, she might never change. But you can make yourself feel better if *you* will change your thoughts about her, and I can help you do that. And remember, you can still act upset if you like, even if you don't feel like it. OK? Willing to give it a try?

Billie: OK! But how do I do this?

Therapist: By seeing that most of your ideas do not make sense—that your mom still loves you; that you don't always have to be number one in her life; that she always comes home from a date loving you as much as she did when she left; that you don't need her to think of you all the time; and that it's not really all that terrible when she is enjoying someone else—and by practicing thinking all this.

Notice that the therapist mixed inelegant ("your mom still loves you") with elegant ("you don't need her to think of you all the time") messages. Even though Billie was a fairly bright youngster, he still was not completely able to make use of the more philosophic insights, although he was quite capable of adopting and using more concrete, yet valid points of view. Subsequent therapy focused on the following: role playing the rational ideas in simulated real life situations (e.g., when Mom is on a date; when Larry is visiting); disputing the validity of the various irrational ideas in therapy; setting up experiments to test out the ideas (e.g., "she's always with him," "she doesn't care anymore"); using imagery to practice rational thinking at home on his own; practicing rational thinking in real life situations; and other interventions. Perhaps one final transcript section from a later session can illustrate this "working through" process.

Therapist: OK, so you're having some good and some not-so-good results with your rational thinking. Let's take one of those times when you got yourself upset and use that to practice. Tell me one.

Billie: When Mom said she was going to come home at eleven, and she was late.

Therapist: OK. What were you doing upstairs to get upset?

Billie: "She promised she'd be home. She lied . . ."

Therapist: ". . . and she doesn't care about me because she's late." Right?

Billie: Yeah.

Therapist: OK. Now what could you have done with that thought? What was silly about it?

Billie: I know she loves me. She's just enjoying herself and that doesn't mean she doesn't love me.

Therapist: Right! And what about the idea that you need her to always be thinking of you and always having you on top of her mind?

Billie: I don't need her to think about me all the time. She always loves me, even when she doesn't think about me.

Therapist: That's correct. And also you could remind yourself that she still loves you when she is with Larry. Now if you had thought that the other night, would you have gotten so upset?

Billie: No.

Therapist: OK, then, Billie, let's use your imagination to practice your rational thinking. Now imagine yourself at home the other night: It's after eleven, your mom isn't home as she said she would be, and you're waiting. Picture that and then, out loud, think the rational thoughts. Go!

So rational-emotive therapy continued with Billie and both his mother and father as described. Through the use of cognitive, emotive, and behavioral techniques, significant attitude changes were brought about in all three of them so that, at the time of this writing, Billie's problems are almost over. He still does not like the fact that his mother is dating Larry, but he is accepting it. Mr. S. has relaxed considerably with Billie, allowing Billie to relate at his own pace; at the same time, Mr. S. has contacted his lawyer to begin final divorce proceedings. Mrs. S. acts much more firmly with Billie in relation to her dating behavior, as well as with other issues, while still communicating a great deal of love to him. She also reports a greater sense of relaxation, self-confidence, and hope for the future. At this point, therapy with the father has terminated, but therapy with both Billie and his mother will continue for a time in order to further habituate rational thinking and acting for each of them.

ANNOTATED BIBLIOGRAPHY

A complete list of texts, pamphlets, tape cassettes for the layperson, and audio and video cassettes and films for professionals can be obtained from The Institute for Rational-Emotive Therapy, 45 E. 65th Street, New York, NY 10021. Annotated below are seven references that provide the next step for the interested reader to further explore RET.

Rational-Emotive Therapy in General

Ellis, A. (1971). *Growth through reason.* Palo Alto, CA: Science and Behavior Books; and Hollywood, CA: Wilshire.

This text provides transcripts of actual RET sessions, with Albert Ellis describing what is taking place and why. Two therapy sessions by Albert Ellis, as well as ones by Drs. Ben Ard, Jon Geis, John Gullo, Paul Hauck, and Maxie C. Maultsby, Jr., are included.

Ellis, A., & Grieger, R. (1977). *Handbook of rational-emotive therapy.* New York: Springer.

This comprehensive text gathers the best and most comprehensive writing in the theory and practice of RET to 1977. Containing both classic and new papers, it covers the theoretical and conceptual foundations of RET, the dynamics of emotional disturbance, basic RET processes and techniques, and RET with children.

Ellis, A., & Harper, R. (1975). *A new guide to rational living.* Englewood Cliffs, NJ: Prentice-Hall; and Hollywood, CA: Wilshire.

An RET classic, this is a book for the layperson outlining the basics of RET as a self-help tool. It is particularly helpful in describing the logical errors and practical pitfalls of the basic irrational beliefs.

Grieger, R., & Boyd, J. (1980). *Rational-emotive therapy: A skills-based approach.* New York: Van Nostrand Reinhold.

The first book presenting the basic skills of RET in an organized, step-by-step manner. It outlines the basic reasons for skills in and common therapist and client roadblocks to rational-emotive psychodiagnosis and goal setting, insight, working through, and re-education. Special chapters outline training methods and techniques in doing RET with women (by Ingrid Grieger).

Rational-Emotive Therapy with Children

Bernard, M. E., & Joyce, M. R. (1984). *Rational-emotive therapy with children and adolescents.* New York: Wiley.

This is a comprehensive guide for practitioners involved in working with children and adolescents utilizing rational-emotive therapy. It provides detailed descriptions of treatment, assessment, and preventative strategies for use with children. This is an excellent reference for practitioners looking for specific intervention strategies.

Ellis, A., & Bernard, M. E. (1983). *Rational-emotive approaches to the problems of childhood.* New York: Plenum Press.

This book presents a wide overview of rational-emotive therapy and cognitive behavior therapy approaches with children. Specific disorders are discussed, and intervention procedures are detailed for these disorders.

Knaus, W. (1974). *Rational-emotive education: A manual for elementary school teachers.* New York: Institute for Rational Living.

This manual outlines an emotional educational program designed to be presented to children as part of their academic curriculum. It presents detailed descriptions of how to conduct exercises whose goals are to help children become aware of their feelings and understand how their thinking causes their feelings, to devèlop self-acceptance, to give up perfectionism, and to overcome a whole host of other childhood problems.

REFERENCES

Abidin, R. R. (1977). *Parenting skills.* New York: Human Sciences Press.

Adler, A. (1931). *What life should mean to you.* New York: Blue Ribbon Books.

Adler, A. (1964a). *Superiority and social interest.* Edited by H. L. Ansbacher & R. R. Ansbacher. Evanston, IL: Northwestern Press.

Adler, A. (1964b). *Social interest: A challenge to mankind.* New York: Capricorn Books.

Albert, S. (1972). *A study to determine the effectiveness of affective education with fifth grade students.* Unpublished master's thesis, Queens College, New York.

Alden, L., & Safran, J. (1978). Irrational beliefs and nonassertive behavior. *Cognitive Therapy and Research, 2*(4), 357-364.

Baker, J. N. (1966). *Reasons versus reinforcement in behavior modification.* Unpublished doctoral dissertation, University of Illinois.

Beck, A. (1970a). Cognitive therapy: Nature and relation to behavior therapy. *Behavior Therapy, 1,* 184-200.

Beck, A. (1970b). Role of fantasies in psychotherapy and psychopathology. *Journal of Nervous and Mental Disease, 150,* 3-17.

Beck, A. (1976). *Cognitive therapy and the emotional disorders.* New York: International Universities Press.

Becker, W. C. (1971). *Parents are teachers: A child management program.* Champaign, IL: Research Press.

Becker, T. M., & Karoly, P. (1979). Cognitive strategies, expectancy, and coping style in the control of pain. *Journal of Consulting and Clinical Psychology, 47*(1), 197-180.

Bersoff, D. N., & Grieger, R. M. (1971). An interview model for the psychosituational assessment of children's behavior. *American Journal of Orthopsychiatry, 41,* 483-493.

Block, J. (1978). Effects of a rational-emotive mental health program on poorly achieving, disruptive high school students. *Journal of Counseling Psychology, 25*(1), 61-65.

Block, J. (1980). Effects of rational-emotive therapy on overweight adults. *Psychotherapy: Theory, Research and Practice, 17*(3), 277-280.

Boyd, J. (1980). Teaching rational ideas. *Middle School Journal, 51*(2), 18-21.

Boyd, J. D., & Grieger, R. M. (1980). Rational-emotive group work with children., In J. A. Duncan & J. Gumaer (Eds.), *Developmental groups for children.* Springfield, IL: Charles C. Thomas.

Brody, M. (1974). *The effect of a rational-emotive affective education approach on anxiety, frustration tolerance and self-esteem with fifth grade students.* Unpublished doctoral dissertation, Temple University, Philadelphia.

Burkhead, D. D. (1966). *The reduction of negative affect in human subjects: A laboratory investigation of rational-emotive psychotherapy.* Unpublished doctoral dissertation, Western Michigan University.

Carmody, T. P. (1978). Rational-emotive, self instructional, and behavioral assertion training: Facilitating maintenance. *Cognitive Therapy and Research, 2*(3), 241-253.

Clark, E. (1973). What's in a word? On the child's acquisition of semantics in his language. In T. E. Moore (Ed.), *Cognitive development and the acquisition of language.* New York: Academic Press.

Cross, N. J. (1964). The outcome of psychotherapy: A selected analysis of research findings. *Journal of Consulting Psychology, 28,* 413-417.

Daly, S. (1971). Using reason with deprived pre-school children. *Rational Living, 5,* 12-19.

Davison, G. C. (1966). Differential relaxation and cognitive restructuring in therapy with a "paranoid schizophrenic" or "paranoid state." *Proceedings of the 74th Annual Convention of the American Psychological Association,* 177-178.

DiGiuseppe, R. (1975). The use of behavior modification to establish rational self-statement in children. *Rational Living, 10,* 18-20.

DiGiuseppe, R. (1981). Cognitive therapy with children. In G. Emergy, S. D. Hollow, & R. C. Bedresian (Eds.), *New directions in cognitive therapy.* New York: The Guilford Press.

DiGiuseppe, R., & Kassinove, H. (1976). Effects of a rational-emotive school mental health program on children's emotional adjustment. *Journal of Community Psychology, 4,* 12-16.

DiGiuseppe, R. A., Miller, N. J., & Trexler, L. D. (1977). A review of rational-emotive psychotherapy outcome studies. *The Counseling Psychologist, 7*(1), 64-72.

DiLoreto, A. O. (1971). *Comparative psychotherapy: An experimental analysis.* Chicago: Aldine-Atherton.

DiNublie, L., & Wessler, R. (1974). Lessons from the living school. *Rational Living, 9,* 29-32.

Dittman, A. T. (1966). Psychotherapeutic processes. In P. Farnsworth et al., (Eds.), *The annual review of psychology.* Palo Alto, CA: Annual Reviews.

Dreikurs, R. (1964). *Children: The challenge.* Des Moines, IA: Meredith Press.

Duncan, J. A., & Gumaer, J. (1980). *Developmental groups for children.* Springfield, IL: Charles C. Thomas.

D'Zurilla, T. J., Wilson, G. T., & Nelson, R. A. (1973). A preliminary study of the effectiveness of graduated prolonged exposure in the treatment of irrational fear. *Behavior Therapy, 4,* 672-685.

Egan, R., & DiGiuseppe, R. A. (1981). *Interpersonal cognitive problem solving skills: A components analysis.* Unpublished manuscript, Hofstra University.

Ellis, A. (1957a). Outcome of employing three techniques of psychotherapy. *Journal of Clinical Psychology, 13,* 344-350.

Ellis, A. (1957b). Rational psychotherapy and individual psychology. *Journal of Individual Psychology, 13,* 38-44.

Ellis, A. (1957c). *How to live with a neurotic.* New York: Crown.

Ellis, A. (1958a). Rational psychotherapy. *Journal of General Psychology, 59,* 35-49.

Ellis, A. (1958b). Case histories: Fact and fiction. *Contemporary Psychology, 3,* 318-319.

Ellis, A. (1962a, August). *Rational-emotive psychotherapy.* Paper presented at the annual meeting of the American Psychological Association, St. Louis, MO.

Ellis, A. (1962b). *Reason and emotion in psychotherapy.* New York: Lyle Stewart and Citadel Press.

Ellis, A. (1965). An answer to some objections to rational-emotive psychotherapy. *Psychotherapy, 2,* 108-111.

Ellis, A. (1967). Phobia treated with RET. *Voices, 3,* 34-40.

Ellis, A. (1968). What *really* causes psychotherapeutic change? *Voices, 4,* 90-97.

Ellis, A. (1969a). A cognitive approach to behavior therapy. *International Journal of Psychiatry, 8,* 896-900.

Ellis, A. (1969b). Teaching emotional education in the classroom. *School Health Review,* November, 1043.

Ellis, A. (1971). *Growth through reason.* Palo Alto, CA: Science and Behavior Books; and Hollywood, CA: Wilshire Books.

Ellis, A. (1973). *Humanistic psychotherapy: The rational-emotive approach.* New York: Julian Press and McGraw-Hill Paperbacks.

Ellis, A. (1975). *How to live with a "neurotic"* (rev. ed.). New York: Crown.

Ellis, A. (1976a.) The biological basis of human irrationality. *Journal of Individual Psychology, 32,* 145-168.

Ellis, A. (1976b). Techniques of handling anger in marriage. *Journal of Marriage and Family Counseling, 2,* 305-316.

Ellis, A. (1977a). Rational-emotive therapy: Research data that supports the clinical and personality hypotheses of RET and other modes of cognitive-behavior therapy. *The Counseling Psychologist, 7,* 2-42.

Ellis, A. (1977b). Rejoinder: Elegant and inelegant RET. *The Counseling Psychologist, 7,* 73-82.

Ellis, A. (1978a). Family therapy: A phenomenological and active directive approach. *Journal of Marriage and Family Counseling, 3,* 43-50.

Ellis, A. (1978b). A rational-emotive approach to family therapy. Part I: Cognitive therapy. *Rational Living, 13,* 15-19.

Ellis, A. (1978c). Rational-emotive approach to family therapy. Part II: Emotive and behavioral therapy. *Rational Living, 14,* 23-27.

Ellis, A. (1979). Rational-emotive therapy. In R. J. Corsini (Ed.), *Current psychotherapies* (2nd ed.). Itasca, IL: F. E. Peacock.

Ellis, A. (1980). An overview of the clinical theory of rational-emotive therapy. In R. Grieger & J. Boyd (Eds.), *Rational-emotive therapy: A skills-based approach.* New York: Van Nostrand Reinhold.

Ellis, A., & Abrahms, E. (1978). *Brief psychotherapy in medical and health practice.* New York: Springer.

Ellis, A., & Grieger, R. (1977). *Handbook of rational-emotive therapy.* New York: Springer.

Ellis, A., & Gulla, J. M. (1972). *Murder and assassination.* New York: Lyle Stewart.

Ellis, A., & Harper, R. (1961a). *Creative marriage.* New York: Lyle Stewart.

Ellis, A., & Harper, R. (1961b). *A guide to rational living.* Englewood Cliffs, NJ: Prentice-Hall.

Ellis, A., & Harper, R. (1975). *A new guide to rational living.* Englewood Cliffs, NJ: Prentice-Hall; and Hollywood CA: Wilshire Books.

Ellis, A., Wolfe, J. L., & Moseley, S. (1966). *How to prevent your child from becoming a neurotic adult.* New York: Crown.

Ellis, A., Wolfe, J. L., & Moseley, S. (1972). *How to raise an emotionally healthy, happy child.* Hollywood, CA: Wilshire Books.

Epstein, N., Finnegan, D., & Bythell, D. (1979). Irrational beliefs and perceptions of marital conflict. *Journal of Consulting and Clinical Psychology, 47*(3), 608-610.

Eysenck, H. (1952). The effects of psychotherapy: An evaluation. *Journal of Consulting Psychology, 16,* 319-324.

Glass, G., & Smith, M. L. (1976, June). *Meta-analysis of psychotherapy outcome studies.* Paper presented at the Annual Meeting of the Society of Psychotherapy Research, Boston.

Glasser, W. (1969). *Schools without failure.* New York: Harper and Row.

Glicken, M. (1968). Rational counseling: A new approach to children. *Journal of Elementary School Guidance and Counseling, 2,* 261-267.

Glogower, F. D., Fremouw, W. J., & McCroskey, J. C. (1978). A component analysis of cognitive restructuring. *Cognitive Therapy and Research, 2,* 209-223.

Goldfried, M. R., Decenteceo, E. T., & Weinberg, L. (1974). Systematic rational restructuring as a self-control technique. *Behavior Therapy, 5,* 247-254.

Goodman, D. S., & Maultsby, M. C. (1974). *Emotional well-being through rational behavior training.* Springfield, IL: Charles C. Thomas.

Grieger, R. (1982). Anger problems. In R. Grieger & I. Grieger (Eds.), *Cognitive and emotional disturbance.* New York: Human Sciences Press.

Grieger, R. M., & Abidin, R. R. (1972). Psychosocial assessment: A model for the school community psychologist. *Psychology in the Schools, 9,* 112-119.

Grieger, R., & Boyd, J. (1980). *Rational-emotive therapy: A skills-based approach.* New York: Van Nostrand Reinhold.

Grieger, R., & Czajkowski, D. R. (1980). *The socialization of irrational thinking through children's television.* Unpublished manuscript, University of Virginia.

Haley, J. (1977). *Problem solving therapy.* San Francisco: Jossey-Bass.

Hamberger, K., & Lohr, J. M. (1980). Rational restructuring for anger control: A quasi-experimental case study. *Cognitive Therapy and Research, 4*(1), 99-102.

Hammen, C. L., Jacobs, M., Mayol, A., & Cochran, S. D. (1980). Dysfunctional cognitions and the effectiveness of skills and cognitive-behavioral assertion training. *Journal of Consulting and Clinical Psychology, 48*(6), 685-695.

Harrell, T. H., & Beiman, J. (1978). Cognitive-behavioral treatment of the irritable colon syndrome. *Cognitive Therapy and Research, 2*(4), 371-375.

Hauck, P. A. (1967). *The rational management of children.* Roslyn Heights, NY: Libra.

Hauck, P. A. (1973). *Overcoming depression.* Philadelphia: The Westminister Press.

Horney, K. (1965). *Collected works.* New York: Norton Press.

Jacobs, M. K., & Cochran, S. D. (1982). The effects of cognitive restructuring on assertive behavior. *Cognitive Therapy and Research, 6*(1), 63-76.

Kanter, N. A. (1975). *A comparison of self-control desensitization and systematic rational restructuring for the reduction of interpersonal anxiety.* Unpublished doctoral dissertation, SUNY at Stony Brook.

Karst, S., & Trexler, L. (1970). An initial study using fixed role and rational-emotive therapies in treating public speaking anxiety. *Journal of Consulting and Clinical Psychology, 34,* 360-366.

Katz, S. (1974). *The effect of emotional education on locus of control and self-concept.* Unpublished doctoral dissertation, Hofstra University, New York.

Kelly, G. (1955). *The psychology of personal constructs.* New York: Norton Press.

Keller, J., Crooke, J., & Brookings, J. (1975). Effects of a program in rational thinking on anxiety in older persons. *Journal of Counseling Psychology, 22,* 54-57.

Knaus, W. (1970, January). *Innovative use of parents and teachers as behavior modifiers.* Paper presented at combined Seventh Annual School Psychology Conference and Second Annual Special Education Conference. New York: Queens College Publications.

Knaus, W. (1974). *Rational-emotive education: A manual for elementary school teachers.* New York: Institute for Rational Living.

Knaus, W., & Block, J. (1976). *Rational-emotive education with economically disadvantaged inner city high school students: A demonstration study.* Unpublished manuscript, Institute of Rational-Emotive Therapy, New York.

Knaus, W., & Bokor, S. (1975). The effect of rational-emotive education on anxiety and self-concept. *Rational Living, 10*(2), 7-10.

Kohlberg, L. (1975). The cognitive-developmental approach to moral development. *Phi Delta Kappan, 56,* 670-677.

Lafferty, G., Dennerll, D., & Rettlich, G. A. (1964). Creative school mental health program. *National Elementary Principal, 43,* 28-35.

LaPointe, K. A., & Crandell, C. J. (1980). Relationship of irrational beliefs to self-reported depression. *Cognitive Therapy and Research, 4*(2), 247-250.

Levant, R. (1978). Family therapy: A client-centered perspective. *Journal of Marriage and Family Counseling, 4,* 42-49.

Linehan, M. H., Goldfried, M. R., & Goldfried, A. P. (1979). Assertion therapy: Skill training or cognitive restructuring? *Behavior Therapy, 10,* 372-388.

Lipsky, M. J., Kassinove, H., & Miller, N. J. (1980). Effects of rational-emotive therapy, rational role reversal, and rational-emotive imagery on the emotional adjustment of community mental health center patients. *Journal of Consulting and Clinical Psychology, 48*(3), 336-374.

Maes, W., & Heinman, R. (1970, October). *The comparison of three approaches to the reduction of test anxiety in high school students.* Final report, project, 9-1-040, Washington Office of Education, United States Department of Health, Education, and Welfare.

Mahoney, M. J. (1974). *Cognition and behavior modification.* Cambridge, MA: Ballinger.

Mahoney, M. J. (1977). Reflections on the cognitive-learning trend in psychotherapy. *American Psychologist, 32,* 5-13.

Malkiewich, L. E. , & Merluzzi, T. V. (1980). Rational restructuring versus desensitization with clients of diverse conceptual levels: A test of a client-treatment matching mode. *Journal of Counseling Psychology, 27*(5), 453-461.

Maultsby, M. C. (1971). Rational-emotive imagery. *Rational Living, 6,* 24-26.

Maultsby, M. C. (1975). Rational behavior therapy for acting out adolescents. *Social Casework, 56,* 35-43.

McGrory, J. (1967). Teaching introspection in the classroom. *Rational Living, 2,* 23-24.

Meichenbaum, D. (1977). *Cognitive behavior modification: An integrative approach.* New York: Plenum Press.

Meichenbaum, D. (1978). *Cognitive behavior modification and the treatment of impulse disorders.* New York: BMA Audio Cassettes.

Merrigan, E., & DiGiuseppe, R. (1981). *The effects of role playing and modeling in the acquisition of interpersonal problem solving skills.* Unpublished manuscript, Hofstra University, New York.

Molesky, R., & Tosi, D. (1976). Comparative psychotherapy: Rational-emotive therapy versus systematic desensitization in the treatment of stuttering. *Journal of Consulting and Clinical Psychology, 44,* 309-311.

Montgomery, A. G. (1971). *Comparison of the effectiveness of systematic desensitization, rational-emotive therapy, implosive therapy, and no therapy, in reducing test anxiety in college students.* Unpublished doctoral dissertation, Washington University, St. Louis.

Patterson, G. R., & Gullion, M. E. (1968). *Living with children: New methods for parents and teachers.* Champaign, IL: Research Press.

Patterson, G. R., & Reid, J. B. (1973). Intervention for families of aggressive boys: A replication study. *Behavior Records and Therapy, 11,* 383-394.

Piaget, J. (1952). *The origins of intelligence in children.* New York: International Universities Press.

Piaget, J., & Inhelder, B. (1970). *The psychology of the child.* New York: Basic Books.

Protinsky, W., & Popp, R. (1978). Irrational philosophies in popular music. *Cognitive Therapy and Records, 2,* 71-74.

Reardon, J. P., Tosi, D., & Gwynne, P. H. (1977). The treatment of depression through rational stage directed hypnotherapy: A case study. *Psychotherapy: Theory, Research and Practice, 14*(1), 95-103.

Ross, A. O. (1974). *Psychological disorders of children: A behavioral approach to theory, research, and therapy.* New York: McGraw-Hill.

Schill, T., & Scott, M. (1978). The effects of self-verbalizations on performance: A test of the rational-emotive position. *Psychotherapy: Theory, Research and Practice, 15*(1), 2-7.

Spivak, G., & Shure, M. (1975). *The social adjustment of young children.* San Francisco: Jossey-Bass.

Straatmeyer, A. J., & Watkins, J. T. (1974). Rational-emotive therapy and the reduction of speech anxiety. *Rational Living, 9*(1), 33-37.

Sutton-Simon, K., & Goldfried, M. R. (1979). Faulty thinking patterns in two types of anxiety. *Cognitive Therapy and Research, 3*(2), 193-203.

Taylor, F. G., & Marshall, W. L. (1977). Experimental analysis of a cognitive-behavioral therapy for depression. *Cognitive Therapy and Research, 1*(1), 59-72.

Tiegerman, S. (1975). *Effects of assertion training, and cognitive components of rational therapy on the promotion of assertive behavior and the reduction of interpersonal anxiety.* Unpublished doctoral dissertation, Hofstra University, New York.

Trexler, L. D., & Karst, T. O. (1972). Rational-emotive therapy, placebo, and no treatment effects on public-speaking anxiety. *Journal of Abnormal Psychology, 79,* 60-67.

VandenBos, G. R., & Pino, C. D. (1980). Research on the outcome of psychotherapy. In G. R. VandenBos (Ed.), *Psychotherapy: Practice, research, policy.* Beverly Hills, CA: Sage.

Vernon, A. (1980). *Help yourself to a healthier you.* Washington, DC: University Press of America.

Wagner, E., & Glicken, M. (1966). Counseling children: Two accounts. *Rational Living, 1,* 26-30.

Warren, R., Deffenbach, J., & Broding, P. (1976). Rational-emotive therapy and the reduction of test anxiety in elementary school students. *Rational Living, 11*(2), 28-29.

Waters, V. (1980). *RET parenting pamphlet series.* New York: Institute of Rational Emotive Therapy.

Watts, F. N., Powell, G. E., & Austin, S. V. (1973). The modification of abnormal beliefs. *British Journal of Medical Psychology, 46,* 359-363.

Wein, K. S., Nelson, R. O., & Odom, J. V. (1975). The relative contribution of reattribution and verbal extinction to the effectiveness of cognitive restructuring. *Behavior Therapy, 6,* 459-474.

Wolfe, J. (1970). Emotional education in the classroom. *Rational Living, 4,* 23-25.

Wolfe, J. L. (1975). *Short-term effects of modeling/behavior rehearsal, modeling/behavior rehearsal plus rational therapy, placebo, and no-treatment on assertive behavior.* Unpublished doctoral dissertation, New York University.

Young, H. S. (1975). *Counseling strategies with working class adolescents.* Paper presented at the first National Conference on Rational Psychotherapy.

Yu, A., & Schill, T. (1976). Rational-emotive therapy as a treatment in reducing vulnerability to criticism. *Rational Living, 11*(2), 12-14.

Zellie, K., Stone, C. I., & Lehr, E. (1980). Cognitive-behavioral intervention in school discipline: A preliminary study. *Personnel and Guidance Journal,* October, 80-83.

Chapter 8

Reality Therapy Approaches

Gerald B. Fuller, Ph.D.
Diane L. Fuller, M.A.

INTRODUCTION

Reality Therapy was developed by William Glasser (1965, 1972, 1976a, 1976b, 1981) when he recognized that existing therapeutic systems did not produce rapid and durable change. The essence of reality therapy is the acceptance of reponsibility of individuals for their own behavior, thus helping them to achieve success and happiness. Concomitant with this responsibility is the importance of personal involvement in all of the therapeutic and growth processes. Reality therapy teaches better ways of fulfilling needs. It stresses the idea that, given an atmosphere of human involvement and supportive confrontation, an individual can learn how to behave in a more responsible and productive manner.

History and Status

Dr. Glasser began the development of reality therapy in 1962 in conjunction with Dr. G. L. Harrington while working at a Veterans Administration hospital in California. During this same period he was the chief psychiatrist at the Ventura School for Girls, which housed 14- to 16-year-old female "incorrigibles." Here the principles of reality therapy were used in developing specific programs for the girls and for the school as a whole. These young women had, understandably, poor self-esteem, and one of Glasser's immediate goals was to build success into their experiences. The school became a place where honest praise was given freely. The girls were put in charge of themselves, thus giving them the responsibility for their own behavior. Rules were clearly defined, as were the consequences for breaking them. The praise and personal responsibility helped shift the girls' attention away from the authority figures against whom they had rebelled.

The title "reality therapy" was officially introduced in an article dealing with juvenile delinquency (Glasser, 1964). The following year his book *Reality Therapy* (Glasser, 1965) appeared. At approximately the same time Dr. Glasser founded the Institute for Reality Therapy. Here therapists do both individual and group counseling and teach the concepts of reality therapy to both laypersons and professionals.

In 1966 Glasser began consulting in the California school system. His experiences in the schools led to the publication of *Schools Without Failure* (Glasser, 1969). Here he applied the concepts of reality therapy to contemporary education. He described the inadequacies of current educational procedures and suggested techniques aimed at reducing school failure. Again, these techniques aimed at the children's involvement in their schooling, giving them a sense of self-esteem and a successful identity. He felt this whole process could best be accomplished by making education interesting and relevant, by retiring the grading system, by showing true concern, and by allowing the children to progress at their own speed. A good classroom, he asserted, should incorporate praise, active listening, and relevant helpfulness.

In 1969, as a result of the popularity of *Schools Without Failure,* the Educator Training Center (ETC) was opened to handle the flood of requests for information and teaching materials. By offering materials such as films, cassettes, and books that emphasized the principles of reality therapy, the Center helped teachers and other school personnel create these *schools without failure.* So many children who appeared to have had adequate advantages (e.g., good homes, security, attention) were responding by failing in school, using drugs, and demonstrating an unwillingness to work for reasonable goals. Glasser's search for an explanation for this phenomenon led to his concept of *role versus goal.* This theory was the impetus for *The Identity Society* (Glasser, 1972). Here he discussed the replacement of a "survival society," where behavior is directed toward keeping people fed, clothed, and comfortable, by an "identity society," where emphasis is placed upon caring, involvement, respect, and satisfaction. Children gain strength and successful identities through involvement with others, and with this strength children can do what is necessary to reap the benefits available in the identity society. Glasser proposed that a person, in looking for ways to gain personal strength or confidence, could become addicted to positive behavior. These positive addictions, the antithesis of negative addictions such as drugs and alcohol which make one weaker, help to make one stronger. Jogging, tennis, or reading could thus become positively addictive. These ideas were set forth in *Positive Addiction* (Glasser, 1976b).

In an attempt to fill the gap that often exists between theory and practice, a case study compilation entitled *What Are You Doing?: How People are Helped Through Reality Therapy* was edited by N. Glasser (1980). A solid neurological and psychological base was added to the clinical approach of reality therapy with the publication of *Stations of the Mind* (Glasser, 1981). Its thesis centers around the idea that people are internally motivated and, thus behavior is purposeful. However, each individual may perceive a different reality, and this idea must be kept in mind when interpreting others' behaviors. What is motivating a particular child and what others think is motivating him or her may be very different indeed.

In *Take Effective Control of Your Life* (Glasser, 1984), Glasser describes his new "control theory" which proposes that people can better their lives through conscious control of their emotions and actions. This is based on his theory that everything a person does, thinks, and feels comes from inside an individual and is not, as most people believe, a response to external circumstances.

In his most recent book, *Control Theory in the Classroom* (Glasser, 1986a), Glasser addressed the need for schools to restructure the classroom environment in order to keep students interested and involved in learning. He contends that students are currently not successful in school because school is not part of the picture in their heads which fulfills their basic needs. Glasser proposed the use of a cooperative learning approach which would satisfy students' basic needs for fun, belonging, power, and freedom. Thus, students would be provided with mental pictures of learning in school that would be "need fulfilling."

The Institute for Reality Therapy teaches the practice and concepts of reality therapy to professional people, interested groups, and organizations. Individuals are taught in one-week sessions which include lectures, discussions, demonstrations, and role-playing situations. Three weeks of instruction are necessary to become certified as a reality therapist. Two of these weeks are spent "in the field" and the third week is spent at the Institute for Reality Therapy in Los Angeles.

The Educator Training Center was created in 1969 to teach reality therapy to educators. The center offers one-week seminars in classroom management. It also offers in-service presentations to schools and school districts with training ranging from basic theory to such specifics as discipline and motivation. In addition, a program called SWF (Schools Without Failure) offers teachers and other school personnel seminars to help develop classroom skills, implement a success-oriented curriculum, and deal realistically with current problems using the resources at hand.

The *Journal of Reality Therapy* was first published in the fall of 1981. This semi-annual publication focuses on theoretical, research-based, and specific descriptions of the successful applications of reality therapy principles in field settings.

OVERVIEW OF THEORY

Basic Theory and Assumptions

COMPONENTS OF A SUCCESSFUL IDENTITY. Reality therapy purports that the driving force for all behavior is the basic, intrinsic goal of having a different, distinct, and unique identity. Each child wants to believe there is no other person quite like him or her anywhere on earth. To attain and maintain this identity, *regardless* of whether it is centered on success or failure, is critical.

Failure-identity children are those who believe, "I can't do it. I'm no good. I'm not successful. I'm worthless." Believing they have little chance to succeed or to be happy, these children appear to have a distressing or negative attitude toward school and life. For them the real world is uncomfortable. These children have given up and, for the most part, have resigned themselves to failure. They often see themselves as losers and lonely and do not care about themselves or others. They are self-critical, irrational, and irresponsible and have little to look forward to. "Apathetic," "indifferent," "uninvolved," and "unconcerned" are some of the terms that are used to describe these children. School failure is personalized and so these children come to view themselves as worthless.

In order for children to acquire the feeling that they are basically successful or good, they must fulfill the following general or basic needs: (1) Love—belonging, friendship, caring, and involvement; (2) Power—importance, recognition, worth, and skill; (3) Fun—pleasure, enjoyment, laughter, and learning; and (4) Freedom—independence, choice, and autonomy.

All people need to be loved and cared for from birth to old age. To love and be loved are necessary ingredients for successful growth and development. The child must learn both to give love and to receive it in return. This necessitates that there must be at least one person who cares for the child and for whom the child cares. The child's need for love and belonging can be seen in the interaction with the members of his or her family and with others in school. In school this might best be reflected in social responsibility. Children must learn to care for, to be responsible for, and to help one another. To the extent that the child becomes involved with others, the child who belongs or is involved is more successful than the uninvolved child who may well be lonely and suffering.

In addition to love, children also need power or a sense of importance. There are ways to satisfy this need for power that are positive and do not interfere with other people's needs. One positive way to meet the need for power is to receive recognition. It is important to remember that it is children's perception of what they do, helped by recognition from others, that gives them that ultimate sense of worth. To feel worthwhile and successful, children must maintain a satisfactory standard of behavior; that is, they must behave in ways that will gain the love and respect of others. It is also necessary for them to behave in a way and to perform so that what they do is worthwhile to themselves as well. To do this they must learn to evaluate and correct that behavior which is wrong, and, most important, to give themselves credit when it is right. Children's being attuned to morals, standards, and values of right and wrong as well as to school behavior, then, is linked to fulfillment of their need for self-worth.

Although belonging and self-worth are separate, children who love and are loved will usually think they are worthwhile. The overindulged child can be the exception. These children are loved too much. Their parents mistake the total acceptance of good or bad behavior for good discipline. Love does not mean blanket approval. When children receive love for behavior that they know is wrong, they do not feel worthwhile and, thus, may act out as a way of asking for limits. A child needs to learn that being the subject of someone's love does not in and of itself give him or her self-worth.

Children need time for fun and time to enjoy themselves and others. This must involve active participation in contrast to passive participation such as is inherent in watching television. Children who do not know how to enjoy life actively, who do not know how to engage in having fun, are often too serious. As such, they tend to stress the aversiveness of a problem and to exaggerate the significance of things. They may also be people who structure their time poorly; the delinquent child often has nothing better to do than to get into trouble. How much fun the child has at home and school is an important variable to evaluate.

Freedom is important to everyone. Reality therapy defines freedom as being able to do and say what you want within the limits of the laws of society and being able to express yourself without discount. Discounts among family members and teachers and children are most destructive. Freedom from criticism does not imply no correction or a laissez-faire attitude. It means refraining from the little extra comments that teachers and parents so often make that chip away at the child's self-concept: "How dumb can you be?";"Don't you ever care about anybody but yourself?"

Criticism of this kind tells children that they are not good people and pushes them toward failure identities. *Criticism should always be directed at the behavior and not at the child or the person.*

When children are not fulfilling their needs, they are unhappy and must do something to reduce their pain and hurt. Often the means they devise are ineffective, and, try as they might to succeed, they view themselves as failures. The concomitant loneliness, pain, and discomfort are often dealt with in four ways: depression and withdrawal, acting out, thinking disturbances, and sickness.

Control Theory

Since 1984, Glasser has integrated reality therapy with control theory which suggests that the above basic needs are part of our genetic structure. Built into our brains are these fixed needs which, if not satisfied, result in stress, tension, and suffering. At the survival level, these needs include food, shelter, and safety, while at the psychological level they include the needs discussed earlier. Consequently all of our behavior is a constant attempt to satisfy one or more of the basic needs that are written into our genetic structure. When there is a difference between what we want (as perceived in our head) and what we are perceiving in the external or real world, there is a mismatch which results in dissatisfaction. Often the child in need of therapy has chosen unsatisfactory behavior which attempts to meet, but does not alleviate, those needs which remain unfulfilled.

From one's general or basic needs, there is a world of specific needs which are not genetic but learned. We usually function at the level of these specific needs although we are also aware of basic needs. We refer to these specific needs as wants—specific perceptions related to a basic need. For example, swimming is a *want* which is related to the basic *need* for fun.

The mechanism through which needs are met is the inner world of wants which is described by Glasser (1985) as a "picture album." Exploring the needs and perceptions in the "picture album" is a means of working with a child in therapy. This is also the first procedure that lends itself to change.

In a theory that explains how we live our lives on a daily basis, the brain is seen as a "control system" which seeks to control, maneuver, and mold the external world in order to satisfy an internal goal. Recently Glasser has brought the theory to a clinical level with practical application (Glasser, 1984).

VIEW OF PSYCHOPATHOLOGY

("The Fruits of a Failure Identity")

DEPRESSION AND WITHDRAWAL. Unable to reduce the pain of failure and loneliness through acceptable and realistic means, the child withdraws into the self-involvement of unhappiness and depression. The child behaves in a way that causes him or her to feel depressed and then uses that feeling as an excuse for an inability to handle problems. In reality therapy terms, a feeling such as depression is called *depressing* because it is viewed as a feeling *behavior.* Depression is not something which comes over children, but rather is something they actively choose and help to create. The child would rather depress than admit to an inability to figure out better behaviors for belonging and getting along. In the child's view it is better to use depression as an excuse than to admit to not knowing what to do. Depressing provides a rationalization for continuing uninvolved behavior. After all, how can anyone expect a depressed child to become involved with others when he or she feels so bad? The successful child, when feeling depressed, realizes that something must be done, whereas the unsuccessful child fights to maintain the depressing behavior because it provides some temporary relief. To give up the depressed state would be to expose oneself to the pain of feeling unloved, a failure, and worthless. To experience this is more than the child wants to do. Depressive behavior may have some value, however, if it can be seen as a child's request for help.

ACTING OUT. Another way to relieve the pain of failure and worthlessness is to act out. Many children strike out in an effort to get rid of pain by hurting the people they believe are denying their needs. They are often indifferent to social rules and reinforce their lack of regard for others by putting the blame on someone else. These children are not afraid of punishment; they often expect it. Having identified and reinforced themselves as failures, they often become antagonistic, breaking home and school rules. Because they feel they will fail anyway, they attempt to gain what they want while expending as little energy as possible. Needing to fulfill this identity, they assert that they are someone—a failure; and they use this as a rationale for their capricious behavior. Consequently, when they are punished, these children often feel victimized or persecuted. Unfortunately, the punishment they receive can serve as a source of involvement because they obtain attention through their acting-out behavior. Punishment is painful, but it is better than being alone.

THINKING DISTURBANCES. Some children, either unable to figure out a satisfying behavior or having tried and failed, attempt to meet their needs by living in a world of their own. They deny reality in an effort to reduce pain. Once self-involved, they do not have to deal with the pain of failing and not being involved. For these children, their own world becomes the real world. All of their seemingly crazy thoughts and behaviors make sense; it is an attempt to avoid a world that they fear they will be unable to control.

SICKNESS. Some children manifest somatic complaints such as headaches, stomachaches, nausea, or dizziness with no physical causes present. It may be better to stay in bed than to face a hectic day at school. If one is too sick, one cannot possibly do schoolwork. For these children, the ache and physical pain are very real, making it impossible to carry on a normal day. By causing the child to be sick and helpless, these behaviors keep anger in check and allow the child to be offered help or to seek it. Probably more than most other behaviors this one allows for sympathy and attention. Somatic illness has the added attractiveness of reassuring the child and his or her teacher and parents that the problem is "physical" rather than social or psychological.

General Therapeutic Goals and Techniques

Although reality therapy places some emphasis on behavioral change, more importance is given to goals that are concerned with values and concepts of individual responsibility. A strong focus is placed on helping individuals understand and accept themselves as they are. An individual's achievements, within the limits of inherited endowment and environment, are what the individual makes of himself or herself. The way a person behaves and whether the person acts responsibly or irresponsibly depends on decisions rather than conditions. Other goals might include developing the ability to express mature and responsible love, the ability to be more aware of both positive and negative feelings, and the ability to give and take. Self-awareness should move toward increasing the client's ability to focus on present concerns and to avoid rehashing the past, particularly mistakes, and dwelling on the distant future. Soon clients will be able to act more responsibly to solve personal crises more effectively and to fulfill their own needs without hurting others or themselves (Glasser & Zunin, 1979).

Reality therapy is a verbally active psychotherapy. A conversational exchange occurs between therapist and client that may include agreements and diagreements. Clients are confronted with their irresponsible behavior. Constructive arguing will focus on showing the client more responsible ways of behaving. The therapist may attempt to "pin down" the client in terms of what the client intends to do about his or her current life situation. A statement such as "I might look for a job" will be met with questions such as "How?" and "When?" with the therapist not accepting excuses. Throughout the therapy process, the therapist directs the client to focus on real-life issues and is concerned with what the client does and what the client plans to do.

The steps for child and adolescent therapy outlined in the next section are essentially similar to the principles (e.g., see Glasser & Zunin, 1979) that guide all reality therapy. Reality therapy begins with the therapist communicating a caring, personal involvement to the client. The focus is on present behaviors and concerns, helping the client make his or her own value judgments on whether the behavior is responsible, and assisting the client in making plans to change "failure behavior" to "success behavior." Then the therapist strongly encourages the client to make a commitment to act on the value judgments and to carry out the specific plans formulated. The therapist does not accept excuses for failure, yet does not punish the client when failure occurs. Throughout, the therapist takes an encouraging, client-advocate stance.

INDIVIDUAL PSYCHOTHERAPY WITH CHILDREN AND ADOLESCENTS

Because the basic approach of reality therapy in working with children and adolescents is essentially the same, no distinction will be made between techniques for these age groups.

Step 1. Involvement

This step has also been referred to as "Be personal" or "Make friends." Because the child who is acting irresponsibly and has a failure identity is lonely and alienated, it follows that an important technique to use is to become involved with him or her. Involvement is a therapeutic prerequisite for anyone who hopes to be helped. Often this step is not given the importance it should have in the therapeutic process. Beginning therapists hear this and agree in principle but are often overly anxious to move on to the "action" of therapy. However, a therapist's skill in dealing with a child depends heavily on this first step.

A child must be made to believe that the person working with him or her is concerned. The therapist needs to be warm, supportive, interested, and genuine in the relationship. Unless this can be done from the beginning to the end, the therapy will seldom be successful. Convincing the child that you want to be involved is demanding, requiring a good sense of humor, patience, and acceptance. The child needs to be convinced that another person cares and is willing to talk about anything that is of interest to the child rather than just focusing on what has gone wrong. This makes it essential that one have a good grasp of child or developmental psychology. It is important to know about the current television programs, movies, records, or books in which children at different ages are interested. In addition, hobbies, recreational activities, and peer relationships should be explored.

What the child says must be respected, although one does not have to agree with it all. If the child makes contradictory statements or is unclear, the therapist should strive for clarification by saying, for example, "I don't understand" or "I'm confused." The therapist should be open and honest with the child.

It should be made clear that the therapist is willing to talk about almost anything the child wishes to discuss. Initially, as little emphasis as possible should be placed on the child's present symptoms or behaviors; this has been done enough in the past. The therapist should not focus on problems or misery first. This only reinforces behavior by giving value to the failure and self-involvement. The less the therapist discusses the problems and instead stresses the possibilities open to the child, the better.

The question of how much time to give the child in therapy often arises. To a child who is lonely and uninvolved, the friendly therapist becomes a much-desired source of needed gratification. It is impossible to be extensively involved with every child in a time-consuming relationship, especially within a school setting. The therapist should never promise more time than can be given. Most children can accept honest statements from the therapist about time commitments once involvement is established. Whatever the amount, it is usually more productive and rewarding than what the child has had previously.

During this first step it is important to ascertain what the child *wants*. The therapist should begin where the child is, not where the therapist thinks the child is. Suggesting what the child might want is counterproductive. Helping the child to examine wants and to establish priorities demonstrates early on that the child needs to begin taking responsibility for his or her actions. A brief summary by the therapist during or at the end of the session helps the child know that the therapist is paying attention. It also gives the child a chance to hear his or her wants, something the child may never have listened to before. In addition, it gives the child an opportunity to correct any misinterpretation. This summarizing technique continues to be valuable throughout therapy.

Step 2. Focus on present behavior

Here the therapist asks the child, "What are you doing?" This question is used in place of the "why" question of conventional therapy. The emphasis is on the present—what the child is doing now and what is planned for the future. Reality therapy sees focusing on the past to be of little use. Dwelling on the past only reinforces the apparent importance of past experiences and their association with the child's present problems. The only way a child can work toward a successful identity is to become aware of his or her current behavior. This approach does not deny that problems can be rooted in the past. But we can basically only deal with current behavior in order to plan a better strategy for the future; we cannot undo what has already occurred. Acknowledge the child's past, believe in it, but focus on the present.

This does not mean that one never asks about the past. If the therapist thinks that knowing something about the past will help plan for more suitable behavior now or in the future, such information should be pursued. However, one should look for the past *successes* to use as building blocks for a better now and tomorrow. Talking about past failures often reinforces the child's use of them as an excuse for present behavior: "My brother was this way and so am I," or "I have a temper like my mother's and that's just the way I am."

Reality therapy purports that a child's behaviors are a combination of his or her actions, thoughts, and feelings. To the child who is upset, it may seem, however, that these feelings are most important. The therapist should not ask the child how he or she *feels* unless the feeling is associated strongly with what the child is doing now or plans to do in the future. Talking about a feeling may temporarily make the child feel better, but it doesn't change anything and is worthless in the long run. *Feelings should be tied to the behavior that evokes them.* This helps the child to understand that one can and must change what one is doing if relief from this present misery is to be found. In essence, behavior is readily observed and responded to; feelings are not. If changes are to occur, it is easier to start with behavior than with feeling. This doesn't mean that the therapist rejects the feelings but tries to point out that the way the child feels may not be as important as the way the child behaves. The therapist might respond, "I believe you; you are upset, you are angry, but what are you doing?" It is hoped that this will redirect the child's attention to his or her responsibility for the behavior. If the child is depressed and is complaining about sitting at home all the time on weekends feeling miserable and thinking unhappy thoughts, the therapist can listen to the upset feelings but stress the sitting-at-home behavior. The therapist might ask, "Is that what you are choosing to do?" The idea is to focus more and more on the activity or the lack of it rather than on the misery and upset conditions. It is easier to change the sitting-at-home behavior than the depressed feeling or miserable thoughts.

Asking the angry, acting-out child about feelings is counterproductive and may produce more anger and hostility. Focusing on what the child is doing and putting less emphasis on feelings may actually reduce frustration. The anger is not the cause of the problem, but rather the result of an inability on the part of the child to satisfy his or her needs.

It is a basic premise that the behavior the child exhibits is chosen. The therapist must keep in mind that children very seldom see their behavior as having anything to do with the problem. Children usually see the world, and not themselves, as needing to change. This has often been referred to as an external locus of control. Also, children may see themselves as victims of things over which they have no control.

Step 3. Value judgment

The important question to be asked here is: "Is what you are doing helping you?" or "Is what you are doing against the rules?" The child must determine if the behavior is good for him or her and for those the child cares for and if it is socially acceptable. Because the child acts by choice, he or she must make the judgment as to whether or not to continue the behavior. This is the child's responsibility. Here the child begins to answer the question, "Is it helping?" The child will not change until it is determined that what he or she is doing does not help accomplish what is wanted. What is actually being asked of the child is, "Are you doing what will help you fulfill your needs?" The therapist should be very careful here to remain nonjudgmental about the child's behavior; the *child* is being asked to make the judgment. The therapist prepares the child for this judgment making by using what was established in the preceding steps—the examination of the present behavior and the trust which comes with involvement. The value judgment may include a decision about what the child wants. "So you really want to quit school? Can a boy of sixteen find a good job? Are you willing to live with the hassle of school?"

Often there is no clear choice about which behavior is the best or most responsible. In some cases, such as obtaining independence from parents, it is difficult for the child to make a choice. If the child is unwilling to make the judgment that what is being done is not helping or that it is against the rules, nothing can be planned or accomplished. No one can make anyone do anything as long as that person is unwilling to accept the consequences of his or her behavior. The most the therapist can do is to continue to strive for increased involvement that will encourage a move away from failure.

Step 4. Planning responsible behavior

Once the child has judged that his or her behavior is not helping and wants to change, it is the responsibility of the therapist to help the child make a plan to do better. This is the time to examine the possible alternatives to the child's present behavior. Both the positive and negative alternatives should be discussed. Children often have a limited repertoire of behavioral responses, making it difficult for them to suggest many alternatives. Initially the therapist may have to generate some ideas. More than one idea or alternative should be presented so that the child can choose the one most acceptable to him or her. In some cases where the therapist must make a plan for the child, it is important to establish that the child thinks he or she can carry it out. Actually, it does not matter who makes the plan as long as it is accepted and becomes the child's plan. It is hoped that the child will learn new behaviors via the plan of action developed. Sometimes, planning proceeds by trial and error; that is, a plan is developed, attempted, and perhaps modified until one is found that fits the situation.

The therapist should be aware that making plans takes skill and that there are critical components which must be considered.

1. A plan must be *small* and manageable, in terms of both time and what the child is going to do. For example, a child might do 15 minutes of homework for each of 4 days. If the plan is too large, it will only reinforce failure. The child needs to feel successful. To allow the child to say, "I will not fight from now on" is setting the child up for future failure. It would be better for the

child to say, "I won't fight in the next 2 hours." Only after initial successes can the time be prolonged.

2. The plan must be *specific,* definite, and detailed. It should be something the child can visualize doing, like completing a math assignment. Key words for the therapist to use here include: what, where, how, when, with whom, and how many. The plan should also depend on what the *child* does rather than what others do. For example, "I will clean my room every Monday if you let me stay up and watch TV" is an unsatisfactory plan; "I will clean my room every week" is better.
3. A plan should be *reasonable.* It should make sense, and the child and therapist should see the value in doing it.
4. The plan should be *positive.* The focus should be on what the child *is* going to do rather than on what he or she is *not* going to do.
5. The plan should begin as soon as *possible.* The longer a child waits to put a plan into effect, the less likely he or she is to do it.
6. The plan should be *repetitive.* It should be something that can be done often or something that can be easily repeated each day. This helps form daily patterns of the new behavior.

If the plan fails, the therapist must have the ability to think of another one or to help the child replan. If, in the attempt to make a new plan, a problem comes up that seems unresolvable, rather than force the issue, it is better for the therapist to relax and just chat with the child about an interesting subject. In time, it is hoped, child and therapist will be able to return to the difficulty during the session and resolve it.

After a plan has been made, it is often wise to return to the value judgment step. The therapist should ask the child if the plan is workable. The therapist might ask the child, for example, "Is the plan reasonable or is it asking for too much?" It is also beneficial to have the child repeat the plan to be sure that the child understands it. This clarification again points out the potential value of summarizing.

If the child carries out the plan, this accomplishment is the beginning of his or her becoming more responsible; and this concept cannot be overly stressed. The therapist will have to emphasize over and over again that the child must take the responsibility, that things in life cannot always be done for him or her, and that one must live one's own life. The child must recognize that the therapist will be of help for a while but that all the therapist can do is to get this process started. The child must come to the realization that eventually all people must assume responsibility for their behavior and live in a world much larger than the restricted world of therapy.

Step 5. Commitment to the plan

After the child makes a reasonable, workable plan, a commitment must be obtained that the plan will be carried out. The child is being asked, "Will you do it?" This is an important stage in plan making because it shifts the responsibility to the child. Commitment is both motivating and binding. It means that the child is no longer alone. What the child does now is not only for him- or herself but also for someone else. This helps provide a sense of strength and purpose.

Getting the failure-identity child to make a commitment is not always an easy task. Having already failed on a number of occasions, these children are often reluctant to commit themselves again for fear of exposing themselves to more painful rejection and consequent feelings of worthlessness. Commitment is also involvement, which may be met with resistance. However, until the child is willing to make a commitment to something or someone else, it is likely that the child will remain self-involved and unable to develop a success identity.

The commitment is made either verbally or in writing. A written commitment is preferred because it is stronger, more binding, and more clear. There is little doubt about the conditions of a commitment when they are written out and signed by the child. It is a good idea for the therapist to sign it also, thus demonstrating involvement. Two copies of the agreement are made, one for the child and one for the therapist as a backup in case the child loses the copy. This approach may sound too businesslike and legal, but it is a fact that a person is more hesitant to escape from a written commitment than from a verbal one. It also avoids disagreements over what the terms of the plan were.

Step 6. Accept no excuses

Plans do fail sometimes, and the therapist must make it clear that excuses are unacceptable because they break the involvement and allow the child an opportunity to avoid responsibility. Excuses, if allowed, do provide temporary relief; they reduce the child's tension and improve feelings on a short-term basis. The excuse undermines the need for action because momentarily the child is off the hook. Too frequently teachers and parents accept apologies such as "I'm sorry" because it is easier to accept the apology than to go through the time-consuming process of assessing responsibility and present behavior. It is also very possible that the child could interpret the acceptance of excuses as a lack of concern. The accepting of an excuse also implies that the child's inadequacy and inability are also accepted.

When the child does not follow through on the commitment to the plan, the therapist asks, "When will you do it?" or "When will it happen?" or "I'm glad you are sorry, but what are you going to do so this same thing doesn't happen again?" It may be necessary to alter the plan. The child is not discounted or punished for failing. Actually, without punishment or rejection, there are no good reasons for excuses.

When the commitment fails, the plan must be reevaluated. If the plan is still reasonable, the child must decide whether or not to commit to it again. At this point a value judgment must again be obtained from the child, and a new plan and commitment formulated. A good way to reduce excuses is to ask for a value judgment every time the child gives an excuse. Often, the making of an excuse is evidence that the child has not fully understood the value judgment that was made. The therapist might say, "Do you want to work at getting along with your teacher or do you want to give up?" Returning to the value judgment often helps put the therapy back on the right track.

A teacher faced with excuses might say, "If you don't do your assignment, I will not punish you, but I do insist we work out a better solution. I don't care why you didn't do the assignment; I will accept your thinking that you have a valid reason. However, we have to solve the problem. We have to find a better way for you to follow the rules and get your schoolwork done."

Step 7. Do not punish

This step probably elicits the most controversy. Many successful people regard the fear of punishment as the prod toward achievement. As a result, punishment has enjoyed a solid reputation in our society. Punishment, while never good, can serve as a deterrent to the success-oriented child who may have strayed momentarily from the path of responsibility. With the child who is a failure, however, punishment often reinforces the failure identity; the punishment only confirms the child's low self-esteem and can even sanction other reckless behavior.

The goal here is not to put more pressure on the child than is now being experienced. This step recognizes and accepts that a child does not function well when he or she is hurting. It proposes that although there is not to be any punishment administered, minimally painful, reasonable consequences (that is, appropriate discipline) have value.

Criticism is also unacceptable. Many children who fail actually expect the therapist to be critical and hard on them and may attempt to provoke this attitude. If the therapist succumbs, the child will use the therapist's behavior to continue excusing inadequacies. This is a popular game played by failing children. A nonpunitive, noncritical therapist will not become involved in the child's inadequate life-style.

Reality therapy defines punishment as any treatment that is intended to cause a child mental or physical pain. Punishment is to be distinguished from natural consequences or discipline. A comprehensive list of the differences (Table 1) between the two is given by Dreikurs, Grunwald, and Pepper (1971).

This step does not imply that reality therapy is a passive, permissive therapy. Discipline is an essential part of reality therapy for children. Reasonable, agreed-upon consequences for irresponsible behaviors are not punishment but discipline. Logical consequences set out the reality of social responsibility. In any given situation, it is necessary that the rules be learned. The establishment of consequences and the understanding of rules help to eliminate the element of the unexpected. Children should

TABLE 1

Punishment	Discipline
1. Not appropriate for (related to) the action. Too severe.	1. Appropriate for the action. Not too severe or meaningless.
2. Unexpected because the punisher has reacted on the spur of the moment.	2. Expected because the individual has been informed of the rules and results of infringement.
3. Often punishment is delayed.	3. Immediate consequences.
4. Expresses power of a personal authority.	4. Based on logical consequences expressing the reality of the social order.
5. Punishment is imposed. Responsibility is that of the punisher (no choices).	5. Discipline is assumed. Responsibility is that of the individual (choices offered).
6. Focuses on stopping past negative behavior.	6. Focuses on teaching present and future positive behavior (e.g., mistakes are seen as chances to learn). Solution orientation.
7. Focuses on external control of behavior.	7. Focuses on reinforcing internal control of behavior.
8. Reinforces failure identity (confirms low self-esteem and may increase rebellion and hostility or withdrawal).	8. Emphasizes teaching ways that will result in a more successful identity.
9. Often is, or is seen as, an expression of anger and hostility.	9. Should be friendly—a partnership.
10. Easy, expedient, and requires little skill.	10. Difficult, time-consuming and requires much patience.
11. Punishment often alienates the individual.	11. Discipline, over time, strengthens the relationship as consistency demonstrates caring.
12. Expression of moral judgment by punisher.	12. Individual makes his or her own value judgment of his or her behavior.
13. Punishment is often seen as linked to the punishee rather than to the act (doer is wrong).	13. Discipline is linked to the act (emphasis is on the deed).
14. Only recognizes *results.*	14. Recognizes *effort* as well as results.
15. Individual has no opportunity to redress wrong.	15. There is an opportunity for retribution or repair.

suffer reasonable consequences when they break the rules. Yelling at children, for example, adds nothing to the learning process and only makes things worse. The child might now suffer what is perceived as the loss of parental or teacher approval and is burdened additionally with the work of reconciliation.

If the child breaks the rules at school or at home, reasonable consequences must follow. The most reasonable of these is deprivation of either a *freedom* or a *privilege*. The child might be asked to sit in a chair at home or school until a plan is worked out. A quiet place to sit, to do schoolwork, to think provides the child with the opportunity to get over the upset and to think about a plan. After an appropriate length of time, the teacher or parent should approach the child in a mild manner offering an opportunity for problem solving. If the child is ready, they then return to Step 4, planning responsible behavior, and continue from there.

Children should not be allowed to criticize themselves unless it is part of a value judgment or is tied to a plan to correct the problem. Even under these circumstances, such criticism should not be accepted but rather dealt with. If the child says, "I'm no good; I never do right," the therapist might reply, "I don't think I can go along with that. You go to school every day on time, and some of the time, from what you say, you do well. You are also here, which shows a willingness not seen in everyone. You are doing some things right."

It is also important that the therapist refrain from criticizing the child. Instead, the therapist might say, "Is what you are doing helping you or anyone else?" or "I think I can suggest a better way; let's discuss it." The child has an option in the second statement and is assured of help in doing better. During all of this, the child is learning a better way to handle problems and to cooperate with another person.

Step 8. Never give up

This step is a reminder to the therapist. No matter what the child does or says, the therapist should continue to convey the attitude of persistence long after the child wants the therapist to give up. Not giving up will, it is hoped, solidify the idea for the child that someone does care. Often the child begins to work only after this assurance has been given.

REALITY THERAPY AND CONTROL THEORY

Glasser (1984) has asserted that the methods of reality therapy are consistent with the concepts of control theory.

The goal of reality therapy in counseling or teaching is to help the child and adolescent gain more effective control over his or her life. In the classroom, teachers can use these same ideas to help the student become aware that it is beneficial to work hard and succeed academically. In either case, the goal is to help the child to become more responsible. To accomplish this, the child is asked to look honestly in the direction the behavior is heading and to determine whether this direction is satisfactory both immediately and in the long run. If either the direction of his or her life or the behavior he or she is choosing in order to move in this direction is not as satisfying or effective as desired, the goal of reality therapy is to help find a more effective behavior, a better direction, or both.

In order to do this, the steps of reality therapy have been expanded and reworked into two major components of reality therapy counseling (Glasser, 1986): *The Counseling Environment* and *The Procedures That Lead to Change.* Both of these components should be used together if counseling is to be effective.

Counseling Environment

The counselor must attempt to develop an environment in which the client feels secure enough to make an adequate evaluation of the effectiveness of his or her present behaviors. The client is then helped both to learn and to attempt different behaviors in an effort to find more effective ways to meet his or her needs. The success of therapy depends upon maintaining this environment throughout the counseling relationship.

The counseling environment needs to be perceived by the child as safe and positive. The child comes or is brought to counseling when some aspect of his or her life is not in effective control. It is critical for the child to see the therapist as a person who is capable and interested in assisting him or her find better choices for behavior. Therapists need to present themselves as persons who are not overwhelmed by the problems of the child and his or her family. To do this, the therapist should show confidence in the child's ability to learn to live life more responsibly and effectively.

The therapist must remember that a client behaves according to the perceptions of his or her own world (as held in the mind). One must realize that what the client perceives may be very different from what the therapist and others close to the client might perceive. Early in therapy, time is directed toward helping the client understand that these differences exist. Learning to deal with these differences becomes the next step in therapy. Unless the client can learn to get along better with those who perceive the world differently, it will be difficult to satisfy needs effectively.

A client is more successful when he or she recognizes and accepts the responsibility for chosen behavior. The role of the therapist is to maintain a relationship with the child which accomplishes the following:

1. Helps the child avoid excuses and accept responsibility.
2. Emphasizes the child's assets and strengths.
3. Provides the child with the chance to learn and to try new and more effective behaviors.

Procedures That Lead to Change

First, the therapist needs to focus on the child's total behaviors; that is, how the child is *acting, thinking,* and *feeling* at the present time. Next, a child must learn that all total behaviors are chosen.

To effect this, ask the client what is wanted now. If the client does not know, continue to focus on the choices and the resultant direction in which those choices are taking the client. The critical question to ask here is, "does your present behavior have a chance of getting you what you want now and will it take you in the direction you want to go?"

If the answer is "no," this implies that the client's direction is reasonable, but that the present behaviors will not get him or her there. At this point, the therapist should help the client plan new behaviors. For example, "I want to improve my grades but to do so I will have to study more."

At times the client is unable to move in the right direction regardless of how much effort is put forth. If this occurs, the therapist should ask the client to consider changing directions.

For example, "No matter how hard I study, my grades do not improve. I may have to consider a tutor." In this case, the plan now focuses more on changing the direction of the behavior than on the behavior itself. If the answer is yes, the behavior will get the client what is wanted now and will achieve the desired direction. Such an answer indicates that the client sees nothing wrong with this current behavior or the direction it is taking.

Before a plan is attempted, both client and therapist should agree that it has a reasonable chance of success, and a commitment should be given for follow-through. Usually the client who makes commitments tends to work harder. With younger children, a written commitment is generally more effective than a verbal one.

The therapist should remember that clients choose their behavior and that the best behavior is always that which the client believes can be accomplished. To this extent the behaviors are "effective" for the client. One must also be aware that a client will not change a behavior until it appears that the present behavior will either not result in what is wanted or will not take the appropriate direction. Change becomes possible only when the client believes that another available behavior will allow him or her to satisfy needs in a more acceptable way.

Reality Therapy Techniques

Specific techniques used in the application of these steps of reality therapy include:

A. *Humor*

Humor may be used to help the child understand that things are not as serious as they appear. It can be used confronting issues such as irrational behavior or lack of responsibility. It also helps the client regain the healthy ability to laugh at him- or herself. The message in humor is that life can be better, that there is hope, and that laughter is good medicine.

B. *Confrontation*

Facing the child with a here-and-now, no-excuses stance is definitely confrontational. Most confrontations require client action: a value is pushed, and the client is challenged to look for alternatives and is encouraged to formulate a new plan. This technique is often used when a child is unable to shake the mistaken ideas or beliefs behind his or her behavior.

C. *Contracts*

A written contract is often used in therapy. A signed contract serves as evidence of the client's intent to change behavior. It also specifies those changes in written form. Completion of a contract, like the fulfillment of needs, promotes feelings of self-worth within an individual. Here is evidence that the child *can* work responsibly toward a goal and succeed. Contracts may be one-sentence agreements such as, "Jack will speak to one new friend by Friday," or they may be quite detailed. The therapist and client each should sign the contract and keep a copy of it.

D. *Instruction*

When a specific skill is needed to formulate a new course of action, instruction may be needed. This can be part of the therapy session if the therapist has the needed competence, or, if not, the child can be referred elsewhere for skill instruction. If at all possible, the client should be encouraged to assume responsibility for the instruction/learning process.

E. *Information*

The child often needs specific and new information for a plan of action and the therapist should be ready to provide it. If the therapist does not have the information the client requires, the therapist should assist the client in finding it. It is the therapist's responsibility to have available a list of probable and reliable sources.

F. *Role Playing*

Role playing is often used when a child is experiencing difficulties in interpersonal relationships or needs to practice a new behavior. Role playing is frequently followed with a feedback session—a discussion of what the client and therapist experienced while playing the roles of others. The session often affords the therapist the opportunity to encourage the client by emphasizing what they did well. Role playing also offers an opportunity to focus on nonverbal behaviors that are part of successful behavioral interactions.

G. *Support*

Support is used to increase the child's awareness, anticipation, and expectation of a positive outcome. Children with a failure identity need much support, especially when putting their plans into action. They have learned to expect failure and do not want to take any further risks. Encouragement and support are paramount if the child is to commit to a new or different behavior. Support can be given by the following means: asking for a child's opinion, requesting the child's evaluaton of his or her present behavior, providing praise for successfully completing a plan, and expressing confidence in the child's ability to change. If successful, this will usually increase the child's motivation and serve to communicate feelings of worth to the child.

H. *Homework Assignments*

Homework is used to build continuity between sessions and to facilitate counseling by encouraging the child to work on problems between sessions. Typical assignments include trying a new behavior, reducing or stopping a present behavior, keeping a record of current behavior, or researching solutions to a specific problem.

I. *Bibliotherapy*

The goals of bibliotherapy include (1) allowing the child to see the similarity between his or her problems and those of others; (2) encouraging free expression concerning problems; (3) looking at alternative solutions; (4) helping the child to analyze attitudes and behaviors. When using bibliotherapy it is important to discuss the readings with the child. Discussion should be focused on feelings, thoughts, behaviors, and consequences. It is important that the child see the relationship between the reading and his or her own life.

Bibliotherapy can be viewed as a form of cognitive restructuring directed toward educating the child about certain areas of concern such as sex, divorce, or death. Suggested books for bibliotherapy can be found without difficulty.

J. *Self-Disclosure*

Some self-disclosure by the therapist is usually needed to obtain involvement with the client. Because reality therapy calls for active and equal participation of both client and therapist, there may be times when the therapist is asked how he or she deals with certain problems. In such circumstances, relevant to therapeutic goals, the therapist can share personal experiences.

K. *Summarizing and Reviewing*

Because clients often give the impression that they are listening when they are not, it is advisable to have the child summarize what was said or discussed in the therapy session. This can be done half-way through the session and/or at the end of it.

GROUP PROCEDURES WITH CHILDREN AND ADOLESCENTS

Once the therapist has established involvement and a relationship with the child, it is still necessary to convince the child that such relationships are also available with others. Reality therapy can be used with groups as well as with individuals. At this point in treatment the advantages of group therapy become apparent. The group offers the opportunity for involvement and provides more support, need satisfaction, and assurance than any one individual can provide. There is also more opportunity for safety in risking or trying new behaviors. Often, too, when the child listens to and becomes involved with other children, he or she becomes less self-involved. The group also allows a wide range of feelings and thoughts to be expressed. Instead of having only the therapist who cares and approves of the child, there is now the potential for the child to experience approval from the whole group. Being part of the group means that the child has an opportunity to get personal, to be warm, to show concern, and to develop more responsible behavior. This gives the child a taste of success and the chance to feel better about him- or herself.

Become Involved

In the initial stages of the group, the therapist takes an active role. Responsibility and caring must be modeled while getting the group members involved with one another. The therapist becomes involved with each member of the group, asking questions, requesting information, and encouraging comments. It is advisable to use games, value clarification, or group projects during the beginning sessions rather than to focus on problems. As in the first step of reality therapy with individuals, being friendly is important to involvement; it may take five or six sessions to get the group running smoothly.

Focus on Reality

The therapist must help the group to focus on reality. After involvement has been established, the attention is focused on present behavior and problems. Events discussed in the group should be kept to a minimum. The children are encouraged to evaluate and analyze, with the therapist asking such questions as: "What are you doing?" "What do you want?" "Is it doing you any good?" "Is it against the rules?" These questions help the children focus on the reality of the situation. The therapist does not evaluate the behavior but rather helps the children to become more aware of the behavior and to reach a decision about it. The other children, however, may evaluate behavior and can also offer specific suggestions concerning how they would handle certain problems.

Make a Plan

Initially the therapist will be very active in plan making. It will more than likely be up to him or her to develop alternative plans or different choices. However, the therapist must always be encouraging the children to become actively involved in this process. The therapist is cautioned to help make a reasonable plan that will have the best opportunity for success. After a plan has been decided upon, a commitment is obtained from the child or children involved. If the plan does not work, the therapist must firmly refuse to accept excuses; no one should be let off the hook. The therapist should be supportive and encouraging by asking, "Are you going to carry it out?" but the therapist must not punish or allow the other children to punish.

Establish Rules

The therapist, together with the children, must see that rules are established and consequences are set up if the rules are broken. For example, it might be established that one must raise a hand in order to speak to the group. The first time this rule is not followed by a child, a warning is given; the second time that child breaks the rule, the child must leave the group until he or she thinks that the rule can be followed; the third time, the child must leave the group and not be allowed to come back until a plan has been established, by the child, to follow the rule.

Group Makeup

Many therapists, because of time demands, put all of their problem children in one group. A group made up solely of children with acting-out behaviors, truants, and/or academically poor students is destined to fail. If one purpose of the group is to help children with failure identities, it makes sense that they should be involved with or come into contact with children who have successful identities. For the most part, children with failure identities learn very little that is responsible from other children with failure identities. A truant child has little that is constructive to offer another truant–if anything, he or she may reinforce and support the truant behavior. A child with a good attendance record may be more likely to help the truant as this child is already living more responsibly and can offer strength, encouragement, and support to the failing child. The successful child may be able to think of several alternatives or different choices for the problem situation and may also help in the development of a plan. It is important to include successful children in the group whenever possible.

Group Size and Duration

The size of the group will depend on the purpose of the group and the setting in which it occurs. However, eight to ten children are more than enough to work with at one time. With younger children, the therapist may want to begin with a smaller number. The group must meet regularly, thus giving the children an opportunity to plan to attend and to assume responsibility for being on time. Age becomes an important variable when a time frame is being considered. Glasser (1969) recommends that primary school children begin by meeting for 10 to 15 minutes per session, increasing to 30 minutes per session. Fourth, fifth, and sixth graders can easily meet for 30 to 45 minutes, and high schoolers for 45 minutes to an hour. The minimum number of meetings for all age groups is once a week; two or three times a week is more desirable.

Time of Day

A morning time is preferable when the children are fresh. Meetings should not be scheduled before recess or lunch.

CLASSROOM AND EDUCATIONAL APPLICATIONS

If one were to poll junior and senior high school-age children concerning their objections to school, many would reply that school has no relevance to the real world and that, although they are forced to go, they simply put in their class time, waiting for the 10 minutes of socialization between classes and the half hour at lunch. Those who do comply with the system often complain that they are learning to memorize, not to think. Or those who have gotten on the memorization railroad, ride it all the way to the perfect "A" report card, the graduation with honors, and the scholarships waiting at the end of the line. Either way there are prevailing feelings among these students that school is something to which one submits, that apathy serves better than taking on the system, and that teachers and the administration don't care as long as they get paid. Although it may be harder to elicit these feelings from the elementary children, they are there, expressed in the child who reaches over and crumples a classmate's paper, or who wanders aimlessly around the room, or who bullies on the playground.

The Classroom Meeting

Fun, freedom, self-esteem, and belonging, the four components of a successful identity, are—if one follows the thinking of reality therapy—for the most part missing in our educational system where an "If you want to pass, you'll do it my way" attitude prevails. It is possible, however, at any level to begin to help students become involved in developing goals of their own, to help them form better relationships with one another and with their teachers, and to help them experience success, gain confidence in their control over their education, and enjoy the process.

The vehicle that has offered students a feeling of belonging and of social responsibility, that has given them an opportunity to both give and receive concern, is the *classroom meeting*. Basically, there are three types: open-ended, education-diagnostic, and social-problem-solving. These meetings serve as an opportunity for the teacher to apply some of the principles of reality therapy in the classroom.

The *open-ended meeting* centers around thought-provoking questions related to the children's lives. The teacher presents hypothetical questions that are designed to enable the children to become involved. The discussion that follows is aimed at stimulating and developing intellectual curiosity. Any topic of interest to the class can be used. There are no right or wrong answers, only alternatives. Topics might include any number of relevant issues (depending, to an extent, on the age of the children) such as war, politics, taxes, or abortion. At no time should the teacher or leader of the group make value judgments.

Education-diagnostic meetings are directly related to what the class is studying. The teacher may use this meeting as a means of evaluating his or her teaching techniques and the current curriculum. This kind of class meeting provides an alternative to objective testing and helps determine whether or not the children are learning the material being taught. The meeting is informational—"How much have my students learned?"—and is not used for grading. It is seen as an efficient method for determining the children's strengths and weaknesses in a given subject. The discussion should provoke individual thinking and allow the children to correct false or misguided information.

The *social-problem-solving meeting* deals with any individual or group problems of the class or school. Problem solving is the major thrust here. Solutions, it should be pointed out, never include punishment or fault finding. This type of meeting gives the children some feeling of having control over their lives. Loneliness, attendance, grades, and individual behavior problems, for example, are very legitimate issues for discussion. The meetings should not strive for perfect answers but should at least work toward clarification of the problems that may very well not have solutions. The child learns that it is beneficial to discuss problems and learns to recognize that there is more than one way of dealing with a problem.

All of these meetings should be conducted with everyone seated in a circle. The circle is intended to provide the children with a feeling of acceptance because they have been allotted an equal amount of space with one another and the teacher.

The initial role of the teacher is to generate questions that will arouse the interest of the children. A basic technique to help stimulate interaction among the children is what has been called a *floater.* This is a statement that does not call for an answer; it is simply a comment sent out for response. The teacher should not feel a need to fill voids or silence; rather another nondirective comment can be offered. Also, the teacher can simply wait for a response. It is critical that the teacher respond to early statements by the children in a way that will not turn them off. This is best accomplished by remaining relatively value free. For instance, even a very good response should not be praised because such praise may inhibit some of the other children from offering what they then believe is a comment of less importance. The teacher should, however, indicate an appreciation for the contribution. Children who fail to volunteer might be brought into the discussion by saying, "You are paying attention; would you like to comment?" or "Think about it and let me know if you come up with an idea or answer." It is important that the teacher be supportive of any child's effort and that no attempt be made to criticize any child. If one child is dominating the group's time, the teacher can handle this situation by saying, "Thanks for your comments; let's hear from someone else now."

When a student behaves in a way that is disruptive to the other students in the class, this student needs to be confronted and helped by the entire class. For this type of situation, the social-problem-solving meeting is held. Here the so-called problem child hears what the other children think of his or her behavior. The teacher needs to be more in control of this type of meeting to insure that it does not become a free-for-all. The reason for the meeting should be explained to the class, e.g., to discuss the fact that a child has been stealing from other children. It is suggested that the group might be able to help the child to act in a more responsible manner. The children are asked to state what this child has been doing which interferes with them personally. The children are encouraged to tell the child directly what the behaviors are and the effects that these behaviors have had on them. After each person in the group, including the teacher, has had a chance to speak, the child with the irresponsible behavior is given a chance to explain what others have done to interfere with him or her. At this point the meeting moves quickly from getting all the facts out on the table to doing something with the information that has been obtained. It might be suggested that the class and the child involved offer some possible solutions to the problem, ones that would be acceptable to everyone. The teacher listens to all the solutions and then tells the group to narrow down the alternative plans and solutions. Last, the child is asked to pick a plan and commit to it. The class members are also asked to commit themselves to doing anything that will help the child carry out the plan. The conclusion of the meeting is an agreed-upon, manageable plan.

These class meetings are basically techniques used by individual teachers in their respective classrooms. A schoolwide approach to discipline or problem solving has been formulated by Glasser (1974) and is presented in the next section.

A Ten-Step Discipline Program

Reality therapy is a commonsense, nonpunitive approach which helps the children figure out what to do when their behavior is displeasing to themselves or interfering with the rights or needs of others. It focuses mainly on personal involvement and is structured toward helping the children plan and commit themselves to plans that will make their lives better. Reality therapy helps children gain a sense of belonging and personal worth.

Based on the principles of reality therapy, a ten-step, schoolwide approach for dealing with problem children has been developed. The approach deals with problems by means of a constructive, no-nonsense but nonpunitive method. It is built upon a positive teacher-student involvement, but it does not accept excuses in place of results. Built into the program are alternatives to consider when something does not work.

As an example, let's take Jack, who has behavior problems in school. It is now February, and despite several conferences with the principal, the school psychologist, and Jack's parents, nothing seems to be working. Perhaps Jack comes from a poor home background or he is an only child or he is the last child of a large family. He has barely learned to read and may never have had much good school experience. Whatever his problems, the teacher now has Jack in the classroom for an entire school year; and if the teacher cannot get him to cooperate, Jack will suffer and the teacher's life will be miserable.

If the following ten steps to better control are followed by the teacher, the child may be helped to change. His or her behavior can become, though not perfect, improved enough to reward all the efforts. No miracles will occur; it is hard, slow work. A period of several months is probably a good minimum time commitment.

This program is divided into three parts. The first three steps look realistically at how the child is dealing with his or her problems and are concerned with what can be done to decrease or reduce these problems. Steps 4 through 6 give the teacher a simple, practical approach to working with the child and getting the child to identify, evaluate, and plan alternatives to his or her unacceptable behavior. Steps 7 through 10 consider what resources within the school and/or community can be used if the child refuses to change the behavior or continues to break the rules.

Steps 1-3: What Am I Doing Here?

Step 1. What am I doing that isn't working? Set aside some time and make a list of the things you currently do when Jack upsets you. Ask yourself the questions, "What am I doing? Do I yell at him? . . . threaten him . . . ignore him?" Be honest and look at the efforts you have made to help the child. For the next few weeks refrain from doing the things you have on the list that have not been working. When you are tempted to use old methods, look at the list and ask yourself: "If they didn't work before, what chances do they have of working now?"

Step 2. A new start. If you have decided that your present techniques are not working, consider stopping these behaviors. Promise yourself that tomorrow, if Jack manifests a problem, you will attempt to act as though this is the first time it is occurring. Stay away from such statements to him as, "You are doing it again," or "I have told you a thousand times, stop it." Do not remind him that his behavior is repetitive behavior. If, on the other hand, he does something right or good, even though he has done it before, reinforce him: "Jack, it's really neat when you sit still," or "I appreciate that." A pat on the head, verbal recognition, or an approving nod is helpful in telling him he is OK. A fresh start for him, if not for you, may make a big difference.

Step 3. A new strategy. Plan at least one thing you might do for Jack that might help him have a better day *tomorrow.* It doesn't have to be a big deal. This step is based on the adage, "An ounce of prevention is worth a pound of cure." Whatever you do should have a positive aspect to it, such as a pat on the back as soon as he comes in, a special errand, or a "Good to see you, Jack." Anything helps that shows your personal concern for him. Fifteen seconds of unexpected recognition can mean a great deal. Commit yourself to these little plans for several weeks. The hope is that Jack will get the idea that he has some value in your class. Don't expect to be repaid with changed behavior immediately. Jack didn't develop his problems overnight nor will he become a pillar of responsibility in just a few days. Initially, he may reject you even more than before. You must stay calm and be persistent. Remember, these first three steps are aimed at changing *your* attitude and strategy.

Steps 4-6: Who's in Control Here?

Step 4. Calm direction. Even if you have some success with the first three steps, at some point Jack is going to demonstrate the problems again. Perhaps when you ask him to pay attention, he will daydream and not respond. Act as if this is the first time he has ever done this (Step 2), and ask him to pay attention and begin his assignment. You might also say, "Please stop it." It is hoped that your improved relationship with him through the first three steps will now help him to do as you ask and he will focus on the task. If he does not respond, walk over to him and help him get started. Do this in a quiet manner, possibly putting your hand gently on his shoulder at the same time. At this point, you might say, "Can you now do your work?" If he doesn't agree to do his work, don't give up; you still have six steps left. You are trying to establish that although he must take responsibility for not doing his work, you are willing to help him get started. If he accepts this, that ends it. You are not blaming, yelling, or threatening. If this step works, say nothing more except to give him some reinforcement such as, "Jack, I knew you could do it."

Step 5. Question time. If Step 4 does not work, ask the child one or both of the following two questions: "Is what you are doing against the rules?" and/or "What are you doing?" Often the child will say nothing or refuse to answer. If this happens, say, "This is what I say you are doing and it is against the rules." In essence, you are saying that Jack should be doing his work. You will have to be insistent. You are telling him that he is breaking a rule. Although he might try to evade the issue, you should continue focusing on the rule. These questions may be all you need to ask to help him begin working. You may also continue by asking, "Can you make a plan to follow the rules?" or "Are you willing to do your work?"

Step 6. Develop a plan. Go through Step 5 briefly, and, if it does not work, tell the child in a very firm voice, "We have to work this out. A plan has to be made that will help you follow the rules or change your behavior." What you are looking for here is more responsible behavior. It will be necessary to make some time available to talk with him about making a plan. If it cannot be done immediately, you might say, "We will work it out later." The time it takes to do this is usually much less than the time you spent with procedures that didn't work. The plan has to be more than "I'm sorry" or "I'll stop it." It has to be a *doing* plan that will help the child move toward more responsible behavior. You might say, "I am glad you are sorry, but what are you going to do so it won't happen again?" The plan should be short, specific, and concrete. At first you may have to put many of your ideas into the plan. Gradually, as he does better, the child may make more contributions to the plan. In Jack's case, you might say, "You do not want to do your work, but there are rules. Can you make a plan with me so you can get your work done? Let's try to work it out. Why don't we take some time and talk this over. It doesn't appear you are having much fun and maybe I can help you." Jack may be quite cautious at first, believing that this will just delay his ultimate punishment.

Tell him he won't be punished and that you'd like to help him work it out. Listen to his complaints; talk with him; get to know him better. Try not to bring up old behaviors or faults but instead stress that rules are important and you believe he can follow them. You may want to put the plan in writing; such a contract helps keep the commitment. You are saying to Jack that he has the power to make a good plan. Developing a plan does take some time, but it is a lot better than the techniques that have failed in the past.

Steps 7-10: Hope at the End of the Rope

Step 7. Someplace close. Assume that Jack still manifests a problem or disrupts again and you are convinced that the previous steps will not work. Now it is time for the child to be isolated, or "timed out." The decision for "time-out" may be made by you or it could have been established as a natural consequence at the planning level in Step 6. This isolation is done right in the classroom. You need to create a place where the child can sit that is comfortable but separate from the class. If this is impossible to do, a desk could be set up in the hallway within viewing distance of the door. This conveys to the child that he is no longer involved in active participation in the class. The child can listen but cannot take part in classroom activities until a plan to follow the rules is worked out with the child. The child needs to inform you of the plan and make a commitment to carry it out. This plan should be mutually agreed upon. If Jack continues his behavior, then say, "Go sit over there." Try not to say anything else. Be firm and quick and send him without discussion. Don't be upset if he spends hours or most of the day there. Isolation has a way of making the everyday class routines look more attractive. It is important that the child learn that rules cannot be broken, and the best way to learn this is through experience. You might, when you think Jack has had enough, ask him if he is ready to return to his seat and participate. If the answer is yes, at your next break, go over the rules and ask him if he has a plan to follow. Remember you are trying to teach him something in a few months that he has not learned over a period of many years. If the child continues the behavior in isolation, the child's only alternative is to be excluded, and yours is to move to Step 8.

Step 8. Somplace farther. In-school suspension is involved in this step. You have tried, you have been patient, but now you have had enough. At this step, there are no questions to be asked. You can make this statement, "Jack, things did not work out for you here. We have both tried hard to work out the problems but now it is time for you to spend time outside the class and maybe talk with some other people. Please report to the Counselor's office [or the Principal's office, or the in-school suspension room]." The room or place should be staffed by a person who can get the idea across to the child that, "We want you in school and class but we expect you to follow the rules. When you have a plan as to how you can return to class and follow the rules, let me know. If you need help carrying out the plan, let me know and I will help you." What you want to get across to the child is that the plan will be different and better than what was used in the past. To get Jack to change his behavior is the task for which a new environment as well as new approaches are necessary. Don't be concerned if he sits there for a time. The whole idea is used to reduce the alternatives to two choices: to be in class and behave, or to be out of class and sit. It is hoped that the class will begin to look better. The point that needs to be communicated to the child is, "Follow reasonable rules, or you are out." However, while he is out, you are not going to hurt or reject the child, which would let the child rationalize his behavior on the basis of his dislike for you. This kind of nonpunitive place may be hard for the school and you, the teacher, to accept, but review Step 1 again—you can see the child has been in the "old" place a long time with no results. Be ready for a lot of excuses from the child; follow them up with, "But you cannot go back to class until you have a plan." When more than one day is required, you should notify Jack's parents that their child is not in class. It may well be that 3 days to a week or more will be required. Perhaps the child's schoolwork will suffer (although he could do schoolwork while in in-school suspension). It is hoped that the child will learn one of the most important things that can be learned: One must be responsible for one's own behavior and one does have the choice to behave in a way helpful to oneself and others.

Step 9. A day off. If Jack cannot be handled in an in-school suspension, the parents should be notified and asked to take the child home. The child will now be put on "a day off" with the idea that he can return the following day. One could say, "We would like your child to return, but he must maintain reasonable behavior. If his behavior goes beyond the rules, he will have to go home again." This means that the child starts again at Step 8, or at in-school suspension, and can stay until his behavior changes for the better or until he reaches Step 9 again. If the child cannot be helped in school at all, then he will have to stay home, which means either his having a tutor at home or the school's proceeding to Step 10.

Step 10. Someplace else. If the child is continually unsuccessful in Step 9, he should stay home and be referred to some other community agency. This may sound tough, but it may take something like this to jolt the child into taking some responsibility for his behavior. If the child is in jail or juvenile detention, perhaps he could return to school for a day to see if he can make it, but not unless a specific plan and commitment have been made to follow the rules.

PARENTING SKILLS

A Parent Involvement Program (PIP) has been designed to help parents gain the necessary reality therapy skills (McGuiness, 1977). Many of the activities demonstrate ways to facilitate increased involvement with one's children. Other aspects of the program attempt to teach parents better listening skills and to reflect to their children the good they see in them.

The program is accomplished in six 3-hour sessions, which can be conducted on weekends or evenings during the week. Each of the sessions has a definite content to provide parents with knowledge about a skill to be used in dealing with their children. The sessions are based on practice after they receive the theory. The sessions are structured to allow the parents to personalize the ideas, share their concerns, and develop a plan to improve things at home.

The objectives of the program for each session contained in the *Idea Book for the Parent Involvement Program* (McGuiness, 1977) are outlined below.

CONTENT OF PARENT INVOLVEMENT PROGRAM

Lesson Objectives	Topics Covered
1. To build trust and support among group members To help parents understand the cultural shift that has occurred since World War II To help parents understand how these cultural changes are affecting their relationship with their children	Group involvement The Identity Society Role vs. goal-activities
2. To help parents realize the importance of building warm, personal, friendly relationships with their children To help parents understand a problem-solving approach (reality therapy) to helping children become responsible	Importance of involvement Successful vs. failing identities Principles of reality therapy
3. To give parents insights that will help them reflect to their children the goodness and beauty which they see in them To share with parents ideas that enhance total family involvement and help create a success-filled atmosphere for the home To develop with the parents a personal plan which incorporates the concepts basic to reality therapy	Practice in using steps of reality therapy Total family involvement How to increase involvement at home
4. To share successes and concerns based on the activities which developed from each parent's personal plan	Successful experiences Communication Components of good listening
5. To help parents improve their communication skills To clarify any misconceptions concerning the understanding and use of the basic steps of reality therapy To expose parents to current authors who have written significant articles in the area of parent/child relationships	Nonverbal communication One-way vs. two-way communication Discipline techniques
6. To help parents gain insights in working with their children, based on articles read and shared with each other To help parents clarify for themselves the basic concepts introduced and to share with their families the spirit of the workshop To receive participant feedback concerning the workshop	Review and feedback

The parents are involved in a number of activities including some of the following:

1. Viewing films and listening to tapes which include:
   a. Identity Society
   b. Reality of Success
2. Using worksheets which include:
   a. Reality therapy planning form
   b. Questions to accompany "Success-Oriented Home Exercises"
3. Reading articles such as:
   a. "Basic Principles in Dealing with Children"
   b. "How to Drive Your Child Sane"
   c. "Rules, Goals, and Failure"
   d. "Your Child and Discipline"
4. Discussing ideas in small and large groups.
5. Making personal plans to meet the needs of the family.
6. Participating in role playing to allow for practice of what is being presented.

FAMILY INTERVENTIONS

Reality therapy does not at present offer a framework for family therapy in the traditional sense. Family therapies usually identify the family as the client and do not focus on an individual, identified client. In family therapies, the focus is on systems, relationships, structures, and interdependencies. Reality therapy emphasizes developing the individual's successful identity and encouraging personal responsibility.

The family therapy focus on environmental influences on behavior is somewhat at odds with reality therapy. Family therapy views individual problems as stemming from a dysfunctional family system or structure, whereas reality therapy views individual problems as resulting more from individual identity and choices. Thus, the two approaches are not entirely compatible.

The reality therapist, however, does have some tools to use with problems that have family components. The first is the Parent Involvement Program, described above. This allows work with families where problems seem centered around a need for more parental involvement with children and a need for the parents to provide more positive feedback to their children. The second tool is marital therapy or conjoint marital counseling (Glasser & Zunin, 1979), to be used when the family problems seem to be a result of marital discord. This type of therapy is often time limited, usually five to fifteen sessions. Reality therapy-based marriage counseling begins by clarifying the couple's goals in seeking counseling. Questions would be directed at determining if the goal of counseling is, on the one hand, to continue in the marriage or, on the other hand, to attempt a last-ditch effort to save the marriage even though a decision to end the marriage has already been made. Attention would also be focused on defining the couple's similarities and differences in opinion and interests, on how the couple seeks friends and other activities, and how much the couple actually knows, as opposed to assumes, about each other. The overall goal is intimacy, not simply familiarity.

EFFICACY

There are numerous favorable case reports in Glasser's writings, a published casebook (N. Glasser, 1980), and a survey of Glasser's work (Bassin, Bratter, & Rachin, 1976). In addition, five books have been written by Ford and others (Ford, 1974, 1987; Ford & Englund, 1977, 1979; Ford & Zorn, 1975) that discuss the techniques and principles of reality therapy as applied to marriage, raising children, and loneliness. A book by Robert (1973) discusses the use of reality therapy in the school situation to deal with loneliness. Two recent books, one on happiness written by Good (1987), focus on knowing what you want and getting what you need, using practical reality therapy techniques in a counseling situation. The methods and techniques and their justification appear reasonable and have been accepted by many professionals in the field. There certainly is no lack of testimony concerning the efficacy of reality therapy. However, in these books there is no adequate statistical evidence or support for reliability and validity. Glasser and Zunin (1973) reported there had been no long-term research on the effectiveness of reality therapy with outpatients. Follow-up work at the Ventura School for Girls, however, indicated that the use of reality therapy in the treatment program had reduced the recidivism rate for that environment (Glasser & Zunin, 1973).

Some studies have focused on classroom meetings and their effect on self-concept, social adjustment, locus of control, and achievement. Matthews (1972) studied the effect of class meetings on the discipline, self-concept, social adjustment, and reading achievement of 221 fourth and fifth graders. Treatment consisted of 16 weeks of a language arts program in the control group and reality therapy in the experimental group. Pretreatment and posttreatment data were collected on three tests. His findings indicated that both treatments increased self-concept scores but neither change was significant. It was also found that neither treatment was significantly better in improving social adjustment. However, reality therapy was found to be significantly more effective in lowering the incidence of discipline problems in the experimental group compared to the control group.

Hunter (1973) reported nonsignificant findings when studying the effects of reality therapy and Rogerian group sessions on math achievement, self-concept, and behavior of 40 fifth grade students. The students were matched on sex and randomly assigned to a Math Remediation, a Rogerian Discussion, a Reality Therapy, or a Control group. Six weeks of treatment (twelve 40-minute sessions per group) resulted in no significant change in math achievement, self-esteem, or behavior in any of the groups.

Tangeman (1973) investigated the effects of a reality therapy program on the achievement and self-esteem of 93 third graders. Four classrooms were randomly assigned to two treatment approaches—reality therapy class meetings and Developing Understanding of Self and Others (DUSO)—and two control groups. Twenty 30-minute meetings were held for each group over a 10-week period. Pretest and posttest data from two tests were analyzed. The results indicated no significant changes for any of the groups on self-concept or achievement.

Hawes (1971) evaluated the use of reality therapy on the locus of control, self-concept, and classroom behavior of 340 third and sixth grade black students. Three tests were administered for pretest and posttest evaluation. Reality Therapy class meetings were employed for a 16-week period, with a control group receiving no treatment. The results showed that the reality therapy program did significantly shift the children's belief system toward an internal orientation. A significant change in behavior was also found, as the reality therapy group demonstrated more appropriate changes on the self-concept measure.

Shearn and Randolph (1978) evaluated the effect of reality therapy class meetings on self-concept and on-task behavior for fourth grade children. In an attempt to construct a "true placebo control" design, the authors randomly assigned four intact classes (27 students in each) into four treatment conditions: pretested reality therapy, unpretested reality therapy, pretested placebo (career education activities), and unpretested placebo (career education). Several tests were administered to all the groups. Pretest and posttest scores were collected for one experimental and one placebo group, while only posttest scores were collected for the other experimental and control groups. The results indicated that neither treatment, pretesting, nor the interaction of treatment and pretesting for posttest scores had any significant effect on self-concept or on-task behavior. The authors concluded that their findings do not support using reality therapy in the classroom. They did caution that the inability to measure the effects of reality therapy empirically in the classroom is a factor which confounds interpretation of research in this area.

Quinn (1979) used seventh and eighth grade children to investigate the effects of class meetings on self-concept and attitude toward school. Three seventh and eighth grade classes were randomly assigned, each to one of the following groups: class meetings, a quasi-experimental group (performing plays), or a control group (no treatment). Pretest and posttest scores were collected on self-concept and school attitudinal scales. The results failed to demonstrate any significant changes in self-concept or improved attitude toward school. Here nonsignificant results may have been a function of insufficient time for behavioral changes to occur.

A study by Grant (1972) used open-ended class meetings to investigate possible changes in self-concept and locus of control of 163 fourth grade pupils. Classrooms were randomly assigned as open-ended classroom meetings. Each treatment group met in twenty-nine 30-minute meetings over a 6-week period. All children were rated by their teachers prior to the treatment on a rating scale as either Normal (N = 78) or Deviant (N = 85). Results of the study demonstrated that the class meetings did influence self-concept somewhat, but had little influence on locus of control. The only significant changes in locus of control occurred in experimental students who had been rated as "deviants" by their teachers. The normal group students accepted responsibility for failure much more than did the "deviant" rated control students. The author concluded that, in general, the open-ended class meetings were of little value in effecting change in self-concept or locus of control.

Rosario (1973) measured the effects of reality therapy group counseling on college students by means of the Nowicki-Strickland Internal-External Scale. The author predicted that extremely external students would show very little change of control orientation, extremely internal students would become slightly less internal, and moderately internal-external students would benefit most from class meetings. A pretest and posttest model, with a follow-up testing 5 months after completion of treatment, was used. Results of the analysis of data for the initial posttest indicated that no significant shift was found for high internals, high externals, or those rated moderately internal-external. After the 5-month follow-up, results indicated that extremely external students did shift toward a more internal stance. The author thought that the change in locus of control for the external males may have been the result of attitude change based on the practice of new behaviors. The study had a number of shortcomings, including the absence of quasi-experimental and control groups. In addition, the use of ten therapists allowed for uncontrolled variability in application of reality therapy techniques.

English (1970) also focused on the use of reality therapy (counseling) in various school environments. He demonstrated that reality therapy was an effective method for reducing disciplinary problems, increasing school achievement, and improving teacher-teacher and teacher-student interactions.

Marandola and Imber (1979) evaluated the effects of classroom meetings on the argumentative behavior (verbal and physical) of ten preadolescent, inner-city, learning-disabled children. Both open-ended and problem-solving classroom meetings were used. During the intervention period, classroom meetings were used daily for 8 days with the focus always related to argumentative behavior in the classroom. Three types of behavior were used for analysis: verbal argument between two classmates, verbal argument involving two or more classmates, and physical confrontation between two classmates. The results of the study provided strong support for the classroom meeting and its role in behavior change. Appropriate behaviors regarding positive interactions were maintained, and inappropriate argumentative behaviors were sharply decreased as a result of the class meetings. The study had some limitations: Nine of the ten children had been with the teacher for 2 years, and strong rapport had been established between teacher and students. The children were also accustomed to having discussions, although they were not the same as Glasser's class meetings.

Poppen and Welch (1976) utilized reality therapy with 16 overweight adolescent girls who volunteered to participate in a weight-loss program. The subjects were evaluated by pretesting and posttesting with a self-concept scale. The treatment program lasted for 6 weeks. The results of the study indicated that reality therapy was effective in producing a significant weight loss; however, no significant changes in self-concept were detected.

Hough-Waite (1980) compared the effectiveness of the Parent Involvement Program with a behavioral program entitled the "Art of Parenting." A group of untreated controls was also included. Participants in treatment groups were 19 randomly assigned parents who volunteered to participate in a parent education group. Eight were assigned to the Art of Parenting Program, and 11 to the Parent Involvement Program. The control group consisted of 14 parents randomly selected from a large population. A Child-Rearing Practices Questionnaire was administered before and after training, which lasted 6 weeks. The results indicated that neither treatment group differed significantly from the controls or from each other. Some factors could have confounded the results, including small sample size, lack of a sensitive outcome measure, and the use of volunteers as subjects.

Bigelow and Thorne (1979) compared client-centered and reality therapy techniques in group counseling at the elementary school level. One group contained six children and the other eight. All children were volunteers for a summer remedial reading program. Six group counseling sessions were conducted with both groups. The Hill Interaction Matrix was administered before and after the six sessions. The results indicated that the reality therapy group performed more efficiently than did the client-centered group in that significantly more therapeutic group member interactions were elicited by reality therapy techniques. It was also concluded that a counselor can direct an elementary age group into defined work areas and maintain it there more rapidly using a reality-oriented counseling approach.

Baskin and Hess (1980) conducted a review of seven affective education programs, one of which was Schools Without Failure. In the area of self-esteem, the authors cited a 2-year evaluation of Schools Without Failure in grades one through six which found no significant impact on self-esteem but did find that the frequency of discipline referrals to the principal decreased with the implementation of the Schools Without Failure program. It was also reported that no differences were found between treatment and control group achievement levels. The authors also discussed the methodological difficulties inherent in evaluating a program such as Schools Without Failure and reality therapy.

Omizo and Cubberly (1983) studied 60 learning-disabled students, aged 12 to 24, who were assigned to experimental and control conditions. The students in the experimental group were exposed to discussions (e.g., obstacles to academic success) by teachers trained in reality therapy. Multivariate analysis revealed that the students in the experimental group attained higher academic aspirations and lower anxiety levels than those in the control group.

Yarish (1986) studied 45 male juvenile offenders (aged 12 to 16 years) to determine whether positive perceptual changes could be brought about by the application of reality therapy. The Nowicki-Strickland Locus of Control Scale for Children was administered to subjects during their first and last week in a treatment facility. A significant difference was found between the treatment and control groups. The subjects who received reality therapy moved in an internal direction and chose to behave better with control of their fate in their own hands. Subjects were treated for an average of 4 months.

Hart-Hester (1986) studied 5 fourth grade students who exhibited behavioral problems such as noncompliance, aggressiveness, off-task behavior, and absenteeism. She tried to improve several targeted behaviors (i.e., on-task behavior, peer interactions, and student-teacher interactions) through the use of reality therapy. Using anecdotal reports from the school principal, classroom teacher, and independent observation by investigation, the data indicated that reality therapy increased on-task behavior but not peer interactions or student-teacher interaction.

Tamborella (1987) investigated how "troubled" adolescents responded to the use of reality therapy procedures in a structured alternative school environment. Twenty students and six staff members were involved in the study. Evaluation was accomplished by using in-depth interview schedules, student permanent records, student attendance reports, student suspension reports, and the Statements About Schools Inventory. The results indicated that the use of reality therapy techniques which govern the types of student-teacher interactions in the alternative school program is effective in producing increased attendance and decreased rates of suspension. Students and staff experienced positive changes in self-perception, and students had positive perceptions regarding personal and academic needs satisfaction. It was demonstrated that significant and positive change in students and staff can be brought about through the impact of reality therapy.

The results discussed in this section that dealt with actual research studies included 19 articles or theses. In fact, the majority were doctoral dissertations. Most of this research has been done with class meetings. The findings with class meetings indicate little effect on self-concept and achievement and mixed results on locus of control. However, most of the studies showed significant decreases in discipline problems.

There were nine studies that used reality therapy in a counseling situation rather than as part of a class meeting. These studies demonstrated that the therapy process significantly decreased discipline problems, aided weight loss, increased attendance, decreased rates of suspension, and increased interaction and involvement. The findings were contradictory for achievement and locus of control, with self-concept showing no improvement.

The above studies share the usual methodological problems encountered when the effectiveness of therapeutic approaches is evaluated. It is very difficult to measure items such as involvement, happiness, fulfillment, and successful identity.

The greatest problems in evaluating reality therapy, class meetings, and other therapies include the following, as discussed by Baskin and Hess (1980):

1. The use of more than one teacher or therapist in either the program or control groups.
2. Assessment of goals is hampered by the complexity of the behaviors to be evaluated. The measures used to evaluate outcomes are not sensitive enough to detect changes that occur as a result of treatment. Bernal and North (1978) suggest that multiple outcome measures, including objective measure of changes, should be used. In addition, the construct validity of self-concept and that of locus of control have not been established.
3. The use of testers who do not know the purpose of the evaluation and identity of treatment and control groups.
4. The usual problems of self-evaluation research, including both the tendency of some subjects to answer questions in a socially desirable manner and the amount of self-disclosure a subject is willing to give to a self-report inventory.

In addition, most of the studies reviewed here utilized small sample size and relatively brief training periods. Also, the amount of time available for actual behavior change to take place is a limitation, because usually several weeks or more need to be spent developing student-teacher or therapist involvement and group cohesiveness. How much experience one has had in the therapeutic technique used is also a variable.

Informal reports and surveys have been made by the Educator Training Center; accounts of them are available in a pamphlet entitled *Glasser's Approach to Discipline.* The pamphlet is full of testimonies from school districts such as: "Discipline referrals dropped by 14% and suspension by 41% in one year." The ETC sent an eleven-question survey to 24 schools that were using reality therapy to handle discipline problems. Of this student population, 6,286 were elementary students, 3,559 were junior high school students, and 4,916 were senior high school students. As reported in the pamphlet, most of the schools report large gains in decreasing fighting, suspension, and vandalism and in increasing attendance.

There is little question that reality therapy has directly or indirectly inspired many individuals and schools. Unfortunately, most applications of the therapy have not been subjected to any kind of formal research program.

The limited research with class meetings and reality therapy counseling does lend some support to its effectiveness in areas such as discipline and lends little support in other areas such as self-concept. Clearly, additional research is needed which will deal with some of the evaluation problems raised in the discussion above to substantitate the validity and usefulness of the reality therapy concepts and principles.

CONCLUSIONS

Reality therapy is based on a commonsense philosophy that can be used by trained persons in a variety of situations. These persons include the teacher in the average classroom, those involved in corrections and mental institutions, clinicians, and parents.

Responsibility is a basic tenet of reality therapy. It is thought that an assuming of responsibility will lead to a heightened sense of self-worth or self-respect and a greater sense of freedom, both of which may, at the same time, help the person experience more fun in life.

Reality therapy emphasizes the rational and the cognitive. A client is asked to describe his or her behavior specifically and to make a value judgment concerning its effectiveness. A specific plan to alter a concrete behavior is then drawn up, and a commitment to follow that plan is elicited from the client. Praise is given for success; no excuses are accepted nor is punishment given for failure. Although the above appears almost simplistic, its success is dependent on an honest and thorough commitment on the part of the therapist to maintain concern and effort in the face of continued failure. As Glasser (1965) wrote: "[the] practice [of] reality therapy takes strength; not only the strength of the therapist to lead a responsible life himself, but also the added strength both to stand up steadily to patients who wish him to accede to their irresponsibility, and to continue to point out reality to them no matter how hard they struggle against it" (p. 23).

Reality therapy follows certain tenets in attaining involvement and influencing responsible, realistic behavior. These tenets include:

1. Personalization–becoming involved.
2. Concentrating on the here and now.
3. Emphasizing behavior.
4. Refraining from asking why.
5. Helping the client evaluate behavior.
6. Developing a different or better plan of behavior.
7. Refusing to accept excuses.
8. Never punishing–only disciplining.
9. Offering little sympathy.
10. Approving and praising responsible behavior.
11. Never giving up.

Testimonials and informal surveys clearly indicate that reality therapy has a positive effect on clients and situations, but new and better approaches to definitive research must be sought. Future research designs must include explicitly defined control and experimental groups and the use of reliable and valid criterion measures.

Reality therapy requires time to be effective. Future research should be oriented toward longitudinal studies of a year or more, and the shorter term studies must include more sessions and subjects if one hopes to measure impact. Use of a formal behavior rating scale, test, or coding instrument to measure the actual behavior change of the client from pretreatment to posttreatment is recommended. It may also prove fruitful to develop an empirical observation system which could help validate the degree to which reality therapy techniques are actually being implemented in the classroom.

Reality therapy focuses on freedom, not license. With loving firmness and respect the child is led away from irresponsibility toward the responsibility and concomitant self-respect that come with true freedom and a successful identity.

CASE STUDY

John, age 10, was referred by his parents at the request of the public school system because of his continued refusal to talk. The difficulty manifested itself in kindergarten, and by the end of third grade he had become a legend in the school system with a multitude of school personnel eager to take on the challenge of making him talk. The previous year he had been diagnosed as having elective mutism and as manifesting anxiety, social withdrawal, and depression both at school and at home. He was passive and withdrawn when confronted with the usual sibling onslaughts from his two brothers and two sisters, and he did not play with the neighbor children. At age 10, he was still an occasional bed-wetter. His mother characterized him as a good boy who was quiet and reserved, who entertained himself well, and who enjoyed playing alone.

Initially, John appeared tense, stiff, immature, and sensitive. He lowered his head to avoid eye contact, and if the situation became too stressful for him, he began scratching his arm and cheek. He was fearfully shy and refused to speak. A beginning relationship was formed with him through playing games, going for walks, or getting some candy at a nearby store. As he gradually relaxed, he began to smile and laugh a bit during the sessions, but when asked a question, he would only shake his head or occasionally write his answer on a piece of paper.

As the relationship became stronger, he was told that he and the therapist would no longer play for the entire hour. Instead, he was told they would talk or sit together for the first 15 minutes. When he came for the next session, this plan was initiated. He was questioned about his happiness and unhappiness and about events at home and at school. Although he didn't speak, he nodded yes that he was unhappy. The problem behaviors that his parents and the school said he was engaging in were stated, and he was asked for his opinion. These behaviors included not talking in school, having no friends, crying a lot, and receiving poor grades. These were written on a piece of paper, and he was asked to check the ones that he agreed with. He checked not talking in school and having no friends. With several of his problem behaviors out in the open, he was asked if they were making him unhappy and if he wanted to do something about them. He nodded. Although some behaviors were identified and a value judgment made by John, he was not yet ready to do something about them. Attempts to elicit a plan from him resulted only in a lowered head and a shrug of his shoulders. At this point, more strengthening of the relationship was needed, and the sessions continued with the initial 15 minutes reserved for conversation. Initially, the therapist talked and John nodded when possible or else they sat in silence. On occasion, the therapist would ask a question and then answer it for him in a manner he wouldn't like. This action made John uncomfortable but did not elicit any speech. The sessions began focusing on his refusal to speak at school. He indicated that he wanted to talk, that he understood that it was important to do so, that he realized his not talking might result in his failing for the year, and yet he refused to speak.

As the relationship grew stronger, it became more threatening to John. He had begun to initiate some silent mouthing that indicated at least some desire to talk. He was now faced with giving up his symptoms. An occasion when the therapist called John's home added to this pressure. Expecting the mother to answer, the therapist was surprised to be greeted by a loud male child's voice. It was John's. At the next session John was confronted with the phone call. John smiled but did not respond. At this point, the therapist tested the relationship by pointing out that John had been coming for 2 months, but that he was contributing very little, and perhaps they should consider termination. He was told to think about these things and that they would pursue the subject at his next session. He agreed to this with a nod of his head.

On his next visit John appeared more uneasy than usual. He started the session by indicating that he wanted to play. This proposal was countered by the therapist's saying that last week's problem had to be discussed. After a brief review of the problem and reconfirmation of John's value judgment, he was asked to talk. Again he refused. In an attempt to force the issue, the therapist suggested that John's mother be called and told that they were terminating. John sat still for several minutes before nodding his head in consent. The therapist immediately said he decided against it, changed the subject, and took John to play. The rationale behind taking such a chance was the risk that the involvement was great enough to keep John from terminating. Strong as it was, however, the involvement was not yet sufficient to help John replace his problem behavior. So with this in mind, the therapist backed off and continued to be friendly and interested in John. Therapy is based on a relationship, and there are times in every relationship when one loses face or gives ground. Frightening as it might have been for the therapist, his move demonstrated to John the important lesson that one can be strong without always being in control.

For the next month, John's presenting problem was avoided and the involvement was focused on. His nonverbal interaction increased and he was more relaxed, laughing and appearing content. At the end of this month he was once again asked what he was doing and whether it was doing him any good. He seemed quicker to agree to his symptoms and to indicate that he was not pleased with them. While joking with him about hearing his voice on the phone, the therapist had the thought that John might talk into a tape recorder. John indicated he would not. He was asked if he would take the recorder home, talk into it there, and then bring it back the next time. He agreed to this, and they shook hands on the plan. He did not, however, follow through. Rather than preaching, the therapist indicated to John that he hadn't carried out the plan as agreed, and John was asked if he wanted to try again. He indicated that he did, and the following week, he arrived with the tape, gesturing to have it put on the recorder which the therapist did. In a whispered tone came the word "Hello." John was praised a great deal for this feat. Over the next several sessions, John continued to make tapes at home and bring them to each following session. John's responses on tape were eventually enlarged into whispered sentences. Each of John's efforts was reinforced, and the therapist often asked him if it felt good to have accomplished this. Always John would smile and nod yes.

But it was time now to move on, and during the next session, it was again indicated to John that he would have to start talking aloud, that using the tapes was a good start and an indication that it wasn't so bad to talk. It was emphasized that it was time for John to demonstrate his contribution to the relationship and to talk because the therapist had been doing most of the work. "Please say 'Hi,'" the therapist said. There were several minutes of silence and finally, with great effort and initial mouthing behavior, John said "Hi" in an audible whisper. This was a special moment for both of them, and it was followed by much praise. On leaving, John whispered, "Good-bye." This incident impressed again how necessary a strong involvement is in therapy and how critical it is in effecting change. How much it must have taken John to say those words!

Expectations for the next session were quickly lowered when John sat and said nothing during the beginning of the hour. Asked if he would talk out loud, he shook his head no. Reminding him of the progress from the last session and the triumph of his success, the therapist asked John whether he would talk if the therapist turned his back to him. He nodded yes and they shook on it. The therapist turned his back and looked out the window. About 5 minutes passed before John spoke loudly enough to be heard. The therapist, continuing to sit with his back to John, then asked him several simple questions and received the answers. Then they talked about John's success during this session, with a lot of praise being given. A plan was made to continue this approach for the next couple of sessions. A written commitment was made. The plan was carried out, with John talking to the therapist in a whisper while the therapist sat with his back to John.

After two sessions, a plan was made that they would talk face to face. When John arrived for the next session, he was more uneasy than usual. He sat down and the therapist said hello. About two minutes of silence followed before John whispered "Hi." They talked about what he had watched on television and what he had done on the weekend and in school, with John responding in whispers. This continued for several sessions, and the therapist then asked him what could be done to help him talk in his normal voice. At first John shrugged his shoulders, but then he said, "Talk louder." This became his responsibility for the next session. At the next meeting, John fulfilled his commitment; he and the therapist talked for approximately 30 minutes.

After this meeting, each session lasted for about 45 minutes, and they were able to talk for the entire time. Up until this point, John's not talking in school had not been discussed. It was important for him to get used to talking in his "loud" (normal) voice over a period of time in order to break his old habit of getting by without speaking. At a certain point, however, it was hoped that John might be able to generalize his success. Consequently, John was asked if the therapist could call his teacher to check on his school progress. John agreed. The therapist learned that John was not talking in the classroom.

At the next session the therapist asked John if this was true and John said it was. When the subject was pursued, John said he did not want to continue not talking in school. He was asked what his plan would be and he said he would talk to his teacher. The therapist indicated that the plan wasn't quite clear in terms of *how, when,* and *where.* After some discussion, it was decided that he would talk to the teacher on Tuesday and Friday mornings. When asked what he would say, he indicated that he would say hello and ask to go to the bathroom instead of just raising his hand. The plan was written up and signed, with each of them receiving a copy.

When John came back the following week, he indicated that he had carried out the plan. Over the next several sessions they worked on increasing the number of days and the things he would say. Indeed, everything seemed to be progressing even better than expected. Each time a plan was formulated, a commitment was made and executed. A phone call from John's mother, however, changed all that.

John's mother called, saying that she had just returned from a parent-teacher conference and was told that John was not talking at school. This news was an eye-opener because previous contacts with her had been encouraging; she had indicated earlier that John was talking more in the neighborhood and in the local stores. John, it turned out, had been telling both his mother and the therapist that he was talking in school when, in fact, he was not. The therapist had taken John's word which on the surface seemed to be the thing to do because a good relationship existed. But John had learned to keep the therapist off his back by quickly setting up a plan and then indicating that he had carried it out.

The next time John came to therapy and indicated that he had executed his plan, he was asked if he had any objections to the therapist's calling his teacher to ask how he was doing. He said yes. When the therapist asked what the objection was, John replied that it wasn't necessary to call the teacher, that he was reporting everything that was happening. The therapist expressed doubt and told John about his mother's phone call. John admitted to not having talked in school and started to make excuses for his lack of success. He was immediately interrupted and asked if he wanted to talk in school; he said he did. Plans similar to the ones used before were then formulated, with the further stipulation that the therapist would call the teacher each week to check on how John's plan was working. The therapist told John he was very much interested in John's talking progress in school and also in knowing how the teacher perceived the progress and whether or not this progress was the same as he, the therapist, thought it was. John agreed to this additional plan.

In an attempt to coordinate their efforts, the therapist saw the teacher before the next session. She was cooperative and interested in helping in any way possible. She was informed of John's progress to date and of some of the techniques that were being used with him. She agreed to read some literature on reality therapy and to carry out some suggestions. The need to praise John's talking and the consequences to be used if the rules were not followed were particularly emphasized.

John was told what took place at this meeting between the teacher and the therapist and what could be expected. It became evident that John was much more likely to talk if he went up to the teacher's desk and whispered than if he attempted to speak from his desk. They started with this approach, and soon he was doing this at least once a day. John would walk to the teacher's desk when he had a question, and, later, the teacher would also ask him questions. Eventually, plans were also made and carried out whereby John talked to his gym and music teachers. Again, he was able to communicate with them in a whisper.

During this period, John was strongly rewarded for his successes, and his feelings of self-worth appeared to increase. He would now admit that school was a better place than before and that he did enjoy it more. John and his therapist discussed John's talking louder and also talking from his desk, but he was still not willing to make a commitment to either of these actions. At this point the school year ended, and because of a number of scheduling problems and summer programs, it was decided that there would be no therapy sessions during the summer. It was agreed that John's mother would contact the therapist in the fall if things were not going well for him.

In the beginning of October, John's mother called and indicated that John had regressed in school and that he wanted to come for therapy. The mother attributed this regression in part to his new teacher, who was older and more authoritarian than the previous one. She reported that he had had a good summer, that he talked to others outside the home, and that he was less shy and more outgoing.

The therapist and John were able to pick up and begin pretty much where they ended in the spring. John was still talking in a loud voice to the therapist and, in no time at all, in a whisper, once again, to the teachers. In a short time the therapist was able to elicit a value judgment and a commitment from John that he wanted to talk out loud in school. It was agreed that John would speak with the teacher alone at her desk. It was also established that if the plan was not carried out, John would have to miss recess. Because he understood and agreed to the outcome before he engaged in the activity, missing recess was seen as a logical consequence of his behavior, not as punishment. When he did not talk out loud to his teacher at her desk the first time, he missed recess. At the same time, it was stipulated that he would have to come up with a plan so that not talking aloud and missing recess would not happen again. His plan was to try it once more with a specific sentence to say, which turned out to be, "Can I have my math assignment?" This time it worked for him. At this point, he and his teacher agreed to his doing this at least three times a week with the days being his choice. The plan was accomplished, and within a short time John was saying something out loud at least once a day. Because the teacher was working so well with him, John and the therapist agreed to meet only twice a month.

There were ups and downs during the school year, but overall John continued to improve. Toward the end of school, John was beginning to talk out loud from his desk, but this activity was still somewhat troublesome for him. The therapist agreed to continue to see him during the summer once a month to help him prepare for a new teacher and grade. In the last several sessions he talked "a blue streak." He was spontaneous, showing no shyness, and was much more confident of his own ability to perform. They went to a store to buy candy and there he asked the clerk several questions and responded to a question asked of him. John and the therapist also talked about alternative strategies and choices—he agreed to talk out loud from his desk when school began in the fall, and he appeared confident about doing so.

During the course of therapy the therapist repeatedly emphasized that he was interested in John's dealing with the present, particularly in John's attempts to succeed and to deal with his problems in an effective and responsible manner. With John it was necessary that he be assured that the therapist would stick with him until his problem was resolved. To this extent the relationship played a major role. When John resorted to "I can't," in discussing certain situations, the therapist converted "I can't," to "You don't want to or you mean you won't—let's explore the choices you have." Until the two were involved and until John realized that he was responsible for his own behavior and that something could be done about his problem, little progress occurred. Through the involvement, he finally did realize that he was responsible for his talking. In this way, he was helped to understand his capacity for more worthwhile behavior in his immediate environment. His decisions to become involved, to change his behavior, and to continue talking were the essence of therapy.

ANNOTATED BIBLIOGRAPHY

Bassin, A., Bratter, T., & Rachin, R. (Eds.). (1976). *The reality therapy reader: A survey of the work of William Glasser.* New York: Harper & Row.

Here the authors present articles on all aspects of reality therapy. The book is divided into various sections, including theory, practice, education, corrections, and role playing. The articles were gathered from books, popular magazines, journals, and original material. Practical tools are provided for all who work professionally with other people.

Ford, E., & Englund, S. (1977). *For the love of children: A realistic approach to raising your child.* Garden City, NY: Anchor Press.

This book provides a new understanding of the basic principles, the "building blocks," essential to raising children. It applies the practical, proven ideas and techniques of reality therapy to raising children, from infancy through adolescence. The authors stress love, responsibility, discipline, work, play, and faith that form the values and the strength of young people. A number of concrete ways are presented for forming a better parent-child relationship.

Glasser, N. (Ed.). (1980). *What are you doing? How people are helped through reality therapy.* New York: Harper & Row.

In this book 25 case histories by therapists who have received certification from the Institute of Reality Therapy are presented. The cases were selected to show as many different kinds of problems as possible. The cases are so varied that anyone using the steps of reality therapy should be helped toward a better understanding of how the steps work in practice. Eight of the cases deal with children and adolescents.

Glasser, W. (1969). *Schools without failure.* New York: Harper & Row.

In this book the concepts of reality therapy as applied to the schools are presented. Many school practices are described that promote a sense of failure in the student, and material is given as to how these practices may be corrected. The three types of class meetings are presented with numerous topics that could be used for each one.

Glasser, W. (1981). *Stations of the mind.* New York: Harper & Row.
This book is an expansion of Glasser's basic reality therapy ideas. The book explains how the brain functions in living—specifically what we do, think, and feel. The main thesis is based on the Control System Psychology of William Powers that indicates that all living creatures are internally motivated. People are driven by internal forces that push them not only to survive but also toward belonging, worthwhileness, fun, and freedom. Glasser points out that what happens outside the person in the real world is of little or no significance unless it relates to what is already inside the person's personal world.

Glasser, W. (1986). *Control theory in the classroom.* New York: Harper & Row.
This book provides a useful analysis of what is wrong with traditional schooling and what needs to be done. The book translates control theory into a classroom model of team learning in the schools. Numerous ideas are given that will contribute to the success of classroom teachers. The book discusses discipline problems and learning team models.

Wubbolding, R. (1988). *Using reality therapy.* New York: Harper & Row.
This book demonstrates the practical uses of reality therapy and the principles of control theory. It contains case studies and exercises for the reader that allow him or her to apply specific reality therapy principles to his or her own behaviors. In addition, the book covers marriage and family counseling, the use of paradoxical techniques, supervision, and self-help.

REFERENCES

Baskin, E., & Hess, R. (1980). Does affective education work?: A review of seven programs. *Journal of School Psychology, 18,* 40-50.

Bassin, A., Bratter, T., & Rachin, R. (Eds.). (1976). *The reality therapy reader: A survey of the work of William Glasser.* New York: Harper & Row.

Bernal, M., & North, J. (1978). A survey of parent training materials. *Journal of Applied Behavior Analysis, 11,* 533-544.

Bigelow, G., & Thorne, J. (1979). Reality versus client-centered models in group counseling. *The Group Counselor,* 191-194.

Dreikurs, R., Grunwald, B., & Pepper, R. (1971). *Maintaining sanity in the classroom.* New York: Harper & Row.

English, J. (March, 1970). *The effects of reality therapy on elementary age children.* Paper presented at the meeting of the California Association of School Psychologists and Psychometrists, Los Angeles, CA.

Ford, E. (1974). *Why marriage?* Niles, IL: Argus.

Ford, E. (1987). *Love guaranteed: A better marriage in 8 weeks.* New York: Harper & Row.

Ford, E., & Englund, S. (1977). *For the love of children: A realistic approach to raising your child.* Garden City, NY: Anchor Press.

Ford, E., & Englund, S. (1979). *Permanent love: Practical steps to a lasting relationship: A reality therapy approach to caring.* Minneapolis, MN: Winston Press.

Ford, E., & Zorn, R. (1975). *Why be lonely?* Niles, IL: Argus.

Glasser, N. (Ed.). (1980). *What are you doing?: How people are helped through reality therapy.* New York: Harper & Row.

Glasser, W. (1964). Reality therapy: A realistic approach to the young offender. *Crime and Delinquency, 10,* 135-144.

Glasser, W. (1965). *Reality therapy.* New York: Harper & Row.

Glasser, W. (1969). *Schools without failure.* New York: Harper & Row.

Glasser, W. (1972). *The identity society.* New York: Harper & Row.

Glasser, W. (1974). A new look at discipline. *Learning: The Magazine for Creative Teaching, 3,* 6-11.

Glasser, W. (1976a). A new look at discipline. In A. Bassin, T. Bratter, & R. Rachin (Eds.), *The reality therapy reader: A survey of the work of William Glasser.* New York: Harper & Row.

Glasser, W. (1976b). *Positive addiction.* New York: Harper & Row.

Glasser, W. (1981). *Stations of the mind.* New York: Harper & Row.

Glasser, W. (1984). *Take effective control of your life.* New York: Harper & Row.

Glasser, W. (1986a). *Control theory in the classroom.* New York: Harper & Row.

Glasser, W. (1986b). *The control theory—reality therapy workbook.* Canogu Park, CA: Institute for Reality Therapy.

Glasser, W., & Zunin, L. (1973). Reality therapy. In R. Corsini (Ed.), *Current psychotherapies.* Itasca, IL: F. E. Peacock.

Glasser, W., & Zunin, L. (1979). Reality therapy. In R. Corsini (Ed.), *Current psychotherapies. Glasser's approach to discipline.* Los Angeles, CA: Educator Training Center. Itasca, IL: F. E. Peacock.

Good, E. (1987). *In pursuit of happiness.* Chapel Hill, NC: New View Publications.

Grant, F. (1972). A study of the effects of open-ended classroom meetings on social and academic self-concept and internal responsibility for academic successes and failures. *Dissertation Abstracts International, 33(10-B),* 1506-B.

Hart-Hester, S. (1986). The effects of reality therapy techniques on the behavior of elementary school students across settings. *Dissertation Abstracts International, 48,* DA 8715124.

Hawes, R. M. (1971). Reality therapy in the classroom. *Dissertation Abstracts International, 32(5-A),* 2483.

Hough-Waite, L. (1980). *A comparison of the art of parenting and parent involvement program.* Unpublished master's thesis, Central Michigan University, Mt. Pleasant, MI.

Hunter, M. L. (1973). Group effect on self-concept and math performance. *Dissertation Abstracts International, 33(10-B),* 5169.

Marandola, P., & Imber, S. (1979). Glasser's classroom meeting: A humanistic approach to behavior change with preadolescent inner-city learning disabled children. *Journal of Learning Disabilities, 12,* 30-34.

Matthews, D. B. (1973). The effects of reality therapy on reported self-concept, social adjustment, reading achievement, and discipline of fourth and fifth graders in two elementary schools. *Dissertation Abstracts International, 33(9-A),* 4842.

McGuiness, T. (1977). *Idea book for the parent involvement program.* Los Angeles, CA: Educator Training Center.

Omizo, M., & Cubberly, W. (1983). The effects of reality therapy classroom meetings on self-concept and locus of control among learning disabled children. *Exceptional Child, 30,* 201-209.

Poppen, W., & Welch, R. (1976). Work with overweight adolescent girls. In A. Bassin, T. Bratter, & R. Rachin (Eds.), *The reality therapy reader: A survey of the work of William Glasser.* New York: Harper & Row.

Quinn, B. (1979). *The efficacy of the open-ended classroom meetings with junior high children on self-concept and attitude toward school.* Unpublished manuscript, Central Michigan University, Mt. Pleasant, MI.

Robert, M. (1973). *Loneliness in the schools.* Niles, IL: Argus.

Rosario, A. C. (1973). The interaction of counseling strategy and locus of control. *Dissertation Abstracts International, 33(10-B),* 5169.

Shearn, D., & Randolph, D. (1978). Effects of reality therapy methods applied in the classroom. *Psychology in the Schools, 15,* 79-83.

Tamborella, E. (1987). The perceptions of staff and students in an alternative high school program using RT behavior management. *Dissertation Abstracts International, 48,* DA 8727114.

Tangeman, J. A. (1973). An investigation of the effect of two classroom guidance programs on self-concept and achievement of third grade students. *Dissertation Abstracts International, 34(8-A, Pt. 1),* 4764.

Wubbolding, R. (1988). *Using reality therapy.* New York: Harper & Row.

Yarish, P. (1986). Reality therapy and locus of control of juvenile offenders. *Journal of Reality Therapy, 6,* 3-10.

Zeaman, R., & Martucci, L. (1976). The application of classroom meetings to special education. *Exceptional Children, 42,* 461-462.

Chapter 9

Systemic Approaches

William B. Gunn, Jr., Ph.D.
Barbara L. Fisher, Ph.D.

INTRODUCTION

The systemic theories of psychotherapy are unique in considering the dynamic relationship between symptomology and the interpersonal context in which the symptoms occur. Systems theorists commonly believe that the system (e.g., a family) maintains the symptoms of its members, and, in fact, is maintained by the symptoms(s). For example, Family A has a 7-year-old daughter who is depressed and withdrawn. A family therapist would view this as a family problem. The depression and withdrawal are viewed as being maintained by the structure, patterns, and beliefs of the family. In turn, the depression and withdrawal permit the family to operate with the least amount of change and the most amount of predictability. This enables a maintenance of the family's structure, patterns, and beliefs. Systemic thinking represents a dramatic epistemological shift from other approaches to psychotherapy, particularly with the premises that etiology and history are significantly less important than understandings of family structure, interaction patterns, and belief systems.

A number of theoretical perspectives have emerged that focus on slightly different dynamics of the general assumption described above. Our overview theory, which integrates three of the major schools of thought (structural, strategic, and systemic), will be described in this chapter as an innovative approach to treating children and adolescents.

Family therapy is much more than an additional technique in the psychologist's bag of tricks. Family therapy represents a new frontier and worldview that encompasses the entire treatment process, including conceptualizing, assessing, and intervening.

Historical Perspective

Most family therapy historians agree that the decade following World War II was formative for the family therapy movement. Goldenberg and Goldenberg (1985) point to five "seemingly independent scientific and clinical developments that together set the stage for the emergence of family therapy" (p. 90). First, they cite the adaptation of psychoanalytic formulations to the study of the family. Nathan Ackerman, a psychoanalyst and child psychiatrist, is first credited with extending this orientation beyond the inner life of the person to that person within his or her family, community, and social contexts. Second, General Systems Theory, proposed by Ludwig von Bertalanffy, was adapted to family systems. This theory created an entirely unique perspective for understanding symptoms. The third scientific development was research into the area of schizophrenia. During the 1950s, three independent research teams (led by Gregory Bateson in California, Ted Lidz at Yale, and Murray Bowen at NIMH) all arrived at a similar conclusion: There is a strong relationship between family processes and the development of schizophrenia. Each team developed different explanations for this correlation, but the basic conclusion helped open the door to family therapy for the treatment of a variety of what were previously believed to be "intrapsychic conflicts." Fourth, the areas of marriage counseling and child guidance emerged early in this century and provided a foundation for family therapy later in the 1950s. The fifth and final development was group therapy, which emerged around 1910 as a new curative approach to intrapsychic conflicts. The extension of group principles to the family (a natural group) was a logical step.

Family therapy is approximately 40 years old. The first two decades (1950s, 1960s) could be characterized as the foundational years. Many "family therapists," beginning as M.D.'s and/or researchers, started questioning traditional approaches at this time. Several treated families without interacting with other professionals for fear of ostracism. Researchers began to speculate about the nature of the relationship between family dynamics and "intrapsychic" pathology. During the 1970s, family therapy proliferated and diversity emerged. Several camps of theories and therapies developed including the intergenerational (Bowen, Nagy, Framo, Paul, Williamson), behavioral (Stuart, Jacobsen, Liberman), structural (Minuchin, Aponte), strategic (Watzlawick, Haley, Madanes), and systemic (Selvini-Palazzoli, Papp) approaches. The late 1970s and 1980s can be characterized by divergence and specialization. However, the 1980s can also be viewed as a period of integration for family therapy. Family therapists work in a variety of clinical settings, integrating family therapy with individual therapy, addictions recovery, and medicine.

The field of family therapy has virtually mushroomed, particularly in the last 15 years. The first journal in the field, *Family Process,* was started in 1962. Today there are well over a dozen journals, and hundreds of books have been published on family therapy. A unique publication, *The Family Therapy Networker,* provides discussion of topical issues and is an excellent resource for upcoming workshops and seminars. The American Association of Marriage and Family Therapy (AAMFT) publishes a clinical/research journal, *The Journal of Marriage and Family Therapy,* and a newspaper, *The Family Therapy News,* which keeps readers informed about national trends and legislative efforts in the field.

There are two professional associations for family therapists. AAMFT is the largest (about 15,000 members) and serves to promote the profession and the practice by credentialed practitioners and by accrediting graduate programs. AAMFT established the Commission on Accreditation for Marriage and Family Therapy Education (COA) in the 1970s. The COA is officially recognized by the Federal Department of Education as the accrediting organization for marriage and family therapy training programs. There are almost 50 programs accredited in North America to teach marriage and family therapy. The second organization, the

American Family Therapy Association (AFTA) is an academy of advanced professionals. AFTA is a "think tank" composed of approximately 500 members who meet yearly to share ideas and develop common interests.

OVERVIEW OF THEORY

Basic Theory and Assumptions

In describing the theoretical differences between systemic or interpersonal therapies and intrapsychic therapies the metaphor of a camera is often used. In individual therapies the lens is focused on the thoughts, feelings, or experience of the client. In all approaches to family therapy the lens is widened from the individual to the relevant context in that individual's life, usually the family. However, family approaches differ in terms of the specific focus of observations, hypotheses, and interventions. This section will describe a comprehensive overview theory which will highlight the important theoretical components of three widely used systemic approaches. These correspond to three important aspects of family functioning: the structure/organization of the family, the patterns by which they interact, and the belief systems the family has developed.

Emphasis on the *structure and organization* of family systems is a crucial factor in the approach developed first by Minuchin (1974). Three key structural concepts are *subsystems, hierarchy* (guidance and leadership), and *boundaries* (closeness and distance).

Subsystems are individuals, dyads, or larger groups who make up a subset of the family. Although some subsystems are natural, such as the parental team or sibling group, the possibilities are endless. For example, a mother and youngest child can form a subsystem such that everyone else is excluded. From the formation of this coalition, problems may develop. A therapist evaluates the functionality of the family in terms of hierarchy and boundaries in these subsystems as well as in the family as a whole.

Families need to maintain some *leadership* function in order to move through normal developmental stages as well as manage acute crises. This usually involves the adults being able to make decisions which are in the best interests of the children and the family. A common problem described in adolescence is an inverted hierarchy (Haley, 1980) in which adolescents are directing the parents.

Boundaries are invisible barriers which surround individuals and subsystems regulating the amount of closeness with each other. Subsystems which are not adequately protected by boundaries may be limited in the quality of interpersonal skills achievable. Boundaries can be described as *internal* (between members or subsystems) or *external* (neighbors, friends, school, society).

Interpersonal boundaries are also described as being on a continuum between *rigid* and *diffuse* (Minuchin, 1974). Rigid boundaries are overly restrictive and permit little contact with other family subsystems or external systems. Families with rigid internal boundaries tend to be *disengaged* from each other. Children in such families often feel isolated or neglected. On the other end of the continuum families with diffuse internal boundaries tend to be *enmeshed,* e.g., overly supportive, and may learn to rely too heavily on each other. Families with rigid external boundaries tend to create overdependence on each other and isolation from others. In families with diffuse external boundaries, it is difficult for family members to feel connected with each other. It is often hard to tell who is a family member and who is not. Figure 1 presents a graphic depiction of this concept.

FIGURE 1: BOUNDARIES

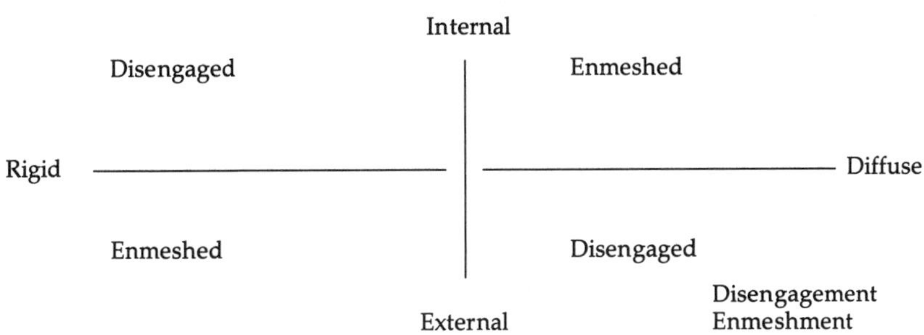

A second aspect of family functioning is the actual problem-maintaining sequences of behavior or *patterns of interaction.* If the sequences which maintain the symptoms can be changed, the symptom is no longer necessary. Thus, symptoms are viewed as maintained by repetitive cycles of interaction. Patterns of interaction are redundant sequences of behavior which may recur across many different content areas. For example, Mom is talking to oldest son when daughter interrupts. Dad criticizes daughter for interrupting and Mom criticizes Dad for being too harsh. Son gets upset about being ignored and leaves the room. This is a simple pattern that may be repeated over and over in this family utilizing different topics to begin the sequence.

In addition to interactions, *rules* and *roles* become part of symptom maintenance. Rules govern power, division of labor, and patterns of interaction in a family. Some rules are overtly stated, for example, a rotation of dishwashing or taking out the trash. However, many family rules are covert and not talked about openly. "Go to your room when Mom and Dad fight" or "If Mom has been drinking, don't talk to her," are examples of such covert rules. Roles are a natural extension of rules. For example, Mother may be "nurturer," Dad the "breadwinner," oldest son the "hero," second son the "troublemaker," and youngest daughter the "peacemaker."

When these patterns prevent the system from accomplishing its tasks, symptoms may develop. The symptomatic behavior, e.g., a child refusing to go to school, is dysfunctional from the school's point of view, but may be logical within the interpersonal network of the family. If the mother of such a child is depressed and suicidal, the child's "protective" behavior may serve to stabilize the system. Thus, the symptom is adaptive for the family system.

In their book *Change, Principles of Problem Formation and Problem Resolution,* Watzlawick, Weakland, and Fisch (1974) emphasize the point that families are always trying to adapt and adjust to changing circumstances while at the same time trying to avoid change and its uncertainties. Thus, when confronted with normal life difficulties, families find solutions to resolve their often conflictual change/don't change position. It is these solutions that become the problems. If the systems or individuals in them can discover new solutions which do not turn difficulties into problems, the symptom would no longer exist.

There are three types of solutions to difficulties that can result in problems and rigid problematic sequences. The first are those in which some action needs to be taken, but the family does not act. From this denial of a difficulty any acknowledgment, let alone an attempted solution, runs the risk of being labeled as madness or badness. An example of this type of problem development would be failure to alter parenting style as a child becomes an adolescent. This can result in increased rebellion and power struggles. A second way problem sequences develop is when actions on a difficulty are taken when there is no need to do so. These are situations where the solution or "cure" is the problem. A couple who have the idea that they will always insist on strict obedience from their children may create a very negative environment by their constant action and unwillingness to "pick their battles carefully." The third way in which problematic sequences can develop is when, although there is a problem and action is taken, it is at the wrong level of intervention, for example, an adolescent who is depressed being "cheered up" by her parents. When these attempts do not meet with success, more vigorous attempts can be made with the result being an increasingly withdrawn and angry teenager who feels controlled and manipulated. Both parents and child can become more engaged in a pattern which does not result in a relieving of the symptoms, but actually leads to an increase in them as a consequence of the misdirected solution.

The final area of this overview theory is the belief system of a particular family. This is the focus of the general systemic theorists from Milan, Italy (Selvini-Palazzoli, Boscolo, Cecchin, & Prata, 1978) and is written about in this country and Canada primarily by the therapists at the Ackerman Institute and by Karl Tomm (1984).

The basic theoretical premise of this view is that family members attribute meaning to behavior within a context and the meaning becomes more important than the behavior. For example, one family may define a child's behavior as cute and amusing whereas another family may define similar behavior as unacceptable. Behavior is far less significant than the meaning attached to it. Behavior is also analyzed through the context in which it occurs. Similar behavior may take on different meaning in different contexts. A child interrupting a parent at a social gathering may draw a punishment, whereas a child interrupting a parent to warn of an approaching danger may be praised. The interpersonal context in which behaviors occur is crucial to a systemic therapist. A child may behave very differently at home when one parent is present compared to when both parents are present. School behaviors may be totally different than at home, and certainly behavior with peers may be even more diverse. An analysis of as many settings as possible and discovering what happens when and who is involved are important in developing hypotheses about the problem and designing interventions.

Family beliefs are constantly evolving. Problems develop when old ways of thinking (beliefs) do not fit the current situation. Moreover, problems develop because of the "meaning" a family attributes to themselves. If new information can be given to the family for them to understand their behavior in a new way, change can occur.

The belief systems of family members are usually linear, that is, they explain events as cause-effect phenomena—Steve did this, then Jenny did that. However, in order to understand the nature and impact of a family's belief system, a circular view of events must be employed. Circularity is the concept that problems are maintained by patterns of interaction between people that have no clear beginning nor end. Circularity maintains a focus on present patterns and emphasizes the reciprocal nature of behavior, thus including all family members in a problem. Behavior problems in a child are not thought of as being "caused" by poor self-esteem or divorcing parents. Circular thinking does not permit individuals in the family to be identified as villains or heroes. There is no extensive search for the cause of a child's misbehavior, only a clear description of what maintains it in the present. A circular hypothesis examines the relationship between the system and provides for interventions that impact the entire system.

In sum, beliefs define the rules, roles, interaction patterns and structure of the family, while these, in turn, define the family's belief. These relationships are graphically depicted in Figure

2. For example, if a parent believes her child cannot be trusted, she may overcontrol the child's behavior, thus making it difficult for the child to learn how to respond to different situations. If the child is given some freedom and acts in a way that displeases the parent, her belief that the child is not trustworthy will be reinforced.

FIGURE 2: IMPORTANT COMPONENTS OF OVERVIEW THEORY

STRUCTURE ⟷ PATTERNS

STRUCTURE	PATTERNS
– subsystems	– rules
– boundaries	– roles
– hierarchy	– interactions

BELIEFS
– meaning
– context

Family Development–Health and Pathology

A cornerstone of this overview theory is the concept that families generally develop through a series of predictable stages requiring the completion of sequential and cumulative developmental tasks. Carter and McGoldrick (1988) suggest there are six stages of the Family Life Cycle. These are outlined in Table 1.

Adjustments are required as the family becomes more complex and matures. The view of family development through stages is very helpful in understanding what is expected or normal for a family at particular stages as well as understanding why a family may be struggling. It is known that disruption in development or inability to complete the tasks of one stage effectively interferes with the ability of the family to complete the tasks of a later stage.

Only in the past 10 to 15 years have family therapists/researchers focused on normal, healthy family processes. As previously shown, one of the foundational areas of family therapy was research into family pathology. Three research studies of the 1970s found very similar characteristics of healthy

TABLE 1: THE STAGES OF THE FAMILY LIFE CYCLE

Family Life Cycle Stage	Emotional Process of Transition: Key Principles	Second Order Changes in Family Status to Proceed Developmentally
1. Between Families: The Unattached Young Adult	Accepting parent-offspring separation	a. Differentiation of self in relation to family of origin b. Development of intimate peer relationships c. Establishment of self in work
2. The Joining of Families Through Marriage: The Newly Married Couple	Commitment to new system	a. Formation of marital system b. Realignment of relationships with extended families and friends to include spouse
3. The Family with Young Children	Accepting new members into the system	a. Adjusting marital system to make space for child(ren) b. Taking on parenting roles c. Realignment of relationships with extended family to include parenting and grandparenting roles
4. The Family with Adolescents	Increasing flexibility of family boundaries to include children's independence	a. Shifting of parent-child relationships to permit adolescent to move in and out of system b. Refocus on mid-life marital and career issues c. Beginning shift toward concerns for older generation
5. Launching Children and Moving On	Accepting a multitude of exits from and entries into the family system	a. Renegotiation of marital system as a dyad b. Development of adult-to-adult relationships between grown children and their parents c. Realignment of relationships to include in-laws and grandchildren d. Dealing with disabilities and death of parents (grandparents)
6. The Family in Later Life	Accepting the shifting of generational roles	a. Maintaining own and/or couple functioning and interests in face of physiological decline; exploration of new familial and social role options b. Support for a more central role for middle generation c. Making room in the system for the wisdom and experience of the elderly; supporting the older generation without overfunctioning for them d. Dealing with loss of spouse, siblings, and other peers and preparation for own death. Life review and integration

From Betty Carter and Monica McGoldrick, *The Changing Family Life Cycle: A Framework for Family Therapy* (2nd ed.). Copyright © 1989 by Allyn and Bacon, Inc. Reprinted with permission.

families. Lewis, Beavers, Gossett, and Phillips (1976) completed extensive studies of families and developed a rating scale to distinguish healthy from disturbed families. They concluded that no single quality identified the healthy family, but that healthy families have the following qualities:

- strong parental coalition
- an affiliative attitude toward encounters
- respect for the subjectivity of others
- open and direct communication
- an understanding of varied and complex human needs and motivations
- spontaneity
- high levels of initiative
- enjoyment of the uniqueness of each individual

Stinnett (1979) studied "strong" families and found the following common characteristics:

- appreciation for one another
- time together that is genuinely enjoyed
- good communication patterns
- commitment to promoting the happiness and welfare of others in the family
- high degree of religious orientation
- ability to deal with crises in a positive manner

Fisher, Giblin, and Hoopes (1982) identified the following aspects as important to healthy family functioning:

- a sense of belonging to the family
- communication that attends to feelings and content
- attentively listening
- expressing feelings and thoughts openly
- enjoyment of one another–doing things that are fun
- acceptance and support for each other's needs

- feeling safe with and trusting one another
- ability to depend on one another

These empirical studies shed light on healthy family dynamics, but "there is a paucity of theoretical and empirical information about normal families" (Gantman, 1980, p. 106).

Likewise, a number of concepts have been elaborated in the literature on dysfunction in families. An attempt to list or catalogue these concepts would result in a confusing laundry list of qualifying characteristics. There is no single qualifying criterion that justifies labeling a family as pathological. "Pathology" is viewed as functional or adaptive. Pathological behavior "makes sense" when viewed in its context.

Thus, family health is context-specific and stage-specific. A family must continue to grow, and rules, roles, structure, beliefs, and interaction patterns must be moderately flexible for its members to stay healthy. Too much or too little flexibility can create problems in a family. Families that change too rapidly encounter confusion and chaos. Families that change too little may be viewed as "stuck" or unable to modify roles, rules, structures, beliefs, and/or interactions. Family therapy seeks to break through the "stuckness" or stabilize the chaos so the family can regenerate healthier patterns.

BASIC TECHNIQUES AND INTERVENTIONS IN FAMILY THERAPY

It would be impossible in this kind of overview chapter to describe completely all the techniques developed from systemic theory. We will briefly outline a few of them which correspond to the aspects of family functioning described in the theoretical section. We will also provide references for a more complete review of techniques.

The interventions a therapist chooses to a large extent depend on which aspect of the overview theory is in focus. With a structural emphasis, a therapist *joins* with the family, *maps* structural dynamics such as hierarchy and boundaries, and has the family *enact* patterns which give them new possibilities for alternative relationships. Minuchin and Fishman's (1981) book *Family*

Therapy Techniques, provides detailed descriptions of interventions into the structure/organization of the family.

Joining is a technique by which a therapist works to understand and accept each person's position in the family. The family often approaches therapy with some anxiety and guilt, and it is important to connect with each member. Failure to join and accommodate to the way things are presently may produce resistance to therapeutic interventions. Joining includes but is not limited to the initial session. It occurs throughout therapy and does not always mean listening and "being nice." Often it involves saying something that is painful but real in the experience of one or more family members.

Mapping the family structure involves two stages. In planning for sessions, the therapist makes some hypotheses about structure. This occurs even before the first session. Questions such as, "Who seems most powerful?" "What relationships might be disengaged from each other?" or "Is the hierarchy functional?" can be asked. These questions or hypotheses continue to be generated throughout therapy. The second stage of mapping involves testing these hypotheses by watching the family interact as well as by asking them to talk to each other. This latter intervention, creating enactments, is a powerful way of allowing the therapist to see what actually happens in the family.

Enactments can also be used to highlight or modify interactions. The therapist encourages family members to behave in new, competent ways. For example, a mother and daughter who are in a constant battle for control may be asked to engage in a different kind of interaction. In a soft tone, sitting in close proximity to the mother, the therapist may ask the mother to talk in a soft tone, sit next to her daughter, and talk to her about her concerns for the daughter's safety.

An emphasis on changing the patterns of interaction involves different kinds of interventions. The therapist is more interested in changing the symptom-maintaining sequences than in changing the structure. Precise questioning about the process occurring around the problem and attempted problem solutions is important. Tasks, either direct or paradoxical, are assigned to alter these sequences.

The questions asked in the initial interviews revolve around who does what, how, and when the problem occurs. This not only provides information about the process, but also about the possible functionality of the symptom for the overall system. Haley (1987) provides an excellent description of such an initial interview.

In these initial sessions, each family member presents his or her view of the problem and of the solutions which have been tried. It is these solutions which often are addressed by therapeutic interventions. After a clear problem definition is agreed upon, the family and therapist set goals for therapy. This is often the most difficult phase of therapy. Presenting problems such as "we want to communicate more" tend to be vague, and families have more ideas about what they don't want than what they do want. However, for the strategically designed interventions which follow to be effective, this problem definition/goal setting is crucial.

Assignment of tasks to be completed outside of the sessions is a primary intervention utilized by therapists focused on altering patterns. These can be direct or paradoxical. Straightforward directives are given with a rationale that is designed to correspond to the goals agreed on in the initial sessions. If therapeutic rapport is developed and resistance to change is low, the family will be able to carry out the tasks. Attention is paid to the way in which they do so. Their level of resistance to change can be gauged by whether they carry out the task exactly, modify the task, or fail to do it at all.

Paradoxical interventions are designed to counter strong resistance to change (Watzlawick et al., 1974). The usual method is to ask the family not to change, to go slow in changing, or to continue the symptom. These directives are given with the intent that the family will be placed in a bind. If they follow the directives, they are exercising control over these symptoms. If they don't comply, the symptoms change. These interventions have been extremely controversial, with proponents arguing they are congruent and respectful of the family's fear of change while others argue that they are tricky and manipulative. The key variable seems to be the rationale which accompanies the directive and the degree to which the therapist believes it to be true.

If paradoxical interventions become routine statements used in every case, they are not likely to be as effective as if they come out of the family's efforts in therapy or if they are designed to have unique meaning to the family.

Cloe Madanes (1981) describes another type of paradoxical intervention. She advocates the use of "pretend" techniques to confront destructive patterns in a playful manner. For example, a symptomatic child is asked to "pretend" to have the symptom and the parents are encouraged to "pretend" to help. The child can give up the actual symptom; pretending to have it is enough. One cannot pretend to have a phobia or throw a tantrum and have a real one at the same time. The intervention can turn a deadly serious struggle which would not respond to a direct approach at change into a playful make-believe game.

The third area of family functioning in the overview theory is in the belief systems of the family. Whereas the focus on structure and patterns emphasizes behavior change first, with a belief change to follow, the systemic therapist emphasizes belief or meaning change as the primary target. Three interventions from this approach are *reframing* (Watzlawick et al., 1974), *circular questioning* (Nelson, Fleuridas, & Rosenthal, 1986; Selvini-Palazzoli, Boscolo, Cecchin, & Prata, 1977; Tomm, 1984) and *family rituals* (Selvini-Palazzoli et al., 1977).

Reframing is an intervention used often by family therapists. The therapist hears the situation as presented by the family and then restates it in a new way. The goal is to change the way reality is perceived so that new behaviors will follow. For example, an anorexic girl who is seen as "sick" by her parents and in need of a great deal of tender loving care can be reframed as being "disobedient" and in a power struggle with her parents. A delinquent boy can alternatively be viewed as sad and insecure, who is in need of firm structure and guidance to feel secure. As with the paradoxical directive, these restatements of the problem must be unique to the particular situation and not seen as standard, to be used in every case.

Positive connotation (Selvini-Palazzoli et al., 1977), a form of reframing, always defines symptomatic behavior in terms of its helfulness to the system. For example, a child's misbehavior may be redefined as helpful to her parents' communication.

Circular questioning is a technique that has received increasing attention in the clinical literature. This form of questioning serves as an efficient process for soliciting information from each member of the family regarding their opinion and experience of (a) the family's presenting concern; (b) the context in which the behaviors occur; (c) sequences of interactions, usually related to the problem; and (d) differences in their relationships over time. Questions such as "Who is the most upset when John throws a temper tantrum?" or "Who feels the most helpless when it happens?" are asked of all family members. The answers are used to generate additional hypotheses about family functioning or additional questions. The questions themselves are seen as interventions in that it is hoped they provide the family with new information about the way things are now and the way they could be in the future. New belief systems can be created which necessitate new behaviors by family members.

A therapist can prescribe family rituals which are usually complex, elaborate tasks involving all family members. The therapist asks the family to complete an action or series of actions sometimes accompanied by verbal expressions. The ritual is prescribed in every detail: the place it must be carried out, who must say and do what action, and the number of times the ritual is to be completed. Often the instructions are given in writing, and the session is ended without further discussion about the assignment. A particular ritual is designed for a family after careful consideration of the unique rules which maintain their problems. The ritual breaks these rules in some way, and the family can experience an alternative belief about themselves.

GROUP PROCEDURES

The family is a small group with a shared history. In some respects, family therapy may be considered similar to group therapy. However, an additional dimension of family therapy is to have multiple families in group programs. Three models of family-group facilitation are described by Hoopes, Fisher, and Barlow (1984). Family education programs are primarily instructional in focus, with the expressed intent of imparting information and skills to family members. Parent education courses are a common type of family education program. One well-developed parent education program is Bevolek and Comstack's (1985) Nurturing Parent Program. This is a 15-week structured program designed to enhance parental self-esteem, parenting skills, social support, and overall healthy family functioning.

Family enrichment programs are designed to enhance skills and healthy family interactions through instructional and experiential activities. Two well-known programs, *Understanding Us* (Carnes, 1981) and *Family Cluster* (Sawin, 1979), bring groups of families together to share experiences, learn new skills, and develop healthier interactions. The purpose of enrichment and education programs is to provide knowledge and skills in a preventive spirit, that is, to assist families in side-stepping or effectively coping with potentially difficult situations and, therefore, maintaining family integrity and cohesion.

Family treatment groups designed to resolve problems encountered and developed by families are, therefore, remedial in nature. Multiple family group therapy involves the treatment of several families together with regular scheduled sessions. A common use of multiple family treatment is in addiction recovery (e.g., substance abuse) and eating disorders. Lacqueur (1976) is well known in this area.

In all three models, family members learn from the facilitator(s) and other families. All models offer a supportive context for the development of new roles and behaviors. In Hoopes, Fisher, and Barlow (1984) several tested enrichment, education, and treatment programs for families with children and adolescents are actually provided.

CLASSROOM AND EDUCATIONAL APPLICATIONS

Systemic theory applies as well to a classroom, a school, or an entire school system as it does to a family. Broadening the lens of analysis to include subsystems such as teacher-student, student-student, principal-staff, or teacher-parents-student can help to provide a more organized way of approaching the problem as well as provide more options for intervention. Once this lens is widened, the choices for intervention can be focused on the organization/structure of the family, the patterns of interaction, or the meaning/belief system.

Children exhibiting behavior problems are often afraid of the power these symptoms have over adults. They may even escalate the problems in order to encourage adults to take charge. Teachers, concerned about this escalation, may call the parents into a conference. After these meetings become adversarial, each looks to blame the other for the child's problem. Principals are sometimes present at these meetings, but are forced either to support the teacher's position or to try to play a mediating role.

This school-family conference is an excellent example of a technique which focuses on the organization or structure of that system. The purpose of these conferences is to "join" with all family members and establish a clear leadership team between the adults. Joining would involve displaying a keen interest in knowing whether problems seen at school are observed in the home context and vice versa. This is done with curiosity about the differences between the two settings rather than projection of blame. One of the important benefits of these meetings is that the child is given a clear role to play. This depends somewhat on the age of the child, but generally the child is asked to observe the discussion and to provide input in a structured way when it is asked of him or her. The child thus observes the important adults in his or her life working together. More detailed descriptions of the possible structure of these interviews can be found in Fine and Holt (1983), Molnar and Lindquist (1984), or Friedman (1969).

A classroom can be thought of in much the same way as a family, with the teacher playing the same role as a therapist. In most therapeutic approaches, a child's misbehavior would lead to a focus on the child and an intervention that was focused on changing the child's behavior. A systemic approach would enble the teacher to focus on his or her part in maintaining the problem behaviors. Outside consultants such as psychologists, social workers, or principals can help teachers to have that perspective and use systemic techniques in addressing the problem.

Interventions can be made by focusing on the patterns or sequence of interactions that occur in a classroom. When teachers are able to look at their students and classrooms as systems, they are able to look at their own beliefs and behavior as part of that system. Instead of looking at the sequence of "teacher yells → child disrupts" or "child disrupts → teacher yells" in a cause-effect manner, both are seen as mutually determining each other. To the extent that the teacher yells, the child disrupts. To the extent the child disrupts, the teacher yells. This dyadic example could be expanded to include complex interactions between groups of students and teachers/administrators.

Another example is as follows: A typical sequence at recess involves one child consistently being scapegoated into trouble by two other students, with the teacher having to enforce punishment on the scapegoat. If the teacher were to change his or her part of the pattern by intervening in a positive manner with all three before recess, he or she might prevent his or her negative involvement later. This example enlarges the context to include the teacher and would require the teacher to embrace firmly the belief that he/she helps to define roles played by the students. This is an alternative to the traditional belief that students are totally responsible for their own behavior.

Reframing or positive connotation is a technique described earlier. It involves a focus on the belief system/meaning of the problem or some aspect of it. Teachers can also use reframing. An "angry, defiant" child can be seen as "extremely sad and desperately seeking to provide structure in his or her environment." Two children "constantly fighting" can be seen as attempting to "work problems out" in the only way they know how. An "annoying" child who is constantly sharpening her pencil can be seen as "anxious to please and perform well on schoolwork." A teacher's response to a child will depend in large measure on his or her belief about the child's behavior. For example, if a teacher sees a behavior as annoying, he or she is likely to become easily irritated and yell at the child. If the same behavior is seen as anxious to please, the teacher may feel more compassionate and help shape the behavior in a more positive way.

PARENTING SKILLS

An awareness and careful assessment of family systems dynamics is extremely important for counselors/therapists who utilize parent educational approaches. Often parent education is begun individually or in groups where each of the parents has a child exhibiting behavior problems in school or in the community. Interactional patterns in the family that might contribute to maintaining these problems need to be explored. Three of these issues are discussed in a recent article by Getz and Gunn (1988).

The first issue is that most current parent education approaches present a one-sided view of the parent-child relationship; that is, parents from a systemic perspective cause their children's behavior. Parents and children are involved in a process of mutual influence. One program, Student Effectiveness Training (Getz & Morrill, 1978), was an attempt to balance the skewedness of parent effectiveness training by teaching the same communication skills to adolescents and parents.

A second issue is the reality that often mothers are the only ones involved in learning new parenting strategies. Levant and Doyle (1981) conducted a review of the literature on parent training and did not find any study which focused on the training of fathers or indicated whether fathers were ever involved in the training. If one member of a family system is changing attitudes and behaviors, there is the danger that the other parent may have difficulty adjusting. A key concept in systemic theory is parental hierarchy which functions in making decisions for the children. Thus, parent education only to the mother may contribute to the disruption of that hierarchy.

Finally, and most important, the same parenting skills are typically taught regardless of the specific characteristics of each of the families. This may aggravate pre-existing patterns. Gunn (1983) developed a training program for parents of children identified as emotionally disturbed and currently receiving special education in the public schools. He interviewed each family separately to assess their strengths and weaknesses in handling positive, as well as conflictual, situations. He then organized a parent training group which used individualized instruction to focus on those weaker areas which could be enhanced with better child-rearing skills. In addition, parents with strengths in certain skill areas served as models for other parents.

Table 2 provides examples of family system issues and parent education approaches which would be important to emphasize.

TABLE 2: SUMMARY OF PARENT EDUCATION STRATEGIES FOR DIFFERENT FAMILY DYNAMICS

Family System Issues	Parent Education Approaches
1. Family communication Dysfunctional communication patterns	Active listening Confrontation and problem-solving skills Examination of irrational beliefs
2. Emotional distance between family members: Enmeshed families (too little distance) Disengaged families (too much distance)	Analysis of children's mistaken goals Use of logical consequences Confrontation skills and "I" messages Communication skills Family meetings
3. Family role structuring Inverted hierarchy (lack of parental authority) Split parental team	Assertive discipline Behavior modification Use of logical consequences Parental communication and negotiation

EFFICACY

As noted earlier, clinical research was one of the key movements that launched the field of family therapy. Since that time, several hundred outcome and process studies have been completed on a broad range of family problems, treatment approaches, therapist factors, and the effectiveness of family therapy. According to Gurman, Kniskern, and Pinsof (1986) "by the 1980s, research had come to occupy a truly significant and undoubtedly permanent place in the field of family and marital therapy" (p. 567).

Family therapy is inherently complex. While seeking to illuminate answers to "what therapy is most effective for what problems treated by what therapists, according to what criteria, in what setting" (Paul, 1967, p. 11), perplexing issues of target outcome variables, measurement, design, control groups, random selection, subject population, and integration of research and practice are complicated by a systemic theoretical foundation. For example, targeted outcome variables may consist of increased healthy family functioning, increased individual functioning, and/or reaching the client's goal for treatment. With regard to increased healthy family functioning, how will this be defined, by whom, and how measured? If increased individual functioning is the target variable, which individual(s) in the family is(are) measured? In studies in which client goals are the outcome criteria, what about those families in which the members do not agree to a common goal?

In spite of these and other difficulties, researchers have provided studies that conclusively demonstrate the efficacy of family therapy. These studies have been notably reviewed by Gurman and Kniskern (1978, 1981), Gurman, Kniskern, and Pinsof (1986), and Todd and Stanton (1983). In general, the following conclusions are some of those that may be drawn from family therapy research:

1. Family therapy is as effective or more effective than individual and other treatment approaches. Gurman and Kniskern (1978) examined 14 comparative studies (family therapy compared to other modalities) and found that family therapy was superior in ten and equal in the remaining studies.
2. Family therapy produces beneficial effects in about ⅔ of cases. In fact, Gurman and Kniskern (1978) estimated the overall improvement rate for family therapy cases at 73%.
3. Family therapy can produce positive results in treatment of short duration (1-20 sessions). Short-term or time-limited family therapy is as effective as longer term therapy (Gurman et al., 1986; Todd & Stanton, 1983).
4. The involvement of the father in family therapy substantially increases the probability of successful outcome (Todd & Stanton, 1983).

5. There is little evidence that one marriage and family therapy approach is superior to another. No systematic comparison of the various "schools" has been completed (Todd & Stanton, 1983).
6. Marriage and family therapy can also cause deterioration in individuals and relationships. Deterioration rates (5-10%) for marriage and family therapy are roughly comparable to those reported for individual and group therapy. Gurman and Kniskern (1978) isolated certain therapist behaviors that were related to poor outcomes, including poor relationship skills, confronting emotionally loaded issues and defenses early in treatment, and little structuring of early sessions.
7. More refined therapist skills seem necessary to yield positive outcomes (Gurman & Kniskern, 1978).
8. The age/developmental level of the "identified parent" (child, adolescent, adult) is not associated with treatment outcomes (Gurman & Kniskern, 1978).

With regard to specific disorders of childhood and adolescence, family therapy research has focused on psychosomatic disorders, juvenile delinquency and conduct disorders, and mixed emotional/behavioral disorders.

Structural family therapy has been studied for the treatment of anorexia, diabetes mellitus, and chronic asthma. Minuchin, Rosman, and Baker (1978) reported an 86% improvement/recovery rate for 53 anorexics and their families. Minuchin et al. (1975) reported a 90% improvement rate for diabetes and chronic asthma. All three populations were treated with a structural approach.

Juvenile delinquency and family therapy has been extensively studied at the University of Utah by James Alexander and associates (Alexander & Parsons, 1973; Klein, Alexander, & Parsons, 1977; Parsons & Alexander, 1973) applying "functional" family therapy. Families treated with this approach significantly improved in communication and showed a lower rate of recidivism (26%) than other treatment modalities (47% for client centered, 50% for untreated persons, and 73% for dynamic-eclectic therapy approaches).

Patterson (1982) studied conduct disorders involving aggressive (e.g., physically violent) and nonaggressive (e.g., stealing, lying) behaviors utilizing "parent management training." This approach has been demonstrated to change child classroom and at-home behaviors.

With regard to mixed childhood and adolescent disorders, no meaningful conclusions may be drawn due to sampling techniques of every study (Gurman et al., 1986).

Family therapy research has continued into such areas as adult schizophrenia, psychosomatic symptoms, addictions, depressions, anxiety, marital distress, and sexual dysfunction. Although the field experiences conceptual and methodological problems, outcome of well-designed studies indicates the effectiveness of family therapy.

CONCLUSIONS

Family therapy is the clinical application of systems theory in working therapeutically with children and adolescents. It has added to the therapist's options of looking at problems and methods of effecting change. The primary orientation is toward evaluating the relevant context in which behaviors occur, what factors within that context maintain the presenting problem(s), and making interventions to increase family members' ability to function in that context. Family therapists are not particularly interested in the historical etiology of problems, but in what factors allow the behaviors identified as problems to continue.

Within the field of family therapy, discussion continues about the aspects of family functioning which are most salient for therapeutic focus. This chapter has described three of these in terms of theory, interventions, group procedures, and educational applications. Assessment covers structure and organization of family hierarchy and boundaries, patterns of interaction, and the belief system of the family as a whole or individual members.

There are several new directions for family therapy. Research will continue to measure outcomes and demonstrate the effectiveness of interventions. These studies will need to state more specific questions such as which theory/technique is effective with what kinds of problems in what kinds of families. For example, questions such as "When should structural interventions be applied?" or "Are tasks given to complete within the session more effective than those given outside the session?" will be asked in future research studies.

Although family theorists may argue about the "correctness" of a given approach, clinical practitioners do not seem to be as concerned. In fact, there has been much more of an integration of approaches in the last few years. The overview theory described in this chapter is an example of this.

Systems therapists are beginning to apply contextual theories in new areas. One example is the training of family medicine physicians. Family therapists have begun to work closely with these physicians in cases involving physical, behavioral, and emotional difficulties (Doherty & Baird, 1983). Another application is in the area of organizational consultation. Schools, businesses, and work teams are systems to which these principles have been applied.

Finally, family therapy has been criticized for losing the "tree for the forest." Intrapsychic dynamics have largely been ignored. The return of the "self in the system" has broadened the thinking of family therapists to be able to consider intrapsychic theories within the systemic perspective.

CASE STUDY

Presenting Problem

Susan, age 8, was identified by her mother, Cathy, and by her teacher as having significant emotional, behavioral, and learning problems. She was attending a small, rural school and engaging in frequent physical fights with peers. She was often defiant and verbally abusive to her teacher. Cathy reported that although these behaviors were not new, negative school reports had escalated this year. In addition, Susan would throw two to three weekly tantrums at home, usually in response to her mother's request to complete a task.

Relevant Background Information/Family History

Susan was the youngest of two girls. Her sister, Elaine, was 11 and had never been in any trouble. Elaine was reported to have been a model child both at home and at school. Susan's father, Tom, had been a long-distance truck driver during his entire 15-year marriage to Cathy. He was home on an irregular and unpredictable basis. Cathy had not been employed outside the home.

Susan began to experience respiratory problems when she was 1 year old. In the following 3 years, the family had her evaluated by a number of medical specialists, and she was hospitalized several times. A diagnosis of atypical asthma was not confirmed until the end of that time. Both parents agreed that this was an extremely difficult time for everyone. They lived in almost constant fear their daughter would stop breathing so she was never left alone. Although Susan had not been sick for several years, the parents admitted to a fair degree of watchfulness due to fear of relapse. Cathy felt that she worried more since Tom was away a large part of the time.

Cathy expressed a great deal of anger and mistrust toward the school system. She moved Susan three times due to her perception of the teachers' lack of understanding of what her daughter needed. She felt the teacher was only interested in making Susan obey and did not allow her to express her opinions.

Assessment

There were two relevant interactional systems to consider in understanding what maintained (not what caused) Susan's problems: the family and family-school systems. During three family interviews and consultation with the school, an assessment was made of (1) the structure/organization of these systems, (2) the patterns of interaction, and (3) the beliefs held about Susan's problems. Beliefs about the implicit rules for interaction between those involved were also explored. This assessment resulted in the following hypotheses:

1. There were poorly defined boundaries within the family, particularly around Cathy and both girls. It was difficult for Cathy to know what level of responsibility

Susan should be given. To the extent that Cathy did things for her, Susan sensed her mother's concern and acted in ways to justify it. The subsystem of mother-daughter could be described as enmeshed. It was difficult to know where "one stopped and the other began."

2. There seemed to be a coalition between the females that, to some extent, excluded Tom. Tom's job requirements were such that he was gone for long periods of time and this helped to maintain the coalition.

3. The following patterns of interaction around the problem were described by the family. If Susan strongly refused to comply with the teacher, she was removed from the classroom and usually Cathy was called. Cathy described feeling threatened by the school and usually responded angrily and defensively to the school, but acted helpless and hopeless in front of Susan. Cathy and Elaine, as well as Susan, expressed the same bewilderment, frequently saying that everything had been tried. The school had developed a role in which they were only the bearer of bad news and had become increasingly frustrated by Cathy's nonsupport and anger toward them. They began to resist calling Cathy except in extreme circumstances. When Tom came home he was told about the incidents in which Susan had been involved at school. He offered counseling and advice as well as established consequences for future misbehavior. These were rarely carried out in his absence, and it seemed that Susan had the worst times when he was away. Mother and daughters felt that Tom was extremely helpful when he came home, suggesting this pattern had a possible function for the system.

4. The family maintained some strong belief systems which were relevant for designing interventions. The first was a certainty on the part of the parents that Susan could get very sick again if she and they were not watchful. Second, was the view that Cathy was the leader and

the glue that held the family together. Her moods set the tone for the rest of the family, and strong fear was expressed about her becoming depressed. Third, the overt view about Tom was that he did the best he could do although covertly there was a great deal of resentment about his erratic work schedule. Finally, Elaine was seen as perfect and needing little attention, guidance, and nurturance to do well. The only problem was a concern that she ate very little and was 15 pounds underweight.

Interventions

Using the assessment data about structure, patterns, and belief systems, the following interventions were among those implemented during the course of therapy:

1. A family-school conference was held with the therapist in charge. The teacher, principal, both parents, and Susan were present. The agenda of developing a unified plan for assisting Susan to succeed at home and school was presented. Susan was asked to leave the meeting for a while during which time a plan was developed for communication and positive and negative consequences of Susan's behaviors. The plan was presented to Susan at the end of the session. This plan involved Tom a great deal, and he expressed a willingness to be more directly involved. This gave Cathy a chance to have a "vacation" from the problem so she did not get overwhelmed.
2. Reframing was begun at the family-school conference and continued in family therapy. The child's patterns of early illness were reframed in a manner that allowed the parents to construe them as a form of protection. Susan was described as becoming stuck at about 4 years of age due to the uncertainty of her medical condition. The normal patterns which developed around the illness were still in place, but not necessary, and were delaying Susan's emotional growth.

3. A concern was raised about Elaine having an eating disorder in the future. Several therapy sessions focused on this possibility, i.e., why she might be at risk and some possible preventive strategies all of which involved more attention paid to her normal development. Cathy was given several assignments to encourage and teach Elaine how to socialize effectively with her peers.

Analysis

The family-school conference was an intervention designed to establish a clear hierarchy and appropriate boundaries between the adults and children in the system. Susan was included in a way that presented the message as clearly as possible. She was put in a student/child role and the talk was in the language of teaching/learning new skills rather than control/punishment of past behavior.

Reframing was used to present an alternative reality/belief system to all involved. Susan was presented as a girl with important developmental tasks to learn rather than an emotionally disturbed or delinquent child. This intervention served to shut the door on guilt for the parents and open the door for new, more competent behaviors to be embraced and practiced.

The structural move to increase Tom's involvement was designed to break up the coalition between Cathy and Susan, give him a more responsible role, and disengage Cathy. Tom found out earlier about any problems and dealt with them more effectively. This replaced the mother's helpless "dance" and may have helped to break the pattern which maintained Susan's problematic behavior.

The focus on Elaine was not solely used to take the spotlight away from Susan although that was one benefit. It also provided a different role and alternative belief system for Elaine and added a more active nurturant dimension to the relationship between her and her parents.

Results

There were immediate dramatic improvements between home and school. There was a significant improvement in collaboration, support, and communication between the adults.

Susan's behavior at school also improved. Tom was able to negotiate his work schedule a month ahead which made family events more predictable. He reported being happy with being in charge of the school-home program and felt successful.

ANNOTATED BIBLIOGRAPHY

Boscolo, L., Cecchin, G., Hoffman, L., & Penn, P. (1987). *Milan systemic family therapy.* New York: Basic Books.

This text was written by two members of the original Milan team and two American Milan therapists. In the introduction, the authors report the evolution of this approach. The remainder of the book is dedicated to case studies of family therapy from a Milan perspective.

Goldenberg, I., & Goldenberg, H. (1985). *Family therapy: An overview* (2nd ed.). Monterey, CA: Brooks/Cole.

This is an excellent overview book for the uninitiated. It covers family systems and family dysfunction, several major theoretical perspectives, techniques of family therapy, and training. It is frequently used as an introductory text at the master's level in marriage and family therapy courses.

Gurman, A. S., & Kinskern, D. P. (1981). *Handbook of family therapy.* New York: Brunner/Mazel.

This is considered one of the major texts in family therapy today. Under one cover, first generation theorists (for the most part) in family therapy have written about their theories in a manner that allows for comparison. Also included are excellent chapters on the history of marriage and family therapy and research into this field.

Haley, J. (1987). *Problem-solving therapy* (2nd ed.). San Francisco: Jossey-Bass.

This is the second edition of a classic book in which Haley first coined the term "strategic therapy." This book is one of the clearest expositions of the basic tenets underlying Haley's approach to family therapy, a combination of structural and strategic concepts. His chapter on conducting the initial interview is particularly good for new therapists who are desirous of a structured way to conduct a family interview. His chapter on ethical issues attempts to address charges that strategic practices are deceptive or manipulative.

Madanes, C. (1981). *Strategic family therapy.* San Francisco: Jossey-Bass.

Madanes, C. (1984). *Behind the one-way mirror.* San Francisco: Jossey-Bass.

These books are clearly written and have been good additions to the scope of strategic family therapy. Madanes emphasizes planning ahead and discovering hidden metaphors in families. The majority of case examples in these books involve children, and her unique "pretend" interventions describe ways for therapists to change patterns in a family more gently.

Minuchin, S. (1974). *Families and family therapy.* Cambridge, MA: Harvard University Press.

This is a seminal text in structural family therapy and an excellent place to begin reading. Minuchin clarified his theory through the use of verbatim therapy transcripts and parallel commentary. Particularly helpful in this book is the description of family mapping, an assessment technique that allows a therapist to place members or involved systems visually in space in order to design structural interventions.

Mirkin, M., & Koman, S. (Eds.). (1985). *A handbook of adolescent and family therapy.* New York: Gardner Press.

The contributions to this handbook cover a large number of topics related to adolescence. The first section of the book covers theoretical issues, while authors of the second explore a variety of settings in which therapy occurs. Finally, the last sections of the book address issues in treatment such as substance abuse and suicide. This book is highly recommended for those working with this age group.

Papp, P. (1983). *The process of change.* New York: Guilford Press.

Peggy Papp, writing from a systemic perspective, provides a very clear approach to treating families. She describes systemic hypothesizing and innovative interventions in practical terms. This is an enjoyable book to read.

Watzlawick, P., Weakland, J., & Fisch, R. (1974). *Change.* New York: W. W. Norton.

Written by the early pioneers in family therapy and based on the work of Gregory Bateson and the Palo Alto project, this book provides the basic assumptions of one version of strategic brief therapy. Innovative interventions are presented that are consistent with these assumptions. Descriptions of how solutions can become problems and the concepts of first and second order change are presented.

REFERENCES

Alexander, J. F., & Parsons, B. (1973). Short term behavioral intervention with delinquent families: Impact on family process and recidivism. *Journal of Abnormal Psychology, 81,* 219-225.

Alexander, J. F., & Parsons, B. (1982). *Functional family therapy.* Monterey, CA: Brooks/Cole.

Bevolek, S. J., & Comstack, C. (1985). *Nurturing program for parents and children: Parents handbook.* Eau Claire, WI: Family Development Resources.

Carnes, P. (1981). *Understanding us.* Minneapolis, MN: Interpersonal Communication Programs.

Carter, B., & McGoldrick, M. (1988). *The changing family life cycle: A framework for family therapy* (2nd ed.). New York: Gardner Press.

Doherty, W. J., & Baird, M. A. (1983). *Family therapy and family medicine: Toward the primary care of families.* New York: Guilford Press.

Fine, M. E., & Holt, P. (1983). Intervening with school problems: A family systems perspective. *Psychology in the Schools, 20,* 59-66.

Fisher, B. L., Giblin, P. R., & Hoopes, M. H. (1982). Healthy family functioning. *Journal of Marital and Family Therapy, 8*(3), 273-284.

Friedman, R. (1969). A structured family interview in the assessment of school learning disorders. *Psychology in the Schools, 6,* 162-171.

Gantman, C. (1980). A closer look at families that work well. *International Journal of Family Therapy, 8,* 106-119.

Getz, H., & Gunn, W. B. (1988). Parent education from a family-systems perspective. *The School Counselor, 35,* 331-336.

Getz, H. E., & Morrill, R. (1978). SET! Student Effectiveness Training. *The Humanist Educator, 16,* 134-144.

Goldenberg, I., & Goldenberg, H. (1985). *Family therapy: An overview* (2nd ed.). Monterey, CA: Brooks/Cole.

Gunn, W. (1983). *The Pulaski project.* Unpublished manuscript.

Gurman, A. S., & Kniskern, D. P. (1978). Research on marital and family therapy: Progress, perspective and prospect. In S. L. Garfield & A. F. Bergin (Eds.), *Handbook of psychotherapy and behavior change* (2nd ed.). New York: Wiley.

Gurman, A. S., & Kniskern, D. P. (1981). *Handbook of family therapy.* New York: Brunner/Mazel.

Gurman, A. S., Kniskern, D. P., & Pinsof, W. (1986). Research on the process and outcome of marital and family therapy. In S. L. Garfield & A. E. Bergin (Eds.), *Handbook of psychotherapy and behavior change* (3rd ed.). New York: Wiley.

Haley, J. (1980). *Leaving home.* New York: McGraw-Hill.

Haley, J. (1987). *Problem-solving therapy.* San Francisco: Jossey-Bass.

Hoopes, M. H., Fisher, B. L., & Barlow, S. H. (1984). *Structured family facilitation programs.* Rockville, MD: Aspen Systems.

Klein, N. C., Alexander, J. F., & Parsons, B. V. (1977). Impact of family systems intervention on recidivism and sibling delinquency: A model of primary prevention and program evaluation. *Journal of Consulting and Clinical Psychology, 45,* 469-474.

Lacqueur, H. P. (1976). Multiple family therapy. In P. J. Guerin (Ed.), *Family therapy: Theory and practice.* New York: Gardner Press.

Levant, R. E., & Doyle, G. (1981). *Parent education for fathers: A personal developmental approach.* Unpublished manuscript, Boston University.

Lewis, J., Beavers, W. R., Gossett, J., & Phillips, V. (1976). *No single thread: Psychological health in family systems.* New York: Brunner/Mazel.

Madanes, C. (1981). *Strategic family therapy.* San Francisco: Jossey-Bass.

Minuchin, S. (1974). *Families and family therapy.* Cambridge, MA: Harvard University Press.

Minuchin, S., Baker, L., Rosman, B., Liebman, R., Milman, L., & Todd, T. (1975). A conceptual model of psychosomatic illness in children. *Archives of General Psychiatry, 32,* 1031-1038.

Minuchin, S., & Fishman, H. C. (1981). *Techniques of family therapy.* Cambridge, MA: Harvard University Press.

Minuchin, S., Rosman, B., & Baker, L. (1978). *Psychosomatic families: Anorexia nervosa in context.* Cambridge, MA: Harvard University Press.

Molnar, A. E., & Lindquist, B. (1984). Demons or angels? A lot depends on how you respond to misbehavior. *Learning, 13*(9), 22-26.

Nelson, T. S., Fleuridas, C., & Rosenthal, D. M. (1986). The evolution of circular questions: Training family therapists. *Journal of Marriage and Family Therapy, 12,* 113-127.

Parsons, B. V., & Alexander, J. F. (1973). Short term family intervention: A therapy outcome study. *Journal of Consulting and Clinical Psychology, 41,* 195-201.

Patterson, G. R. (1982). *Coercive family process.* Eugene, OR: Castalia.

Paul, G. L., (1967). Outcome research in psychotherapy. *Journal of Consulting Psychology, 31,* 109-188.

Sawin, M. (1979). *Family enrichment with family clusters.* Valley Forge, PA: Judson Press.

Selvini-Palazzoli, M., Boscolo, L., Cecchin, G., & Prata, G. (1977). Family rituals: A powerful tool in family therapy. *Family Process, 16,* 445-453.

Selvini-Palazzoli, M., Boscolo, L., Cecchin, G., & Prata, G. (1978). *Paradox and counterparadox.* New York: Jason-Aronson.

Selvini-Palazzoli, M., Boscolo, L., Cecchin, G., & Prata, G. (1980). Hypothesizing-circularity-neutrality. *Family Process, 19,* 73-85.

Stinnett, N. (1979). In search of strong families. In N. Stinnett, B. Chesser, & V. DeGrains (Eds.), *Building family strengths.* Lincoln: University of Nebraska Press.

Todd, T. C., & Stanton, M. D. (1983). Research on marital and family therapy: Answers, issues and recommendation for the future. In B. Wolman & G. Stricker (Eds.), *Handbook of family and marital therapy.* New York: Plenum.

Tomm, K. (1984). One perspective on the Milan systemic approach: Part I: Overview of development, theory and practice. *Journal of Marital and Family Therapy, 10*(2), 113-125.

Watzlawick, P., Weakland, J., & Fisch, R. (1974). *Principles of problem formation and problem resolution.* New York: W. W. Norton.

Chapter 10

Counseling and Psychotherapy with Handicapped Children and Adolescents

Harriet C. Cobb, Ed.D.

INTRODUCTION

In providing therapeutic intervention with the handicapped, the most important characteristics therapists and counselors must take into consideration are the child's thoughts, feelings, and individual strengths and weaknesses. In this respect, intervention is similar to that provided to nonhandicapped individuals. Given this framework, there are some special needs of handicapped children of which the child therapist, to be effective, must be aware. These include a number of special cognitive and physical characteristics which differentiate handicapped children from nonhandicapped.

Describing children on the basis of their handicapping conditions is a difficult task. Each of the groupings under the rubric "exceptional" dealt with in this chapter (mentally retarded, learning disabled, and physically handicapped) is extremely heterogeneous. Children must be recognized as individuals, each with many facets, with their handicap being only one facet of their personalities. The reader is directed to the reference section for additional information regarding specific characteristics of each handicap.

An important issue for child therapists is their own attitudes and feelings regarding the handicapped. Many studies have examined the perceptions of professionals toward disabled individuals (Cook, Kunce, & Getsinger, 1976; Greer, 1975; Ross, 1964; Yuker, Block, & Young, 1966). These studies show a clear relationship between the attitudes a given therapist holds for the handicapped and the effectiveness of the therapy he or she does with this population. The therapist's thoughts and feelings about a given handicapping condition have significant impact upon the behavior of the client. Nathanson (1979) describes several beliefs commonly held by professionals working with the disabled that can inhibit therapeutic intervention. First, a problem may arise if the therapist views the child only in terms of the label (e.g., mentally retarded, learning disabled, or physically handicapped) and provides treatment to the child based on preconceived notions related to that label. The counselor/therapist may tend to evaluate the child primarily on the basis of a unitary dimension, which may be related to a single aspect of the handicap such as lower intelligence. This perception may result in a disregard for other attributes of the child including interests, positive personality characteristics, social skills, and adaptive behavior. The uniqueness of the child as an individual may be undervalued, and stereotypes of what the handicapped can and cannot do may be imposed. The child may be wrongly assumed to conform to various limitations and potentials that have been imposed by the therapist as characteristic of a given label.

One of the most common feelings that many people, including professionals, have toward the handicapped is pity. The therapist's attention may be directed only toward the negative aspects of the child's life instead of the positive. The counselor may see the child as a "victim" in a despairing situation, and this attitude may prevent the child from focusing on his or her strengths and capabilities as well. The well-intentioned therapist may assume that the child or adolescent is less able to cope with frustrations and crises than he or she really is. Such an assumption may subsequently foster dependency—something the counselor would not instigate with a child considered to be nonhandicapped. Goals in therapy may be set too low, with the counselor/therapist projecting the attitude that, "If this were me, I don't know how I would manage."

The therapist may unconsciously reject the child because of a feeling of revulsion toward the handicap. These feelings may be manifested in avoidance or impatience and will interfere with establishing rapport. If the therapist has not had previous experience with handicapped children, feelings of anxiety and uncertainty may be present in the therapist despite the fact that the therapist may be quite competent to deal with other types of children.

It is not unusual for the child therapist to experience feelings of anxiety or pity when first encountering a handicapped child. As has been indicated above, these feelings are the prevailing attitudes held by society toward the disabled. It is, therefore, important for the therapist to examine his or her own attitudes about the handicapped and to modify them accordingly. In order to work effectively with handicapped children, therapists must monitor their own behavior in order to prevent beliefs from interfering with therapeutic efficacy. A primary step in this direction is for the counselor/therapist to acquire a basic working knowledge of the various handicapping conditions. It is also beneficial for therapists to undergo peer review of their therapeutic interventions for the purpose of receiving feedback regarding projections of attitudes in the therapeutic setting.

Within the therapeutic process itself, providing basic information about the handicapping condition to the child may be the most important component of the counseling process. This includes comprehensive information on the handicap itself—what it is and what it is not. Some children may be reluctant to voice their questions, and it is appropriate for the therapist to say something like, "Children who have a learning disability often ask . . ." This serves the dual purpose of helping the child put his or her thoughts into words, perhaps expressing the "worst fears," as well as letting him or her know that other children have similar questions and similar problems.

The conclusions that handicapped children formulate about their handicap have a profound impact on their total self-concept. These conclusions are usually based on the reactions of parents, peers, teachers, or others to the handicap, reactions that may vary from complete acceptance to total rejection. These children may experience feelings of unhappiness in relation to any limitations imposed by the handicap. In addition, they may have unrealistic goals, and it may be a slow and painful process to assist them in coming to terms with any real limitations. In some children, the unhappiness about the handicap may become so severe that the behaviors exhibited can be considered manifestations of depression. Depression often occurs in children who experience a personal loss. The knowledge regarding limitations imposed by a handicap may constitute a severe loss of certain goals and opportunities for these children.

Although knowledge of the categorical condition, such as mental retardation or learning disabilities, is necessary, it is not sufficient for providing effective intervention. The special learning, emotional, or behavioral characteristics accompanying the handicap, in addition to the unique attributes of the individual child, are critical aspects in providing therapy. Knowledge of normal developmental changes experienced by children is crucial in working with handicapped children as well as with the nonhandicapped. However, in addition, therapists must accommodate their own approaches to the special needs of handicapped children.

As an example, let's consider how this accommodation would apply in the case of a mentally retarded child. A mentally retarded child will possess more limited cognitive ability, and, therefore, a more concrete approach may be required. Mentally retarded individuals learn at a slower rate, and their overall maturity level may be lower than that of their nonretarded peers. The child's experiential background and vocabulary may be restricted, and thus the expressive vocabulary utilized by the therapist must be adjusted. Attention span is often shorter, and this fact, in combination with distractibility, may limit the length of therapy sessions. In addition, the therapist may need to make a concerted effort to reinforce the child's attending behaviors and to provide additional structure in order to manage other unwanted behaviors exhibited by the child.

The use of role playing and behavior rehearsal is often more appropriate with the retarded in order to facilitate the attainment of therapeutic goals such as the acquisition of social skills. Skill in social interaction may be the most important affective goal for some handicapped children. The perception by others of their relative level of impairment is directly influenced by their set of social skills.

Similar considerations must be made when the therapist is dealing with the learning disabled and physically handicapped. Attention span, distractibility, physical stamina, neurological impairment, and perceptual disorganization are all factors which will require modification in the therapeutic process. The ability of the therapist to estimate the impact of these disabilities on personality functioning is a major aspect of the diagnostic process prior to therapeutic intervention. The remainder of this chapter will be devoted to detailing specific considerations in providing therapy to handicapped children and their parents. In addition, a number of therapeutic interventions will be discussed.

SPECIAL NEEDS OF HANDICAPPED CHILDREN

Neely (1982) has listed four issues that commonly arise in the counseling of handicapped children. These issues are self-other relations, self-conflict, maladaptive behavior, and a need for vocational counseling. These concerns may be experienced by nondisabled children as well but are particularly pertinent to the handicapped. As DeBlassie and Cowan (1976) pointed out, handicapped children face greater numbers of frustrations, are misunderstood and rejected more often, and have greater difficulty developing positive self-concepts.

Handicapped children may be confronted with prejudice and stereotypes about their disability and may be subjected to excessive teasing by classmates. Counselors must be prepared to assist these children in learning to cope with attitudes that may be cruel or that impose unnecessary limitations on opportunities for certain experiences. Facilitating the development of a healthy self-concept in these children may be a major task of the therapist. Helping them accept the handicap and see themselves as capable human beings often allows them some "immunity" from ridicule or the results of stereotyping. Therapists may find it necessary to involve the parents in learning to accept these children's handicaps and in learning to communicate confidence in their capabilities. Whether or not these children have been mainstreamed with nonhandicapped peers, the awareness of being "different" or perceived as different may take its toll on building positive relationships with others. Group counseling can provide the ideal situation for helping handicapped children develop skills in relating to others as well as experiencing the feeling of not being alone. In some cases, including nonhandicapped children in the group can further the process of normalization because it exposes normal children to the handicapped and simultaneously provides a shared experience. Through social learning, handicapped children learn more normalized forms of behavior.

Group counseling can also offer the opportunity for learning appropriate social skills such as tact, assertiveness, or making conversation (Staggs, 1979). Because maladaptive behaviors are often associated with certain handicaps, social skills training is a commonly used approach among counselors and others who work with mentally retarded or learning disabled children (Brannigan & Young, 1978; LaGreca & Mesibov, 1979; Zigmond & Brownlee, 1980).

Maladaptive behaviors such as impulsivity and distractibility may not only be characteristics of some handicapped children but may also be targeted for modification and counseling. Meichenbaum (1977) described a cognitive behavioral method of decreasing impulsivity using verbal rehearsal and fading. These techniques are discussed in detail in Chapter 6.

Making the appropriate match between therapeutic method and the specific problem while taking into consideration the implication of the handicap itself can be a challenge to the counselor. It is important for the therapist to keep in mind that any learning situation, even with a trusted adult, can be anxiety producing for children who have experienced failure with academic or other tasks that involve learning something new. Furthermore, therapists must be aware that because of the special characteristics of mentally handicapped children, many situations will be new and unfamiliar to these children (Shontz, 1980). Guaranteeing success by proceeding in small steps, along with keeping expectations for change realistic, is an appropriate approach not only for teachers and parents but for therapists.

Self-conflicts experienced by handicapped children referred to by Neely (1982) include anxiety, frustration, lack of motivation, and depression. Often these problems are a result of feelings of inadequacy brought about by repeated failure experiences. Although handicapped children have the same fears as other children, worries about being accepted by others or doing well in school can be exacerbated for disabled children. Therapists can draw from a variety of techniques found to be successful in coping with anxiety. These include relaxation training, RET, and other behavioral techniques. Frustration is often experienced by handicapped children who have repeatedly had their goals thwarted. Sometimes this frustration results from misinformation or lack of information provided by adults. It may also result from unrealistic expectations that these children may have for themselves. Although children respond differently to frustration – some with aggressiveness, others with depression or apathy – all need to acquire skills to cope with frustrating events. It is often in this context that therapists must provide basic information about handicapping conditions to the children as well as to the parents. For example, in the case of the mentally retarded or the physically handicapped child, sexuality may be an issue avoided by well-meaning adults who feel uncomfortable with this topic. Specially written materials about sexuality can be used as part of the information-giving process (Gordon, 1975).

Handicapped children may feel overwhelmed by the implications of their handicaps and will need help in removing barriers to success, as well as support in learning how to tolerate obstacles that cannot be removed. If at first handicapped children feel that any goal is impossible to attain, this may be reflected in "unmotivated" behavior. Again, helping the child to formulate realistic goals (assuming the goals of parents and teachers are not unrealistic either) is the appropriate course to take.

Depression in handicapped children may be manifested in feelings of unworthiness, apathy, and withdrawal; or it may be masked, manifesting itself as aggressive behavior, just as it occurs in nondisabled children. Children who fail to come to terms with any limitations imposed by their handicap may experience a sense of personal loss. The therapist can be in a position to help these children through the stages of grief that may be associated with this sense of loss.

Once children have accepted their handicaps, the need for acquiring decision-making skills is usually apparent, particularly when the time for choosing a career approaches. The counselor should be aware of instruments specifically designed for individuals with handicaps to measure interests and abilities, such as the Reading Free Vocational Interest Inventory (Becker, 1975) or the Social and Prevocational Information Battery (Halpern, Raffield, Irvin, & Link, 1975). Vocational counseling and teaching decision-making skills are important components of therapy with handicapped adolescents. Career satisfaction is a major part of emotional stability. For the retarded, career choices are limited and must be carefully examined.

Furthermore, handicapped children or adolescents will encounter the same developmental changes and/or life stressors that nonhandicapped individuals experience, such as the birth of a sibling, moving, a divorce, or a death in the family. Handicapped children may need extra assistance in understanding and coping with such crises. Deutsch (1985) reminds us that handicapped individuals develop attachments and experience losses throughout their lives, too. Like other individuals, they will enter a period of mourning for which they are completely unprepared. Their poorer adaptive skills make it difficult enough to cope with everyday stress, let alone the loss of a significant interpersonal relationship. The therapist can be helpful in assisting handicapped clients through the grief process with educative counseling, catharsis, and specific cognitive-behavior techniques (Deutsch, 1985).

THE LEARNING-DISABLED CHILD

The current definition of a learning disability found in Public Law 94-142 (Education for All Handicapped Children Act), is as follows:

> Specific Learning Disability means a disorder in one or more of the basic psychological processes involved in the understanding of language, spoken or written, which may manifest itself in an imperfect ability to listen, speak, read, write, spell, or to do mathematical calculations. The term includes such conditions as perceptual handicaps, brain injury, minimal brain dysfunction, dyslexia, and other developmentally caused disorders. The term does not include children who have learning problems which

> are primarily the result of visual, hearing, or motor handicaps, or mental retardation, emotional disturbance, or environmental, cultural, or economic disadvantage.[1]

Although there is some controversy over the exact nature and etiology of learning disabilities, a child is generally diagnosed on the basis of school performance as evidenced by a problem with academic achievement. If achievement level falls significantly below that which would be predicted by aptitude measures, a learning disability is suspected of being the cause. Incidence figures for learning-disabled children range from 1% to 15%, but most professionals consider 2% to 3% to be the most realistic estimate.

Several characteristics have been included in the symptomology of learning-disabled children. The most frequently cited, according to Bryan and Bryan (1978), are:

1. Hyperactivity.
2. Perceptual motor impairment.
3. Emotional lability.
4. General coordination deficits.
5. Attention disorders (either distractibility or perseveration).
6. Impulsivity.
7. Memory or thinking disorders.
8. Specific learning disabilities in reading, arithmetic, or spelling.
9. Difficulty in understanding or remembering spoken language.
10. Equivocal or "soft" neurological signs.

Ross (1974) suggests that learning-disabled children may be classified into two groups. The first group consists of children who have long-term, chronic disabilities which are secondary

---

[1]Federal Register 42, number 250, December 29, 1977, 65083.

to other conditions such as infantile autism and childhood schizophrenia. This group must receive instructional remediation directed both toward the specific learning disabilities and toward their more global emotional disturbance. The second group consists of children who develop specific learning disabilities after they have entered school. These disabilities may be associated with other emotional stress reactions such as separation anxiety, school phobia, and mild depression.

Although not all learning-disabled children will possess the characteristics described above, most will exhibit at least one or more of these behaviors. The child therapist must make modifications in technique in order to accommodate the special needs of learning-disabled clients. As Morse (1977) pointed out, specialized knowledge of specific learning disabilities and the ability to be flexible and creative are essential skills for working with the learning-disabled child. As with the mentally retarded, a shorter attention span and distractibility mean that it may be necessary to hold briefer sessions. The sessions may also need to be more structured and to include a greater amount of "activity-oriented" material. Depending on the nature of the learning disability, the therapist may need to identify the best means of communicating with these children. For example, with a child who is distractible with auditory short-term memory deficits, it may be helpful to make notes or list in writing the major points covered in each session. These should be commensurate with the child's vocabulary level and reviewed with the child. If the child has difficulty reading, it is possible to use pictures of objects, rebus symbols, signs, or letters, which suggest words or phrases in place of the usual written word. If, for example, the therapist is attempting to work with the child in meeting the goal of completion of household chores, it might be helpful to use a series of pictures representing various chores. For the child with memory or organizational problems, using a written list of chores may be helpful. This list can be attached to the child's desk or bedroom door as a visible reminder of his or her commitment.

Because learning-disabled children are often emotionally labile and erratic in their behavior patterns, progress in therapy may be somewhat slower than with nonhandicapped children.

Therapists may see gains made one day only to watch these children regress by the time the next session is held. Although this seesawing can be true of all children in a therapy situation, it is especially common with the learning disabled. The fact that learning-disabled children have difficulty with attention span, concept formation, motor control, and communication skills hinders many common therapeutic interventions. Often intervention must focus on these variables at the same time that counseling occurs.

CASE STUDY OF A LEARNING-DISABLED CHILD

Timmy was a 9-year-old fourth grader who had been identified as learning disabled. Timmy was very bright and creative, but his extreme distractibility and lack of organizational skills negatively affected his daily classroom performance. Furthermore, although family relationships were quite positive, Timmy was rather manipulative and had become a management problem at home. The school psychologist saw Timmy on a regular basis for 4 months. In addition, monthly sessions were held with his parents over that period of time.

The goals of the intervention were to increase Timmy's "on-task" behavior in the classroom and to reduce some of the parent-child conflict which occurred in the home. A checklist for keeping track of acceptable behaviors was developed with the parents. In addition, the teacher's and Timmy's active participation were also solicited. Points for on-task behavior were accumulated and spent on extra art time, one of Timmy's favorite activities. A separate checklist was made for home that included jobs such as helping to set the table and going to bed without a fuss. The parents were also advised to participate in a STEP group (Systematic Training for Effective Parenting, described in Chapter 4), which they were able to join during the latter part of the intervention period.

Timmy began each session very excitedly, talking about whatever was on his mind (the subject usually did relate to the goals of the intervention). After a brief period set aside for "catch-up" talk, Timmy was then taught progressive relaxation in order to acquire calming behavior. He was encouraged to use this in the classroom when he was feeling particularly jumpy and restless. Like many learning-disabled children (and many non-disabled children), Timmy had difficulty remembering to use his new skill of relaxing, which he had learned rather quickly. The teacher agreed to give Timmy a discreet hand signal for when it was time for him to "calm down." In addition, Timmy was taught self-talk strategies as described by Meichenbaum (1977), which he used with a worksheet in order to increase accuracy. After 3 months of weekly sessions practicing relaxation and self-talk, as well as setting new goals, Timmy had significantly increased his on-task behavior in the classroom. Participation in the STEP program enabled his parents to learn to avoid power struggles with Timmy, and he was able to reach his weekly goals by the third month fairly easily.

The intervention program with Timmy was implemented with full knowledge that his distractibility and lack of organization would interfere. Sessions were kept quite brief (20 minutes) although most 9-year-olds are capable of maintaining concentration for longer periods of time. Timmy's catch-up talk time was structured, and a timer was set so Timmy could see when it was time to work. The checklists at school were taped to his desk, and at home they were displayed on the refrigerator door. Both his parents and teacher had additional copies, so losing a checklist did not interrupt the weekly goals nor cause time to be lost in looking for a list. Toward the end of the session, points were given to Timmy for not losing checklists. The teacher's hand signal for relaxation was needed throughout the intervention period. Although she used it less frequently as the school year progressed, it still continued to be needed occasionally.

The counseling sessions were held in the school psychologist's office, and it was necessary to remove materials from the office desk in order to minimize distractibility for Timmy. The long-term goal for the intervention was to fade many of the cues utilized for calming behavior gradually and, concurrently, to increase the level and quality of Timmy's attention span.

THE MENTALLY RETARDED CHILD

The definition of mental retardation given by the American Association of Mental Deficiency (AAMD) (Grossman, 1973) is as follows:

> Mental retardation refers to significantly subaverage general intellectual functioning existing concurrently with deficits in adaptive behavior, and manifested during the developmental period. (p. 122)

Within this general definition there are four levels of retardation recognized by the AAMD: mild, moderate, severe, and profound; educators usually refer to the terms *educable, trainable,* and *severe/profound.* Approximately 3% of the U.S. population is considered mentally retarded. There are specific characteristics of retarded children that do have implications for counseling.

A primary difference between retarded and nonretarded children is the speed and efficiency with which they learn (Robinson & Robinson, 1965). Attention span and memory are two components of the learning process which may be particularly affected. In addition, the adaptive behavior of a retarded child is significantly below that of comparable chronologically aged peers. This is particularly evident in the areas of social interaction, self-help skills, motor development, and affective development. Furthermore, the acquisition of basic concepts by the retarded is significantly slowed and may be totally absent in the more severely involved individuals. It is this lack of concept development that limits the therapeutic interventions which may be utilized with the retarded.

Mentally retarded children often have difficulty focusing their attention on a given stimulus and may exhibit hyperdistractible behavior. Their memory processes tend to be limited and unpredictable. Short-term memory processes which fluctuate erratically may prevent or slow down the learning of new tasks and skills. The long-term memory of a retarded child may be as good as that of a nonhandicapped child, but the presence of short-term memory deficits results in much slower acquisition of new material.

Mentally retarded children experience the same emotional and social problems as other children. Parental pressure, peer conflicts, sibling rivalry, and other childhood stresses are common among the retarded. However, the retarded child's cognitive ability limits the variety of responses to these situations. The level of "formal operations" characterized by abstract thinking which begins to manifest itself in adolescence may never be attained by a retarded child. Thus, complex cognitive solutions to social interaction problems are beyond the capability of most retarded individuals. Because their thinking is more concrete, problem-solving skills must concentrate on areas which can be easily remembered. Solutions which have a focus far into the future will not be easily acquired by a retarded person. This difficulty means that coping with developmental changes or unexpected crises is a much more difficult process for the retarded child than for the normal child. The ability of the retarded child to predict the future is severely limited by his or her lack of conceptual development.

Language deficits are much more common in the retarded than in normal children. Verbal expression is less elaborate, and repetitive or perseverative language is quite common. Commonly, receptive language is significantly better than expressive language. The social and emotional development of the retarded child often lags behind his or her nonretarded peers. Although physical development may not differ, the retarded child's ability to understand and cope with physiological changes or limitations may be limited. Adaptive behavior deficits are an integral part of the definition of mental retardation. Therefore, the child's level of independence from adults in the areas of self-help and vocational competence may be significantly delayed. The role of the parents in therapy is even more critical for retarded children and adolescents than it is for young nonretarded clients.

Selwa (1971) suggests several considerations for psychotherapy with retarded children. Therapeutic interventions must be structured around concrete situations and elements. The verbal comprehensive and expressive abilities of the child must define the parameters of the language used by the therapist. This means that time must be spent in formally evaluating the expressive and receptive language skills of the child *prior* to therapeutic intervention. The use of materials and play media such as clay, painting, toys, and puppets may be appropriate even for adolescent retardates in order to help them dramatize problems, fears, and anxieties which they feel.

A more directive approach is often recommended for clients with cognitive limitations. As Hurley and Hurley (1986) point out, the therapist sets the agenda, and generally provides more structure than necessary with a nonhandicapped child. During the initial interview, the therapist needs to take extra care in introducing him- or herself and explaining what counseling is in language the child will understand. The therapist must educate the client as concretely as possible regarding (1) how often the sessions will take place, (2) what generally will occur during the sessions, (3) what will be expected of the client between sessions, and (4) under what circumstances the child can request an emergency session.

The therapist must be careful to ascertain how the child is conceptualizing his or her problem. This determination may involve actually teaching the child vocabulary words such as those related to emotional expression. Because of the child's attention and short-term memory deficits, the counselor may find it necessary to apply the principle of "overlearning." This means that complex tasks will need to be segmented and rehearsed over a long period of time before they are finally mastered. The use of repetition is critical in assisting the child in generalizing newly acquired coping skills to situations outside the therapy room.

Sessions may need to be shorter and more heavily structured around activities than with the nonretarded child. Because retarded children usually learn more slowly, the frequency of sessions may need to be increased and actual behavior change may take longer to establish.

A long-standing stereotype of the mentally retarded suggests that group counseling and therapy are not appropriate intervention techniques. Several studies have indicated, however, that the retarded can benefit from this method of intervention. Humes, Adamczyk, and Myco (1969) found that group counseling resulted in better adjustment for educable mentally retarded adolescents, as seen in teacher ratings on a behavioral scale. Blohm (1978) found that self-concept can be as difficult to change in the mentally retarded as it is with other children. However, group counseling did improve three of thirteen personality factors for moderately retarded elementary school children. Welch and Sigman (1980) also recommended using group therapy with mentally retarded adolescents. They specifically suggest that the therapist take a very active role in structuring therapy and that this therapy include nonverbal activities. They cite the advantages of group therapy as providing the mentally retarded adolescent contact with peers and a sense of belonging to a peer group, the availability of behavioral models, greater opportunities for feedback, and improvement in participants' verbal skills. Selwa (1971) suggests using homogeneity in intellectual level in the grouping of retarded children for therapy, because retardates of the same chronological age may differ significantly in mental maturity. The therapy session should concentrate on a series of operationally defined objectives. In addition, the length of sessions should be shorter than those normally used with nonretarded children.

Group work should be concrete, focused in the present, and realistic (Wells & Allan, 1985). As with nonhandicapped clients, group counseling can teach members to express thoughts and feelings, understand themselves and others, and learn new behaviors. It affords the handicapped child or adolescent the opportunity to feel a sense of "belongingness" to a group, reducing feelings of isolation and loneliness. Wells and Allen (1985) describe a group counseling program in a school setting for secondary-aged mentally retarded students. The program specifically addressed the issues of experiencing failure and how to cope with it. Activities were divided into two types: listening and memory games, and discussions of memories around a set topic, such as "feeling embarrassed." These sharing-of-memories sessions were preceded by a discussion with the leader always modeling the first response. At one point, nonhandicapped students were invited to share difficult experiences, which demonstrated the potential benefits of self-disclosure in a supportive setting.

Although most efficacy studies with the mildly retarded utilize behavioral and directive approaches, at least two studies (Davidson, 1975; Hayes, 1977) used a psychoanalytic approach in an effective manner with the mentally retarded. This approach was developed on the basis of Anna Freud's developmental theory rather than traditional Freudian therapy.

CASE STUDY OF A MENTALLY RETARDED ADOLESCENT

Tracy was a 14-year-old girl identified as mildly mentally retarded who was referred for counseling by the social services department. A number of incidents regarding sexual abuse had been brought to their attention. Tracy had become withdrawn in school, and her mother complained that Tracy "didn't listen to her the way she used to."

Tracy was seen by the psychologist for a period of 6 months on a regular basis for individual counseling; she also participated in group counseling. Tracy was quite withdrawn at first, avoiding eye contact and rarely speaking. It became apparent that she was operating on a very concrete level and was extremely confused about the incidents of sexual abuse which had precipitated her referral. Although she had attained sexual maturity at the age of 12, her knowledge of sexuality and reproduction was almost nonexistent. Her verbal expressive skills were extremely deficient and this lack, in combination with her reluctance to talk, made developing communication with her a very slow process. Because of her limited verbal skills, drawings were used extensively as a means of communicating. In order to elicit expression of feelings it was easier to request that she draw a picture of "what was on her mind." Large portions of the early sessions were spent in attempting to expel some of the misperceptions Tracy had about sexual abuse. For example, she believed that because she was first molested at the age of 7, pregnancy could ensue at any time. She also believed that these incidents had caused one of her breasts to be larger than the other. A sex education booklet that was intended specifically for mentally retarded adolescents was used to aid in explaining relevant points about sexuality to Tracy. Role playing was also a frequently used technique in helping Tracy to acquire coping and social skills. Conflict resolution methods were role-played, and Tracy was encouraged to use them at home (a social worker was working closely with Tracy's parents during this time). Coaching and social reinforcement were effective in facilitating the development of the skills in Tracy, although it took several months before any noticeable changes were made. When Tracy appeared to be ready for further peer interaction, group counseling was initiated. Tracy and four other girls (with cognitive functioning in the mildly retarded to borderline range) met with the psychologist for eight sessions on a weekly basis. At least one of the other girls had been sexually abused; the others had not has this experience. However, as with nonretarded adolescents, the major issues dealt with in the sessions were parent conflicts and relationships with peers. Feelings of universality and cohesiveness developed rather quickly in the group. Tracy participated somewhat reluctantly at first but soon responded positively to the others and developed a close relationship with one of the other group members. Tracy maintained friendships with the girls in the group after the sessions had ended. For Tracy, a major turning point in her progress occurred when one of the girls invited Tracy to spend the night at her house. Although conflicts with her parents continued to exist from time to time, Tracy's mother reported that they were getting along better and Tracy had become more cooperative at home.

THE PHYSICALLY HANDICAPPED CHILD

The term *physically handicapped* includes several different conditions which are congenital, accidental, or disease related. These conditions result in the individual being physically limited. Physically handicapped children are those whose nonsensory physical limitations or health problems interfere with their school attendance or learning to such an extent that special services, training, equipment, or materials are required (Hallahan & Kauffman, 1978). The incidence of physically handicapped school-age children is approximately 0.5%, as estimated by the U.S. Department of Education. Causes may be prenatal, associated with perinatal or maternal factors, genetic factors, accidents, or infections, or in some cases there may be an idiopathic etiology.

The physically handicapped are such a heterogeneous group that generalizations are impossible to make. As Neely (1982) points out, these children may have normal intelligence or may be mentally handicapped as well as having other sensory impairments. Some physically handicapped children have adapted well to their disability, although others experience considerable difficulty in this regard. Therefore, with this population, particular care must be taken by the counselor to view each child in relation to the specific handicapping condition and to generate the therapeutic approach which focuses on strengths and coping strategies commensurate with the handicap.

The developmental process of disengaging from the family may be especially difficult for the physically handicapped adolescent because the issue of dependence/independence becomes more complicated than is the case for teenagers with no limitations. The therapist needs to be sensitive to the ambivalent feelings of the adolescent as well as of the parents. This is particularly important if the handicapped adolescent acquired his or her handicap adventitiously as opposed to congenitally. Family involvement may be crucial at this stage in the intervention process.

CASE STUDY OF A PHYSICALLY HANDICAPPED ADOLESCENT

Betty was a 16-year-old girl who had recently been in an automobile accident. The accident resulted in her being paraplegic and confined to a wheelchair. She had previously been extremely active in sports and in the high school drama club. In the first year after the accident, she received instruction at home in addition to physical therapy. Betty's family was extremely supportive, and several members of the community as well as her friends visited her frequently. Betty and her family appeared to be adjusting to the handicap very well for the first two years. As time went on, however, Betty became increasingly demanding of attention and was referred for counseling by her parents when she began to display "childish" temper tantrums. The psychologist saw Betty and her family on a regular basis for a period of 2 months.

It became apparent rather quickly that much of the problem was related to Betty's complete dependence on her family. The accident occurred at the time when normally an adolescent would be establishing independence from the parents as part of adult behavior. Betty's family had fallen into the role of anticipating every need for her and had begun doing things for her that she was quite capable of doing for herself. In addition, her sense of personal identity and autonomy were diminished. These issues were dealt with openly in the family session, and roles were modified with Betty taking more responsibility for herself and contributing her share to running the household. During individual sessions, Betty was given information about vocational opportunities based on her expressed interests and capabilities. Counseling was terminated when Betty began contracting her services with a local store which sold crafts and artwork.

PARENT EDUCATION

It has been pointed out elsewhere in this book that the child therapist must always acknowledge the parent role in therapeutic intervention. Regardless of theoretical orientation, the etiology of many childhood disorders involves parent-child and parent-parent interactions. With handicapped children, the role of the parent may be even more significant. For example, parents of retarded children often have difficulty accepting realistically the limitations placed on their child by this condition. In addition, some parents may feel responsible for the child's disability. This situation places an added burden of guilt on these parents and increases the degree of family involvement which may be necessary in order to work effectively with the individual handicapped child.

A major component of the counseling relationship with parents of the handicapped is that of information giving (Burggraf, 1979). This information can be provided within the context of a group parent training session or on an individual basis. Answering questions regarding the assessment process and current developmental functioning of the child, and explanation of unfamiliar terminology, is very helpful. In addition, the procedures for gaining access to other resources such as advocacy groups are usually perceived as very useful by parents. This information can be incorporated into training sessions intermittently in order to avoid overloading parents with too much data at one time. The therapist must be prepared for the ventilation of frustrations and complaints about other professionals and be able to handle such outpourings appropriately. Comprehensive knowledge about handicapping conditions is essential for the therapist to work effectively with parents and families of handicapped children. Therefore, the therapist must have training and expertise in the etiology and psychoeducational implications of various handicapping conditions. It is particularly helpful for the therapist to have a thorough knowledge of community resources and facilities for this population.

Parents of handicapped children experience a number of unique problems associated with their children. Murray (1973) has described six of the most common difficulties experienced by parents. These include:

1. Accepting that the child is handicapped.
2. Coping with the increased financial responsibility associated with certain physical handicaps.
3. Coping with stress built up by carrying a burden that cannot be adequately shared with others.
4. Facing the conflict and ambivalence they may have regarding their handicapped child.
5. Planning for the education and perhaps lifetime care of their handicapped child.
6. Coping with attitudes and sometimes ill-timed or inept advice that they may receive from others.

Training needs for the parents of the handicapped are often more extensive for the above reasons. Parents want specific information about how to foster cognitive and/or social development in order to have their child's behavior approach that of other, nondisabled children. They often want to know the relationship of personality characteristics and cognitive abilities to the specific handicap. Some parents want information about aiding their child in developing as much autonomy and independence as possible. They may want information about realistic alternatives that may aid their child in making decisions about vocational training, careers, and other independent living concerns.

Improving parent-child communication and behavior management training are often major needs of parents with handicapped children. Approaches to parent training described earlier in this book have been applied to parents of handicapped children with considerable success. One parent involvement project utilized a group discussion with an Adlerian approach in dealing with the parents of the mentally retarded and multihandicapped (Yura, Zuckerman, Betz, & Newman, 1979). School personnel observed the group discussions in order to align home and classroom behavior management strategies closely. The participants attended eight biweekly sessions which focused on understanding child behavior and developing democratic parenting skills. The examination of pre- and postbehavior checklists indicated that parents showed more positive attitudes toward their children and had fewer problems with behavior as a result of this training.

Yura and colleagues (1979, p. 219) have designed a specific training program for parents of exceptional children that includes eight structured sessions. The content of these sessions is presented below.

Session 1: Introduction to the parent study group.

Topics

A. Philosophy of study groups.

B. How your parent study group will run.

C. Ground rules of your parent study group.

D. Setting your goals.

Learning Activity:

A. Goal chart to emphasize goal writing (specifies family goals as well as goals pertaining to the exceptional child's behavior).

Session 2: Basic principles in child development.

Topics:

A. Child-rearing in contemporary society.

B. Development of behavior patterns in children.

C. Characteristics of exceptional children.
D. Behavior patterns of exceptional children.
E. Characteristics of parents of exceptional children.
F. The exceptional child: Effects on other children.

Learning Activities:

A. Parental feeling chart (helps the parent identify non-constructive feelings that interfere with developing a positive parent-child relationship).
B. Chart identifying characteristics of handicapped that influence misbehavior (helps the parent be aware of factors that affect the child's misbehavior and, therefore, factors that may affect remedial procedures).

Session 3: Basic principles in dealing with exceptional children.

Topics:

A. Purpose of misbehavior.
B. Encouraging positive behavior.
C. Logical consequences.
D. Natural consequences.

Learning Activities:

A. Chart identifying purpose of misbehavior (helps parent understand purpose of child's actions).
B. Chart developing a logical or natural consequence (helps parent plan corrective measure).
C. Encouragement chart (helps insure positive parental recognition of child).

Session 4: Implementation of basic principles.

Topic:

A. Review previous week's learning activity.

Learning Activity:

A. Chart developing a logical and natural consequence

(helps parent clarify or modify previously established corrective measure).

Session 5: Guidelines to raising exceptional children.

Topics:

A. Avoid drastic routine change.

B. Consistency: A key factor in changing misbehaviors.

C. A stitch in time saves nine.

D. Actions speak louder than words.

E. The bathroom technique: A lesson in positive withdrawal.

F. Avoid reinforcing negative behavior.

Learning Activity:

A. Parent encouragement chart (a self-monitoring method designed for parents to encourage themselves).

Session 6: Positive parental attitudes.

Topics:

A. Good parents are allowed to say no.

B. Encourage independence.

C. Children's greatest handicap: Overprotection.

D. How to communicate with children.

Learning Activity:

A. Communication diagrams (provides parents with a visual representation of how certain parental responses maintain a child's mistaken goal and what parental responses will not reinforce this mistaken goal).

Session 7: Family atmosphere.

Topics:

A. Include the other children.

B. Have fun as a family.

C. The weekly family council meeting.

D. Enjoy your child.

Learning Activities:

A. Encouragement chart (same as Session 3).

B. Initiate a family council checklist (assists parents in following democratic guidelines during initial council meeting).

Session 8: Re-examining goals.

Topic:

A. Re-examining goals from Session 1.

Tavormina (1975) found that both behavioral and reflective group counseling were effective with parents of mentally retarded children. Several outcome criteria, including direct observation, attitudinal scales, maternal reports, and frequency counts, were used to measure success. Although both approaches had beneficial effects as compared with untreated controls, the behavioral method resulted in a significantly greater degree of improvement. This approach used the programmed text *Parents Are Teachers: A Child Management Program* by Becker (1971). The group leaders emphasized using praise, focusing on positive behaviors exhibited by the children, and the need to identify and observe clearly behaviors targeted for change. The leaders structured the group around discussion, role playing, and modeling. Each mother was encouraged to try these new techniques and was given feedback to assist in developing improved parenting skills.

Each parent in Tavormina's reflective group received a copy of *Between Parent and Child* by Ginott (1965). The discussion centered around communicating empathy, acceptance, and understanding when relating to children. The leaders also focused on reflecting feelings, setting limits, and providing appropriate alternative activities. Each mother within the group was asked to share her experiences and problems with other group members and to apply Ginott's principles to her own situation at home.

Brown and Cobb (1978) have developed a parent training module for training foster care parents of the retarded. The program is designed to train foster care providers of the mentally retarded in basic behavioral principles. This includes fundamental behavior management, social skills training, and affective intervention. The program is divided into six training sessions which cover such areas as basic concepts of mental retardation, the needs of the mentally retarded, and a comprehensive practicum experience for application of didactic content. A number of criteria are utilized to select potential foster care trainees. These include acceptance of the mentally retarded, previous experience with exceptional populations, a reasonable level of cognitive development, and the ability to be patient, consistent, and warm toward their foster child. Unlike many other foster care programs, continuous follow-up after training is provided in order to assure that behavioral principles are being carried out consistently and accurately.

Group counseling is part of Bricklan's approach to working with parents of learning-disabled children (1970). She suggests grouping parents who have similar-aged children and who are having similar problems. Within the group, parents are able to see their child from a different (in some cases, more positive) perspective. Furthermore, they are given the opportunity, perhaps for the first time, of knowing that they are not alone in experiencing these problems. Bricklan provides parents with basic information about various sources of stress for children and parents. After reviewing this information, parents become more aware of the causes of stress and are able to deal with them more effectively. In addition, a major goal of this activity is to demonstrate to parents that they are not entirely responsible for their child's behavior. Bricklan advocates using the group as a forum for assisting parents in learning how to set appropriate limits, communicating effectively with their children, and influencing their children's behavior in a positive manner. Critical to Bricklan's approach is the provision of basic information to parents about the nature, etiology, and prognosis of learning disabilities. Additionally, the parents are encouraged to express their feelings about their child, the school, and other aspects of their lives that have been influenced by their learning-disabled child. Specific listening and observing skills are taught to the participants in order to help them develop improved parenting techniques.

Another method of counseling parents of learning-disabled children is described by Adamson (1979). He advocates a three-dimensional model which focuses on helping parents direct the individual habilitation of their child.

"Educative counseling," the first dimension, instructs parents in the methodology of structuring their home in order to provide the child with external controls until the child is able to develop internal controls. Adamson recommends stressing routine, regularity, and repetition, as well as reducing the child's role in decision making until he or she is ready to handle this process. The structure is imposed in order to break what Adamson refers to as the "inadequacy cycle." In this cycle the child attempts various tasks and fails, which reinforces feelings of inadequacy. The child's frustration results in efforts to manipulate his or her parents, either by becoming aggressive or by expressing excessive dependency toward them. The parents may respond by increasing demands, and the family system may become distorted with feelings of despair, anger, or overinvolvement. The objective of educative counseling is to break this cycle.

"Interpretive counseling," the second dimension, emphasizes acceptance and expression of feelings on the part of both parents and the child. The primary focus is on developing awareness and skill in positive communication. Parents are encouraged to work through the emotions they have experienced and to focus on the present.

"Habilitative input," the third dimension, encourages parents to become involved in their children's education in a supportive manner. The parents are discouraged from overinvesting in their children's learning. They are strongly encouraged to hold realistic expectations regarding their children's potential progress. The overall goal of Adamson's technique is to develop responsibility within the handicapped child through the three-dimensional approach described above. This is accomplished by intervention with both parents and child but with the major focus being that of modifying parental patterns which reinforce cyclically destructive behavior on the part of the child.

PARENT COUNSELING/FAMILY THERAPY

The birth or later acknowledgment of a handicapped child, particularly if the impairment is severe, often has a significant impact on the entire family as well as the parents of the child. The degree to which it is seen as a crisis depends on whether or not family members perceive the event as changing their lives in an undesirable manner (Turner, 1980). Parents have been described as progressing through the stages of grieving for personal loss of a perfect child and of experiencing "chronic sorrow" (Olshansky, 1970). Parents usually need assistance in working through their reactions to their child's handicapping condition. Most agencies (especially the public schools) serving handicapped children are primarily child-centered and may inadvertently neglect the needs of the parents. It is especially important for the professional involved to provide follow-up over an extended period of time to the parents. It is not realistic to expect the parents to go through the process of adjustment in one session or even several sessions in a brief time span.

It is the long-term nature of the issue for parents to which Schild (1982) refers, and the need for recurrent counseling. Many of the questions regarding the handicapped child simply cannot be answered until considerable time passes after the initial diagnosis has been made.

Although families of the handicapped are more similar than dissimilar to other families, there are special dimensions to routine parental tasks such as discipline, guidance, and nurturance. It is unrealistic to advise parents to treat their handicapped child just like the other children in the family. Parents may need periodic counseling in relation to such issues as expectations, value conflicts, and life transitions.

In their initial shock, parents may experience a period of denial in which they seek advice from a multitude of sources and may move from professional to professional seeking a more hopeful diagnosis. Denial serves as a defense against the anxiety produced by the discrepancy between the desired healthy baby and the reality of the disabled child. It may be relatively easy to continue denial while the child is young and comparisons with other, normal children can be avoided. This denial may result in unrealistic expectations for achievement because there is "nothing wrong" with the child (Ross, 1964).

Anger usually follows denial, and this anger may be directed toward the child in the form of rejection or as envy of other parents who have normal chidren. Feelings of anger may also translate into guilt or resentment of one parent toward the other which may lead to marital conflict.

Bargaining is often the next stage of the grief process in which the parents may believe that if they work hard enough and long enough in some special program, the child will be normal. When it becomes increasingly apparent that their child is still handicapped no matter what program they work at or which professional they consult, depression may result.

The grief may remain unresolved to a certain extent because of the recurring crises that center around the different stages in the life of the handicapped child. These crises may include informing other family members and friends of the child's handicap, coping with the educational needs of the child, dealing with special medical problems, and maintaining the child at home through adulthood. Attempts on the family's part to meet each new crisis may evoke the same feelings of sadness, anger, and grief (Turner, 1980).

In order to cope with overwhelming feelings of guilt and depression, parents either may become overprotective or may cause their child to avoid interaction with other children. Either move exacerbates the problem. In this regard the therapist can play a major role in aiding the family toward resolution of these issues.

In some instances, parents will attempt to cope with the stress caused by a handicapped child in different ways. These differences may increase the conflict between the parents as a couple. One parent may become overinvolved and the other withdrawn and distant from the family. Other siblings may attempt to take over the parenting role, and their needs for attention and nurturing may be neglected. The family may become totally enmeshed in this process, resulting in confusion about roles and a failure on the part of the handicapped child to develop appropriate self-concept and individuation.

Interventions can take the form of either primary parent education or family therapy. Turner (1980) proposed a list of suggested interventions for families of mentally retarded children that are applicable to families of children with other handicaps.

1. An accurate assessment of family functioning is essential, including the strengths and weaknesses of the family system.
2. The family should be assisted in redirecting its focus from the handicapped child to examining the entire family's method of coping with change.
3. Attention should be directed to the communication network within the family and expression and acceptance of feelings encouraged.
4. The family should reinforce responsibility by supporting effective coping behaviors and encouraging their use.
5. The family should be provided with basic information about the child's handicap and on how to locate additional resources as they are needed.

Multiple-family sessions may be helpful in facilitating the individual family's ability to cope. These sessions would provide the opportunity to families for sharing feelings, modeling effective coping skills, exchanging possible solutions to common problems, and increasing the knowledge base and awareness of future developmental crises. Depending upon the nature of the handicap, the child can be included in family therapy. If the child is moderately to severely retarded, the role may be quite limited, as is usually the case with children under the age of 3.

As with families without a handicapped member, some families with a disabled child may be very dysfunctional and require significant professional assistance. This may occur for a number of reasons, such as the psychopathology of individual family members. Munro (1985) cites several characteristics of these dysfunctional families such as:

1. Chronic complaining—Any minor problem is perceived as a major crisis.
2. Program sabotage—Attempts to assist the family are blocked.
3. Extreme overprotectiveness—Attempts for individuation of any family member are thwarted.

Therapists are advised to focus on specific "here and now" strategies, while working on developing a trust relationship with the family.

Because of the unique stresses placed upon the families of handicapped children, the teaching of coping mechanisms is an important aspect of therapy and can aid families in a better understanding of their handicapped child's needs. If developmental limitations are taken into account, family therapy can be a most successful intervention for the retarded.

SUMMARY

Although handicapped children have the same fundamental needs as their nonhandicapped peers, the techniques for therapeutic intervention must be modified in order for the therapy to be effective. Consideration must be given to the child's learning style, including cognitive abilities, length of attention span, and memory processes. Language and communication skills must also be considered; the level of language development is a key factor in the designing of interventions. In addition, the presence of any physical limitation is a factor in the designing of an intervention. The setting of objectives must be tempered by knowledge of the child's developmental level relative to his or her chronological age. When dealing with the handicapped, therapeutic interventions are generally more concrete and involve the family.

Other special problems occur in the designing of interventions for the handicapped:

1. The child's acceptance of the handicap.

2. The child's relationship with his or her peer group.
3. The degree of parental acceptance or rejection of the handicapping condition.
4. The level of knowledge about the handicapping condition expressed by both parents and child.
5. The level of helplessness experienced by the child as a result of the handicap.

A key goal for therapy is to provide detailed information about the handicapping condition to both the child and parents. This often aids in acceptance of the handicap and dispels various myths generally surrounding the perception of the handicap by all concerned. The therapist must also concentrate efforts on determining the dynamics of the family as a result of having a handicapped child. The early rearing strategies employed by parents with their handicapped child may be a key variable in explaining current modes of behavior. Clearly, the intervention process must concentrate on the entire ecosystem, cutting across individual, family, and institutional settings. The current intervention literature on the handicapped tends to stress the need for the therapist to have an awareness of the special characteristics of handicapped children and adolescents. Many goals are cited for the counseling process. Paramount among these are the development of appropriate social skills and the "normalization" of the handicapped person.

ANNOTATED BIBLIOGRAPHY

Baruth, L., & Burggraf, M. (Eds.). (1979). *Counseling parents of exceptional children.* Guilford, CT: Special Learning Corporation.

This book is a series of reprinted articles on counseling exceptional children including the learning disabled, mentally retarded, behaviorally disabled, orthopedically disabled, and visually/auditorily disabled. The volume also contains theoretical perspectives for counseling the handicapped.

Buscaglia, L. (1975). *The disabled and their parents: A counseling challenge.* Thorofare, NJ: Charles B. Slack.

This book covers the knowledge base on counseling the handicapped and their parents. It is extremely useful to practitioners for formulating strategies for counseling with the handicapped.

Cruickshank, W. M. (Ed.). (1983). *Psychology of exceptional children and youth.* Englewood Cliffs, NJ: Prentice-Hall.

This book is a comprehensive reference on exceptionality. It covers in an in-depth fashion psychological impairment resulting from a variety of handicaps including orthopedic handicaps, visual impairment, hearing impairment, and chronic medical disorders. Chapters of particular interest include the one by Shontz on "Theories About the Adjustment to Having a Disability" and the one by Knoblock on "Psychological Considerations of Emotionally Disturbed Children."

Neely, M. A. (1982). *Counseling and guidance practices with special education students.* Homewood, IL: Dorsey Press.

This book is a comprehensive text on counseling techniques for use with the handicapped. It covers both individual and group interventions in a wide variety of settings including the schools. Parent counseling is also reviewed in depth.

Strohmer, D. C., & Prout, H. T. (Eds.). (1989). *Counseling and psychotherapy with mentally retarded persons.* Brandon, VT: Clinical Psychology.

This is a comprehensive overview of counseling with the mildly mentally retarded. Included are sections on psychopathology, assessment, individual therapy, behavior therapy, group therapy, family therapy, and vocational counseling. An excellent resource for the practitioner.

REFERENCES

Adamson, W. C. (1979). Helping parents of children with learning disabilities. In L. Baruth & M. Burggraf (Eds.), *Counseling parents of exceptional children.* Guilford, CT: Special Learning Corporation.

Becker, R. L. (1975). *The Reading Free Vocational Interest Inventory.* Washington, DC: American Association of Mental Deficiency.

Becker, W. (1971). *Parents are teachers: A child management program.* Champaign, IL: Research Press.

Blohm, A. L. (1978). Group counseling with moderately mentally retarded and learning disabled elementary children. *Dissertation Abstracts International, 39,* 3362A. (University Microfilms No. 7824128). East Texas State University, *DAI* 39/06A, p. 3362.

Brannigan, G. G., & Young, R. C. (1978). Social skills training with the MBD adolescent: A case study. *Academic Therapy, 13,* 401-404.

Bricklan, P. M. (1970). Counseling parents of children with learning disabilities. *Reading Teacher, 23,* 331-338.

Brown, D. T., & Cobb, H. C. (1978). *Family care providers handbook.* Richmond, VA: Virginia State Department of Mental Health and Retardation.

Bryan, T. H., & Bryan, J. H. (1978). Social interactions of learning disabled children. *Learning Disabilities Quarterly, 1*(1), 33-38.

Burggraf, M. Z. (1979). Consulting with parents of handicapped children. *Elementary School Guidance and Counseling, 13,* 214-222.

Buscaglia, L. (1975). *The disabled and their parents: A counseling challenge.* Thorofare, NJ: Charles B. Slack.

Cook, P., Kunce, J., & Getsinger, S. (1976). Perception of the disabled and counseling effectiveness. *Rehabilitation Counseling Bulletin, 19,* 470-475.

Cruickshank, W. M. (Ed.). (1980). *Psychology of exceptional children and youth.* Englewood Cliffs, NJ: Prentice-Hall.

Davidson, C. D. (1975). Psychotherapy with mentally handicapped children in a day school. *Psychotherapy: Theory, Research and Practice, 12,* 13-21.

DeBlassie, R. R., & Cowan, M. A. (1976). Counseling with the mentally handicapped child. *Elementary School Guidance and Counseling, 10*(4), 246-253.

Deutsch, H. (1985). Grief counseling with mentally retarded clients. *Psychiatric Aspects of Mental Retardation Reviews,* 4(5), 17-20.

Gardner, R. A. (1975). Techniques for involving the child with MBD in meaningful psychotherapy. *Journal of Learning Disabilities, 8,* 272-282.

Ginott, H. G. (1965). *Between parent and child.* New York: Avon.

Gold, P., & Richmond, L. J. (1979). Counseling parents of learning disabled children. *Elementary School Guidance and Counseling, 14,* 16-21.

Gordon, S. (1975). The disabled are also sexual. In L. Buscaglia (Ed.), *The disabled and their parents: A counseling challenge.* Thorofare, NJ: Charles B. Slack.

Greer, B. G. (1975). Attitudes of special education personnel toward different types of deviant persons. *Rehabilitation Literature, 36,* 82-184.

Grossman, H. J. (Ed.). (1973). *Manual on terminology and classification in mental retardation.* Washington, DC: American Association of Mental Deficiency.

Hallahan, D. P., & Kauffman, J. M. (1978). *Exceptional children: Introduction to special education.* Englewood Cliffs, NJ: Prentice-Hall.

Halpern, A., Raffield, R., Irvin, L. K., & Link, R. (1975). *Social and prevocational information battery: Testbook, user's guide, examiner's manual, technical report, answer key, class record.* Eugene, OR: University of Oregon Rehabilitation Research Training Center in Mental Retardation.

Hayes, M. (1977). The responsiveness of mentally retarded children to psychotherapy. *Smith College Studies in Social Work, 47,* 112-153.

Humes, C. W., Adamczyk, J. S., & Myco, R. W. (1969). A school study of group counseling with educable retarded adolescents. *American Journal of Mental Deficiency, 74,* 194-195.

Hurley, A. D., & Hurley, F. J. (1986). Counseling and psychotherapy with mentally retarded clients: The initial interview. *Psychiatric Aspects of Mental Retardation Reviews, 5*(5), 22-26.

LaGreca, A. M., & Mesibov, G. B. (1979). Social skills intervention with learning disabled children: Selecting skills and implementing training. *Journal of Clinical Child Psychology, 8,* 234-241.

Meichenbaum, D. (1977). *Cognitive-behavior modification: An integrative approach.* New York: Plenum Press.

Morse, D. (1977). Counseling the young adolescent with learning disabilities. *The School Counselor, 77,* 8-15.

Munro, J. D.(1985). Counseling severely dysfunctional families of mentally and physically disabled persons. *Clinical Social Work Journal, 13,* 18-31.

Murray, M. A. (1973). *Needs of parents of mentally retarded children.* Washington, DC: National Association for Retarded Children.

Nathanson, R. (1979). Counseling persons with disabilities: Are the feelings, thoughts, and behaviors of helping professionals helpful? *The Personnel and Guidance Journal, 58,* 233-237.

Neely, M. A. (1982). *Counseling and guidance practices with special education students.* Homewood, IL: Dorsey Press.

Norton, F. H. (1976). Counseling parents of the mentally retarded child. *The School Counselor,* January, 200-205.

Olshansky, S. (1970). Chronic sorrow: A response to having a mentally defective child. In R. L. Noland (Ed.), *Counseling parents of the mentally retarded: A sourcebook.* Springfield, IL: Charles C. Thomas.

Robinson, H. B., & Robinson, N. M. (1965). *The mentally retarded child: A psychological approach.* New York: McGraw-Hill.

Ross, A. O. (1964). *The exceptional child in the family.* New York: Grune & Stratton.

Ross, A. O. (1974). *Psychological disorders of children: A behavioral approach to theory, research, and therapy.* New York: McGraw-Hill.

Schild, S. (1982). Beyond diagnosis: Issues in recurrent counseling of parents of the mentally retarded. *Social Work in Health Care, 8*(1), 81-93.

Schontz, F. C. (1980). Theories about the adjustment to having a disability. In W. M. Cruickshank (Ed.), *Psychology of exceptional children and youth.* Englewood Cliffs, NJ: Prentice-Hall.

Selwa, B. T. (1971). Preliminary considerations in psychotherapy with retarded children. *Journal of School Psychology, 9,* 12-15.

Staggs, A. M. (1979). *Group counseling of learning disabled children in the intermediate grades enrolled in the public school special education program: Training in cognitive behavior modification.* Ann Arbor, MI: (University of Michigan, No. 8012141).

Tavormina, J. B. (1975). Relative effectiveness of behavioral and reflective group counseling with parents of mentally retarded children. *Journal of Consulting and Clinical Psychology, 43,* 22-30.

Turner, A. (1980). Therapy with families of a mentally retarded child. *Journal of Marital and Family Therapy,* April, 167-170.

Welch, V. O., & Sigman, M. (1980). Group psychotherapy with mildly retarded, emotionally disturbed adolescents. *Journal of Clincial Child Psychology, 9,* 209-212.

Wells, L., & Allan, J. (1985). Counseling the mentally handicapped student. *Guidance and Counseling, 1*(2), 13-21.

Yuker, H., Block, J., & Young, J. (1966). *The measurement of attitudes toward disabled persons.* (Resource Study No. 7). Albertson, NY: Human Resources Center.

Yura, M. T., Zuckerman, L., Betz, M. J., & Newman, S. S. (1979). Parent involvement project. *The Personnel and Guidance Journal, 58,* 290-292.

Zigmond, N., & Brownlee, J. (1980). Social skills training for adolescents with learning disabilities. *Exceptional Education Quarterly, 2,* 77-83.

Chapter 11

Summary and Comparison of Approaches

Douglas T. Brown, Ph.D.
H. Thompson Prout, Ph.D.

In an area such as psychotherapy, it is critical that a definitive analysis of the adequacy of each therapeutic approach be done. Some therapeutic approaches demonstrate excellent efficacy but with relatively narrow groups and confined techniques. Others provide a detailed framework for conducting their therapy. The purpose of this chapter is to evaluate the underlying therapeutic framework for each therapy approach as it has been specified by the individual chapter authors. Table 1 provides a summary of the basic theoretical and clinical tenets of each approach. No attempt is made to evaluate the efficacy or general worthiness of each therapy based on other external sources of data. However, it should be noted that each of the theoretical approaches in this volume was selected because it offered a significant body of literature for dealing with the child and adolescent client. Other approaches were not included because they offered little in dealing with nonadult clientele. In effect, this chapter is a critical review of the data presented in this volume. Further, it is important to note that the authors of this chapter have undertaken to evaluate each therapy based on the adequacy of the presentation in each chapter relative to a series of predefined criteria.

TABLE 1: SUMMARY OF THE BASIC PRINCIPLES OF APPROACHES

Approach	"Causes" of Disturbance or Deviance	Core of Theory	Treatment Focus	Techniques
Psycho-analytic	Intrapsychic conflict resulting from imbalance among id, ego, and superego. Importance of unconscious and psychosexual forces.	Topographical (e.g., conscious, unconscious, and preconscious) view of mind. Dynamic and structural views.	Insight, rather than symptom relief. Bringing repressed material to the surface.	Use of transference, interpretation of projections, working through of conflicts, interpretation of patient-therapist axis.
Adlerian	Mistaken beliefs, discouragement, and faulty private logic lead to disturbance. Emphasis on goals of misbehavior.	Behavior is purposive and goal-directed. Behavior has social meaning, and individuals seek to "belong."	Understanding of beliefs, feelings, motives, and goals that determine one's life-style. Changes in these yield behavior change.	Life-style analyses which assist in development of insight into self-defeating behavior. Interpretations of behavior goals and offering alternative ideas and beliefs.
Person-Centered	Incongruence between self and experiences in which individuals try to please others, leading to low self-regard.	Striving toward self-fulfillment and self-actualization. Emphasis on self-theory, humanistic view, and phenomenology.	Changes in self-understanding, self-concept, attitudes, self-directed behavior.	Emphasis on "core conditions" and client-therapist relationship. Communication of empathy and respect; reflection of feeling; active listening; etc.
Behavioral	Abnormal behaviors learned through same mechanisms as "normal" behaviors; influence of environment.	Operant and classical conditioning; observational learning and, more recently, cognitive variables.	Change in observable or measurable behaviors. Modifying environmental factors that lead to behavior change.	Systemic data collection and behavioral assessment. Wide variety of learning-theory based techniques, e.g., desensitization, reinforcement, modeling.

TABLE 1 (CONTINUED)

Approach	"Causes" of Disturbance or Deviance	Core of Theory	Treatment Focus	Techniques
Rational-Emotive	Irrational beliefs and cognitions and absolutistic thinking lead to emotional disturbance.	Thoughts, beliefs, and behaviors overlap and influence each other. Emphasis on role of person's thoughts.	Change in disturbance-producing irrational ideas and beliefs.	Challenging irrational beliefs; teaching new styles of thinking; encouraging client to engage in activities and behaviors that refute irrational beliefs.
Reality Therapy	"Failure" identity leads to pessimistic and negative attitudes toward life and a resignation to failure.	Basis for behavior is intrinsic goal of having different, unique, and distinct identity.	Behavior change based on changes in values and concepts of individual responsibility; increases in self-understanding and self-acceptance.	Confronting client with irresponsible behavior; helping client make plans to change failure behavior to success behavior.
Systemic	Dysfunctional behavior patterns resulting from distortion of boundaries within the family which produces either disengagement or enmeshment among group members.	Focuses on the ecological context, usually the family, rather than the individual.	Insight into dysfunctional family or group patterns.	Use of family therapy methods such as joining, mapping, reframing, and restructuring.

Thus, our personal and theoretical biases have been omitted from this discussion. The overall concern is to rate the degree to which the theory is operationalized for the practitioner.

In order to accomplish this task, each theory was rated on the basis of the following eight criteria:

1. *Definition of Psychopathology:* Whether the theory provides an adequate explanation of disturbed behavior; whether the theory provides an operationalized framework for the explanation of emotional disturbance.
2. *Individual Work with Children:* The adequacy of the theory in detailing specific approaches and techniques for dealing with children under age 12.
3. *Individual Work with Adolescents:* The adequacy of the theory in presenting a detailed framework for dealing with children over the age of 12.
4. *Group Procedures:* Is there an adequate framework for dealing with groups? Does the therapy describe specific, detailed, structured programs for work with groups?
5. *Classroom and Educational Applications:* Does the therapy provide specific techniques for use and implementation by school personnel?
6. *Parenting Skills:* Does the therapeutic approach provide specific techniques and programs for dealing with parent counseling? Does the therapeutic approach provide specific programs and techniques for dealing with parent training?
7. *Family Intervention:* Does the therapeutic approach provide specific skills and techniques for dealing with family therapy, i.e., treating individual families as a group?
8. *Efficacy:* Is there a significant body of research literature demonstrating the efficacy of the therapeutic approach?

All therapeutic approaches have been rated on each of the eight criteria specified above. The quasi-ordinal rating scale which was utilized for this purpose is presented below. (Note: Any resemblance between this rating scale and a well-known restaurant guide is coincidental.)

* * * * * = Excellent
* * * * = Very Good
* * * = Good
* * = Fair
* = Marginal

It is important to note again that these ratings are based on the ability of each of the therapies to meet or exceed each of the eight operationalized criteria specified above. These ratings in no way reflect on the overall worthiness of the therapeutic techniques. Additionally, some narrative evaluation will be provided to explain the various ratings.

PSYCHOANALYTIC APPROACHES

1. *Definition of Psychopathology:* (* * * * *)
   Psychoanalytic therapy has the most detailed description of psychopathology among the theories presented here. This is the case with both the etiological descriptions and the theoretical rationale. The therapy is also clearly interfaced with a developmental framework.

2. *Individual Work with Children:* (* * * *)
   Because of the developmental framework and individual therapy techniques with children, the psychoanalytic approach offers a detailed set of guidelines for working with younger children. Numerous specific techniques are available.

3. *Individual Work with Adolescents:* (* * *)
   Although the analytic approach details many of the variables operating within individual therapy with adolescents, a set of specific techniques does not appear as well developed. Many of the aspects discussed would seem to be relevant with numerous other therapeutic approaches utilized with adolescents.

4. *Group Approaches:* (* * *)
   The psychoanalytic approach does appear to consider

developmental aspects in group formation and function. However, a well-delineated set of group techniques is not in evidence.

5. *Classroom and Educational Applications:* (* *)
   The psychoanalytic approach does recognize the schooling experience as being important to emotional development. However, these techniques do not appear as applicable to the regular classroom environment and are more directed at a therapeutic school situation.

6. *Parenting Skills:* (* *)
   Although the psychoanalytic approach places greater emphasis on the role of the parents in the development of their children, there does not appear to be a well-defined set of techniques for working with parents. There do not appear to be any structured parent programs available within the psychoanalytic approach, although there are applications to parent counseling.

7. *Family Intervention:* (* *)
   There do not appear to be well-developed family intervention techniques in psychoanalytic therapy, although familial variables are considered in treatment.

8. *Efficacy:* (*)
   The psychoanalytic approach does not lend itself well to empirical examination and evaluation. Few empirical studies supporting the efficacy of this approach with children and adolescents are presented.

Psychoanalytic therapy has a very well developed theoretical structure. Through this structure pathological behavior is easily identified and categorized. The structure lends itself to individual work with children and provides a developmental framework for therapy, particularly with younger children. Techniques for use with adolescents have not been as well developed. Although school and educational techniques are presented, they do not appear to be applicable for general classroom use. Generally, psychoanalytic therapy does not provide techniques for family intervention nor for parenting skills training. The psychoanalytic approach does not lend itself to empirical evaluation in the traditional sense.

ADLERIAN APPROACHES

1. *Definition of Psychopathology:* (* * *)
   Adlerian therapy discusses both cognitive (mistaken beliefs) and behavioral (i.e., the goals of misbehavior) components of emotional difficulties in children. However, the system appears relatively weak in elaborating the descriptions of various emotional-behavioral disturbances as found in other theories.

2. *Individual Work with Children:* (* * *)
   Adlerian approaches provide a good framework for working with a child within a family context. The Children's Life Style Guide appears to be a useful technique in structuring counseling with children. However, the general techniques of working with children do not appear to be especially well operationalized.

3. *Individual Work with Adolescents:* (* *)
   Although Adlerian therapy does address the unique aspects of adolescent dilemmas, it does not appear to provide a specific set of techniques for dealing with them.

4. *Group Procedures:* (* * *)
   Whereas the Adlerian chapter does offer guidelines in terms of formation and functioning, these guidelines do not appear to be significantly different from general group process guidelines. However, it must be recognized that the DUSO procedure is a group procedure as well as a classroom procedure.

5. *Classroom and Educational Applications:* (* * * *)
   The Adlerian approach does present some relatively well-developed classroom approaches. An educational philosophy has been developed and several programs exist for helping teachers refine their teaching style (e.g.,

STET). The DUSO program is one of the most widely used and accepted affective education techniques available.

6. *Parenting Skills:* (* * * *)
   Adlerians present considerable material to help parents in understanding their children's behavior. The STEP program is a well-accepted parent education and training technique.

7. *Family Intervention:* (* * *)
   Much of Adlerian theory relates to the individual within the family context. However, a well-defined set of family therapy techniques has not been developed.

8. *Efficacy:* (* * *)
   Considerable research appears to be available on the effectiveness of the various structured programs provided by Adlerian therapy. The child and adolescent counseling research appears to be largely case study in nature.

Adlerian therapy is especially strong in defining approaches and procedures for utilization in home and educational settings. A comprehensive theory of emotional disturbance is provided together with assessment techniques. The area of teaching parenting skills is especially well addressed, with numerous programs provided for the purpose. Adlerian therapy is not able to differentiate some techniques for utilization with adolescents. Adlerian therapy does not fully operationalize many of the procedures which are recommended. The efficacy literature, however, does tend to support the effectiveness of the structured approaches presented.

PERSON-CENTERED APPROACHES

1. *Definition of Psychopathology:* (* *)
   Person-centered therapy provides neither a strong structure for describing disturbance nor a comprehensive base for understanding the wide range of psychopathology.

2. *Individual Work with Children:* (* * * *)
   Person-centered therapy has a relatively well-defined set of techniques for face-to-face therapy with children. The major principles of direct work with children are well described and also lend themselves to use by other therapeutic mediums. Further, the use of play is developmentally appropriate for the younger child.

3. *Individual Work with Adolescents:* (* *)
   Person-centered therapy has not developed a distinguishable set of techniques which specifically address themselves to adolescents' needs. Thus, it does not attune itself to turbulent behavior patterns normally associated with adolescence. The approach appears somewhat too passive to be effective with this group.

4. *Group Procedures:* (* *)
   There do appear to be some general guidelines for conducting group procedures with children and adolescents. However, there do not appear to be any structured and well-operationalized group programs.

5. *Classroom and Educational Applications:* (* * * *)
   Across the variety of techniques presented in the chapter, person-centered therapy details a number of school applications. A number of structured techniques are available for self-esteem building activities and affective education. However, person-centered approaches do not appear particularly strong in classroom management techniques.

6. *Parenting Skills:* (* * * *)
   Person-centered therapy does lend itself well to applications with parenting skills training (e.g., Parent Effectiveness Training). The approach also lends itself well to the affective aspects of parent counseling.

7. *Family Intervention:* (* *)
   Although person-centered practitioners recognize family variables, family therapy in the traditional sense is an underveloped area.

8. *Efficacy:* (* *)
   Although there is a body of efficacy literature presented which reflects interventions with adults, the efficacy literature under child and adolescent therapy is not well developed.

Person-centered therapy has well-developed techniques for one-to-one therapy with children and adults. It does not address itself well to working with the problems presented by adolescents. It is, however, applicable to parenting skills training and parent intervention. Person-centered therapy has an especially well-developed set of classroom intervention procedures for use in affective education. Although the therapy does not provide a clear structure for describing emotional disturbance, it is well suited to children with a variety of affective disorders. The research literature in person-centered therapy is not well developed with children and adolescents.

BEHAVIORAL APPROACHES

1. *Definition of Psychopathology:* (* * *)
   Behavioral approaches by virtue of their theoretical underpinnings avoid examining psychopathology. However, a very exact framework is provided for operationally defining those behaviors which are dysfunctional in a given environment.
2. *Individual Work with Children:* (* * *)
   Behavioral approaches are particularly strong in certain areas such as phobic reactions, desensitization, and specifically defined behavior problems. However, the technique falls short in providing an overall framework for direct, individual therapy with children. Behavior therapy tends to address itself to the manipulation of a series of environmental factors that will indirectly influence child behavior rather than to the provision of highly individualized, one-to-one therapy.
3. *Individual Work with Adolescents:* (* *)
   A wide variety of techniques have been developed for

utilization with adolescents. These include both operant and cognitive interventions, some of which have been used with adults.

4. *Group Procedures:* (* * * *)
   Behavior therapists have developed a significant number of approaches and techniques for utilization with groups. Techniques such as behavior rehearsal, group relaxation, and social skills training are a few examples. Several structured, packaged programs are available for the practitioner.

5. *Classroom and Educational Applications:* (* * * * *)
   This area is clearly behavior therapy's forte. Numerous classroom application packages have been developed and are available for use. Furthermore, behavior therapy provides an excellent framework for the development of individualized classroom interventions by numerous school personnel.

6. *Parenting Skills:* (* * *)
   Behavior therapy is quite strong in providing a framework for parenting skills training. However, it is not particularly adequate in providing a framework for parent counseling and affective intervention. Numerous parent training packages are available.

7. *Family Intervention:* (* *)
   A family therapy approach distinctive from parenting skills and marital counseling does not exist in this technique per se.

8. *Efficacy:* (* * * *)
   Behavior therapy, by its nature, is empirically based. A plethora of supportive research has been generated for this technique. However, most research tends to focus on behaviors which are narrowly defined. Although no therapy presents consistently favorable efficacy data, behavior therapy comes the closest.

Although behavior therapy does not utilize the classical approaches to the identification of pathology, it is strong in delineating the specific behaviors which constitute disturbance. It has shown remarkable success in dealing with behaviors which stem from conditioned reflexes or operant learning. These include phobic reactions, somnambulism, anxiety states, and a host of other behaviors which were formerly difficult or impossible to treat using other therapeutic approaches. Behavior therapy's most widespread utilization has been in educational settings. It forms the basis for numerous programs which attempt to shape or modify behavior patterns. It has been successfully used with large groups of children such as in Lindsley's precision teaching (Lindsley, 1972). Perhaps behavior therapy's major weakness lies in the fact that it does not provide an adequate framework for developing affective intervention. It is, however, the most thoroughly researched of the therapeutic techniques discussed in this volume.

RATIONAL-EMOTIVE APPROACHES

1. *Definition of Psychopathology:* (* * * *)
   RET provides a well-defined framework which explains the cognitive basis of disturbance. Further, some of the patterns of disturbed thoughts are identified as well as the underlying cognitive mechanisms related to common behavioral and emotional disturbances.

2. *Individual Work with Children:* (* * *)
   RET does provide a comprehensive framework for dealing with children. However, this framework does not differ significantly from that provided for adults and adolescents. It considers the developmental characteristics of children but does not appear to adapt its techniques specifically to them.

3. *Individual Work with Adolescents:* (* * * *)
   The nature of the RET techniques is well adapted to the more cognitively mature adolescent. Given the adolescent's propensity toward irrationality, RET is particularly effective in dealing with adolescent disturbance.

4. *Group Procedures:* (* *)
   The RET approach is not well suited to utilization with

groups of younger children. However, there is a framework which has been established for teaching rational-emotive therapy techniques to middle school and older children.

5. *Classroom and Educational Applications:* (* * *)
Classroom techniques exist for teaching rational-emotive concepts, yet few structured curricula or classroom management procedures exist. The Institute for Rational Living in New York City runs a school that utilizes rational-emotive concepts.

6. *Parenting Skills:* (* * * *)
RET has identified a number of specific dysfunctional parenting styles. Additionally, two packaged programs for parent training based on RET are available.

7. *Family Intervention:* (*)
Although RET does recognize familial aspects of disturbance, it remains substantially an individually oriented therapy.

8. *Efficacy:* (* * *)
At this point, although there is a sizeable body of research on RET for adolescents and adults, a more limited body of research exists involving the efficacy of RET for child applications and Rational-Emotive Education. Most of the data presented are anecdotal in nature but tend to be supportive of this therapeutic approach.

Rational-emotive therapy provides a clear and concise framework for the cognitive aspects of emotional disturbance which lend themselves to therapeutic intervention. It is well suited for use with adolescents and adults who are intellectually mature. Thus, rational-emotive therapists have shown considerable success in dealing wth adolescent disturbance. RET, however, has not been sufficiently well developed for utilization with younger children. It is also not particularly well suited for use with groups. Thus, RET should be treated as a narrowband therapy which has shown substantial success with certain groupings of people. However, new research is emerging in the area of utilizing RET with middle school and younger children. Also, substantial work has been done in the area of dysfunctional parenting styles.

REALITY APPROACHES

1. *Definition of Psychopathology:* (* * *)
   Reality therapy does provide explanations of common childhood emotional problems. However, it does not seem to exhibit a very elaborate and detailed system of delineating and explaining emotional disturbance. The system appears similar to that of RET but is not as well developed at this point.

2. *Individual Work with Children:* (* * *)
   A fairly systematic approach is presented for working with children. However, little attempt is made to distinguish developmentally the utilization of this approach across various age levels of children.

3. *Individual Work with Adolescents:* (* * * *)
   Many of the publicized applications with reality therapy have been directed toward adolescents. This technique is also well adapted to dealing with the more cognitively mature adolescent and particularly the many life problems encountered by the adolescent.

4. *Group Procedures:* (* * *)
   Although a framework for group therapy work does exist, it does not appear to be a very elaborate methodology in contrast with the individual procedures presented.

5. *Classroom and Educational Applications:* (* * * *)
   Reality therapy provides one of the best systematic approaches to classroom discipline and management. Further, a well-defined educational philosophy is provided in *Schools Without Failure.* It does not, however, address itself well to affective education.

6. *Parenting Skills:* (* * *)
   One program for parent training (PIP) is presented

which seems fairly well conceptualized. However, a framework for parent counseling of a more general nature is not addressed.

7. *Family Intervention:* (*)
   Although some methodology borrowed from parent training and marriage counseling is utilized, reality therapy does not address family therapy well. Reality therapy, like RET, remains substantially an individually oriented therapy.

8. *Efficacy:* (* * *)
   A growing body of research appears to support generally the efficacy of reality therapy. Anecdotal reports, controlled case studies, and more elaborate group studies have been reported.

Like RET, reality therapy is directed at more cognitively mature children. However, reality therapy presents a highly systematic approach to classroom intervention and management. It is also well suited to teaching parents parenting skills and to doing individual work with adolescents and children. The major weakness of reality therapy, like RET, lies in its failure to discriminate therapeutic procedures utilized across various developmentally different groups. Thus, there is no clear differentiation between the treatment of young children and that of older children or adolescents. However, the efficacy research tends to support the utility of this approach, particularly with adolescents.

SYSTEMIC APPROACHES

1. *Definition of Psychopathology:* (* * * *)
   Systemic theory has a clear definition of pathology rooted in the ecological environment of the child. The theory clearly delineates the types of dysfunctional interactions that are possible.

2. *Individual Work with Children:* (NA)
   Systemic theory does not specifically provide procedures for individual work with children other than through family and group therapy.

3. *Individual Work with Adolescents:* (NA)
   Systemic theory does not provide specific techniques for individual work with adolescents other than those described for family and group therapy.
4. *Group Procedures:* (* * * * *)
   Systemic theory has a rich and varied array of group procedures available to group practitioners. This is, perhaps, the strongest aspect of this theoretical approach.
5. *Classroom and Educational Applications:* (* * *)
   Much of systemic theory has been applied to the classroom, because the classroom also represents an ecological system. However, research in this area is still in its infancy.
6. *Parenting Skills:* (* * * *)
   Systemic theory has a wide array of parent education strategies available. A variety of specific interventions are prescribed by this theory.
7. *Family Intervention:* (* * * * *)
   Much of systemic theory is focused on family interventions. Together with group interventions, this is the strongest and most developed aspect of systemic theory.
8. *Efficacy:* (* * * *)
   Systemic theory has a particularly well developed body of literature on efficacy, especially given the complexity of the variables with which it is dealing. The amount of research being generated in this area is equaled only by the area of behavior therapy.

Systemic theory has a well-developed theory of normal and abnormal behavior as it relates to family and group dynamics. As such, the structure of the theory lends itself well to intervention with families and small groups. A wide array of techniques for intervention is also provided by this theoretical approach. However, the complexity of these interventions makes evaluation of their effectiveness more difficult than in the other therapeutic approaches.

TABLE 2: COMPARISON OF RATINGS OF THERAPEUTIC APPROACHES ACCORDING TO EIGHT CRITERIA

Rating Scale:
* * * * * = Excellent
* * * * = Very Good
* * * = Good
* * = Fair
* = Marginal

	Therapeutic Approach						
Criterion	Psy	Adl	PC	Beh	RET	Rlt	Sys
1. Definition of psychopathology	*****	***	**	***	****	***	****
2. Individual work with children	****	***	****	***	***	***	NA
3. Individual work with adolescents	***	**	**	**	****	****	NA
4. Group procedures	***	***	**	****	**	***	*****
5. Classroom and educational applications	**	****	****	*****	***	****	***
6. Parenting skills	**	****	****	***	****	***	****
7. Family intervention	**	***	**	**	*	*	*****
8. Efficacy	*	***	**	****	***	***	****

Note: Psy = Psychoanalytic; Adl = Adlerian; PC = Person-Centered; Beh = Behavioral; RET = Rational-Emotive; Rlt = Reality; Sys = Systemic.

SUMMARY

Inspection of the seven therapeutic approaches presented in this volume reveals a comprehensive array of techniques that can be utilized by the practitioner. The editors are biased in the direction of an *intelligent eclecticism* in approaching these therapies. No single therapy is able to meet the eight criteria established above adequately. (See Table 2.) A number of the therapies are able to provide an adequate definition of pathology or emotionally disturbed behavior. Rational-emotive therapy, systemic, and psychoanalytic therapy are especially adept in this area. Certain therapies are better developed for work with children. These include behavioral, person-centered, Adlerian, and psychoanalytic. Others are more suited for work with adolescents, including rational-emotive and reality therapy. Behavior and systemic therapy appear to be particularly well suited for use in group settings. Adlerian therapy and reality therapy are also useful in this area. Classroom and educational applications have been developed extensively by behavior therapists. Reality therapy and Adlerian therapy also lend themselves to classroom applications. Parenting skill approaches have been comprehensively developed within the framework of Adlerian, behavior, and systemic therapy. Reality therapy has also been directed in this area but to a lesser extent. Adlerian and systemic therapy in particular address themselves to family intervention. The majority of the other therapies discussed do not provide specific techniques for family therapeutic interventions.

A major weakness of many therapies is their failure to provide a developmental framework for differentiating techniques across various groups. Thus, for example, rational-emotive therapy has a well-developed cognitive system for use with older children and adolescents who have reached "formal logical operations." The theory, however, does not provide a downward extrapolation for use with adolescents who have not reached this level of conceptual development, with younger children, or with the mentally handicapped. Conversely, behavior therapy presents an excellent operant framework for utilization with these groups. Although theorists such as Meichenbaum have developed elaborations of behavior therapy using cognitive structures, the theory is marginally adequate in explaining highly complex types of emotional disturbance. Psychoanalytic therapy perhaps comes closest to providing a detailed developmental framework for behavior, and this developmental framework is carefully interfaced with the therapeutic procedures provided. Generally, the therapies discussed are more adequate in presenting specific techniques for utilization with children than they are in presenting a developmental rationale for the utilization of these techniques. The editors can foresee that future refinements of some of the approaches will entail integration of developmental considerations into the theories.

A number of the therapies presented appear to be more suited for use in specific environments. Behavior therapy, Adlerian therapy, reality therapy, and systemic therapy all appear to be well suited for application in school settings. All four of these therapies provide structured packages or techniques which can be utilized either by trained psychologists or counselors, and, in some cases, by teachers. Systemic theory is particularly well suited to application in ecologically complex classroom settings. To a lesser extent, person-centered therapy is also applicable in small group settings within the schools. This has been particularly the case in instances where counselors have been available to provide affective education. Each of these therapies requires a somewhat different level of training and experience in order to implement it effectively.

Rational-emotive therapy and psychoanalytic therapy are less applicable to group and classroom settings. These approaches lend themselves to traditional clinic settings where one-to-one individual therapy is practiced. Behavior therapy and person-centered therapy may also be utilized in this way but are not limited to one-to-one situations. Basically, factors which determine the utility of a given therapy in multiple settings include:

1. The extent to which the therapy hypothesizes an underlying theory of learning.

2. The ability of the therapy to define developmentally various stages of cognitive development and to differentiate techniques on that basis.

3. The ease with which nonprofessionals can learn and implement the fundamental techniques of the therapy.
4. The ability of the therapeutic technique to handle both adolescents and children.
5. The extent to which the therapy has operationalized techniques.

In summary, many of the therapies reviewed are significantly stronger in their technology than in their theoretical underpinnings. Each therapy possesses various strengths and weaknesses, many of which tend to be complementary as one moves across the therapeutic techniques. Some are more applicable to adolescents, such as RET and reality therapy. Others are more applicable to group settings, including Adlerian, behavior therapy, reality therapy, and systemic therapy. Psychoanalytic, Adlerian, person-centered, and behavior therapies are especially strong in dealing with disturbance in young children. Of these, psychoanalytic therapy provides the best theoretical rationale, whereas behavior therapy provides the most empirically based treatment system. Reality therapy and RET are relatively weak in dealing with young children and essentially attempt to apply to younger children the principles developed with adolescent and adult populations.

A number of therapies (e.g., behavioral, RET, person-centered, Adlerian, and systemic) are quite strong in parent training applications. The diversity of parent training programs which have been developed through these therapies is truly impressive. Among the therapies discussed, only systemic theory provides a comprehensive set of procedures for family systems interventions. This is a unique feature of this therapeutic approach, one which requires extensive training and experience. An excellent discussion of family therapy techniques may be found in the *Handbook of Family Therapy* (Gurman & Kniskern, 1981).

RESEARCH ISSUES

The ability to perform empirical research on the effectiveness of a given therapy is highly contingent upon the extent to which its various techniques have been operationalized. Therapies which have as their major goals the promotion of "client growth," "personal self-esteem," and "general well-being" do not lend themselves to definitive research on their effectiveness. With the exception of the behavior and systemic therapies, the majority of the therapies reviewed are not especially strong in research efficacy. Reality therapy and Adlerian therapy have been significantly researched. However, much of the data collected is either of an anecdotal nature or has resulted from experimental conditions which do not meet the control requirements normally associated with parametric research. Weiss and Benoit (the authors of the chapter on psychoanalytic therapy) freely admit that psychoanalytic therapy does not lend itself to empirical research. This makes it especially difficult to conclude what impact the implementation of psychoanalytic techniques might or might not have on a given population of children. Of the therapies discussed, behavior therapy is probably the most easily operationalized. This fact has facilitated a virtual plethora of research demonstrating its efficacy. However, most of this research is $N = 1$ (single subject) based and thus does not meet parametric research requirements. In addition, the strong link that behavior therapy has with Skinnerian learning theory has tended to narrow its conceptualization of human behavior and to disregard developmental variables affecting therapeutic interventions.

Several directions for future research should be considered. First, procedures which are not sufficiently operationalized cannot be researched for effectiveness. This has been a chronic problem in adult psychotherapy. This problem is further exacerbated when these same adult therapies are extrapolated for use with children. The fact that many childhood interventions occur in ecologically complex settings (e.g., schools, child development centers) further complicates research methodology. Thus, a more clearly delineated set of operationalized interventions must be developed for virtually all of the therapeutic techniques discussed. Second, a large percentage of the research that does exist tends to be anecdotal in nature. Although anecdotal records do provide relatively concrete behavioral data, they do not meet the rigorous research requirements necessary to determine under which circumstances a given therapy is most effective. Third, extensive research needs to be performed on the relative merits of particular therapies with specific diagnostic categories of disorders. For example, the question might be asked, "Does rational-emotive therapy work more effectively with anxious and depressed clients than behavior therapy does?" It is clear that many of the therapies discussed were designed for specific applications (e.g., parent interventions, classroom intervention, anxiety reduction). Research needs to be performed which demonstrates that these therapies are more successful at treating the specific disorder for which they were designed than are other comparable therapies. For example, it is not possible to determine at this juncture whether psychoanalytic therapy might be better in treating childhood psychosis than behavior therapy. The extent to which variations in settings affect the adequacy of a given therapeutic technique should also be explored thoroughly. Fourth, although group techniques are employed in a number of therapies (e.g., Adlerian, behavioral, systemic, person-centered), they have not been extensively researched. The largest body of research exists in systemic therapy. However, more research should be done to determine outcomes of group therapeutic techniques with children. Research centering around many of the packaged programs presented is proceeding at a relatively steady rate. Programs such as DUSO, STEP, STEP/Teen, and PIP have generated a considerable body of data related to their effectiveness. Although these data suggest evidence of short-term success using these intervention programs, long-term studies are needed in order to determine the efficacy of all of the above therapies. Finally, research must continue to address the methodological complexity of studying the psychotherapeutic process. Many who have reviewed the various efficacy studies that show little or no effectiveness dismiss these findings because of methodological problems. It is possible that therapeutic change is so individualistic that "genuine" change in a group is not shown on group measures. Of particular importance in future research and practice is the continued development of measures of behavioral and affective change. Given that most referred children present multiple problems, unitary measures of change (e.g., an anxiety scale) might mask actual therapeutic change.

In order to generate the research data required, additional continued professional development for practitioners will be necessary. It is through those professionals who work with children on a day-to-day basis that the primary research data for various therapeutic techniques will be collected. Because social workers, counselors, and school and clinical psychologists engage in long-term therapeutic interventions, a virtually unlimited and diverse array of data could be available for ascertaining the differential impact of various therapeutic techniques. It is clear that more specific techniques for younger children in the 5- to 8-year-old range will need to be developed and tested. With the exception of play therapy, few techniques exist for use with this age group. This situation is complicated by the fact that few of the therapies presented provide an adequate framework for affective intervention wth young children. A concerted effort must be undertaken to interface existing knowledge and developmental psychology with the affective needs of these children. For example, structured techniques for anxiety reduction and amelioration of depression are urgently needed by school systems and other agencies dealing with children. Although many therapies address these areas, they do not provide techniques for use with children who are entering the state of concrete operations. In this regard, a more complete understanding of the relationship of language to affect in young children would be helpful.

Many of the techniques which are currently available are underutilized in the schools and family settings. The need for therapy in these settings is well documented (Guidubaldi, 1980). However, the paucity of efficacy research has made it difficult to persuade school administrators that therapeutic interventions can be of significant benefit. The drastic increase of emotional disorders being reported in the public schools will produce an ever-expanding demand for effective and cost-efficient therapeutic prodedures. If modern developmental theory, such as that of Piaget, can be integrated with the most efficacious aspects of the various existing therapies, then an eclectic framework might be developed for providing meaningful services to a wide array of children. It is the editors' suggestion that no one therapeutic technique can adequately treat the vast array of possible disorders. It is also clear that none of the therapies presented provides a totally adequate theory of the development of atypical behavior in children. Thus, future research will be in order to delineate these relationships. For the time being the individual therapist would be well advised to employ techniques from various therapies based on their usefulness with various age groups.

REFERENCES

Guidubaldi, J. (1980). The status report extended: Further elaborations on the American family. *The School Psychology Review, 9,* 374-379.

Gurman, A. S., & Kniskern, D. P. (Eds.). (1981). *Handbook of family therapy.* New York: Brunner/Mazel.

Lindsley, O. R. (1972). From Skinner to precision teaching: The child knows best. In J. B. Jordon & L. S. Robbins (Eds.), *Let's try doing something else kind of thing: Behavioral principles and the exceptional child.* Arlington, VA: Council for Exceptional Children.

INDEX

G

H